Reporting and Publishing Research in the Biomedical Sciences

Peush Sahni • Rakesh Aggarwal
Editors

Reporting and Publishing Research in the Biomedical Sciences

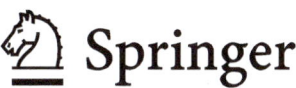

Editors
Peush Sahni
Department of Gastrointestinal Surgery and
Liver Transplantation
All India Institute of Medical Sciences
New Delhi, Delhi
India

Rakesh Aggarwal
Department of Gastroenterology
Sanjay Gandhi Postgraduate Institute of
Medical Sciences
Lucknow, Uttar Pradesh
India

ISBN 978-981-10-7061-7   ISBN 978-981-10-7062-4   (eBook)
https://doi.org/10.1007/978-981-10-7062-4

Library of Congress Control Number: 2017964264

Printed on acid-free paper

This Springer imprint is published by the registered company Springer Nature Singapore Pte Ltd.
The registered company address is: 152 Beach Road, #21-01/04 Gateway East, Singapore 189721, Singapore

Foreword

Medicine is both an art and a science. Progress in medical science enables improvement of existing methods of diagnosis and treatment and, at times, leads to breakthroughs in treatment of diseases that were hitherto beyond remedy. Such progress depends on research—in the laboratory, in the ward and in the field. Vital information gained through research is of little use unless it is shared among the peer group. This book addresses the methods by which such information can be disseminated effectively—and in a manner that even the humblest professional or research student is stimulated to imbibe and use for the benefit of patients or for further study.

Many of us in India are educated in schools and work in institutions where English is a second language. Expression in this language does not come easily as we may think in our mother tongues and translate our thoughts into English each time we are required to communicate. This often leads to difficulties in understanding what we wish to convey. Special efforts are necessary to gain fluency in English and familiarity with its idiosyncrasies. This book has chapters that could help such aspects of communication.

Transmission of research-related information for permanent record is principally through journals and books. We also transmit information through papers read at meetings, seminars and conferences. Each mode has its own preferred style that must be mastered for successful communication. These styles have evolved over time. Currently, we disfavour long-winded sentences and opt for brevity and crispness. It is important to get to the point and convey the gist of our data, conclusions and suggestions as effectively as possible.

Most books and journals on biomedicine published in India have a long way to go before they reach international standards. We are also prone to look upon ethics in relation to writing and publication with indifference if not disdain. The consequent malpractices make our publications unwelcome to local and international scholars of repute.

The book you hold in your hands brings together principles and guidelines that will help you transmit your scientific findings and suggestions to your peers in a manner that is at once easy to understand and effective. The editors and authors have taken care to incorporate the latest advances in publication and have done their best to make this volume comprehensive. The standards laid down are those followed the world over.

When you have something important to communicate—that is, when you need to put pen to paper or start tapping your keyboard purposefully—this compilation of essays will stand you in good stead.

Sunil Pandya
Jaslok Hospital
Mumbai, Maharashtra
India

Indian Journal of Medical Ethics
Mumbai, Maharashtra
India

Editors' Note on the Revised Edition

We believe we owe an explanation to our readers as to why a revised edition of this book is being issued so soon after the appearance of the first edition in October 2015.

The first edition was released by Dr. George Lundberg (the former editor of *JAMA*) during the first conference of the World Association of Medical Editors (WAME), held at New Delhi in October 2015 and attended by several contributors to this book. A limited number of copies were produced digitally, in time for release at the conference and distribution among the contributors and a few others. Our intention was to print more copies shortly thereafter.

However, on publication, two of our well-wishers (John Mackrell and Dinesh Sinha, who had assisted with the editing and production of the original edition) submitted the text to analysis that might almost be described as forensic. They proposed substantial revisions, and we asked our contributors to review their chapters in the light of those suggestions. While some updated their contributions, others went along with much of what had been suggested. We now have a book with greater conformity across chapters and many more cross-references between them.

For the limited number of readers who have access to copies printed for the conference, this book may be perceived as a revised edition. But for most of you, this will be the first version of the book now open (as indeed we are) to your valuable criticism.

June 2016

Peush Sahni
Rakesh Aggarwal

Editors' Note

Biomedical research is essential for humankind. In the past century, it has played a major role in increasing average human longevity by more than two decades. In addition, it has made it possible for us to eradicate some diseases (e.g. smallpox), brought us to the verge of eradicating others (e.g. polio) and has changed the outcome of several others (diabetes, cardiovascular disease, human immunodeficiency virus infection and hepatitis C). Dramatic as these successes are, new diseases are still emerging, for instance, H1N1 influenza and Ebola. Though the diseases we investigate may change, biomedical research will stay with humankind as long as it exists.

Communicating research findings to peers—at meetings and, more importantly, through publications—is an integral part and the final step of the research cycle. As has been said about scientific research, 'If it ain't published, it never happened'. However, it is quite common to come across research studies that fail at this step. Though the fate of some may be due to the poor quality of science, many fail due to problems faced during writing and publishing, particularly in low- and middle-income countries.

Medical schools and science faculties in universities give their students a good grounding in science, medicine, scientific experimentation and research methodology. However, they often do not prepare them well for the task of writing and publishing research. Thus, when biomedical scientists start writing up their research findings, they often find themselves adrift and rudderless. This book, *Reporting and Publishing Research in the Biomedical Sciences*, attempts to bridge this gap.

The late Professor S.R. Naik was in many respects a mentor to both of us. He was editor of the peer-reviewed *Indian Journal of Gastroenterology*, one of the few MEDLINE-indexed medical journals published in India at that time. He realized that a major impediment to running a journal in India was the poor quality of manuscripts, mainly because physicians and scientists had little training and poor skills in writing. He decided to take the problem 'by the horns' and organized workshops for authors in the science, and art, of writing their research work. Of course, he could not conduct the 1- to 3-day workshops alone. So he 'coerced' us and others (some of whom have written chapters for this book) to join him. He would at times spend his own money to travel to these workshops, just as we often spent ours. Thus, we participated in several workshops with him—teaching skills in writing and publishing to young and old alike while learning the ropes and catching the bug of 'conducting writing workshops'.

As we moved from one workshop to another, we realized the need for a book which would consolidate all the information in one place. Indeed, Professor Naik, too, had felt such a need. After being diagnosed with terminal cancer at an early age, he spent his remaining few months editing *Communication for Biomedical Scientists*. The volume was published by the Indian Council of Medical Research and distributed free of cost. However, it has been out of stock for quite some time now, and we hope that this book will fill the vacuum. In a sense, this work is our tribute to Professor Naik and an expression of our gratitude for all that we learnt from him, in scientific writing and otherwise.

We have tried to get experienced writers, editors and researchers to write the chapters and have aimed to cover some of the recent developments in publishing that often stump the fledgling researcher. We are very grateful to all the authors, who have been so cooperative over the long gestation of this project. Their willingness to share their contributions with other authors has enabled us to bring information right up to date and avoid unnecessary duplication. We applaud their response to the consequent late changes and tight deadlines.

Praise, if any, is due entirely to our collaborators. The responsibility for any faults rests entirely with us, the editors. We will value any reader suggestions and try to incorporate them in subsequent editions of this book.

If this book eases the task of converting your research work into a manuscript, we will consider that our efforts have been worthwhile.

Last, but not least, we wish to acknowledge the support of Mr. Dinesh Sinha of Byword Editorial Consultants without whose help this project might never have come to fruition.

4 September 2015   Peush Sahni
                                                                   Rakesh Aggarwal

Preface

My personal experience with courses and books on biomedical communication began around 1986 at the All India Institute of Medical Sciences (AIIMS), New Delhi, when Stephen Lock, who was then editor of the *British Medical Journal (BMJ)*, brought with him three colleagues—Jane Smith, William Whimster and Alex Paton—to conduct a workshop on 'better medical writing'. We had invited people interested in writing up research and were astonished when about 100 turned up. They sat through the day absolutely enthralled by the proceedings.

The *BMJ* team in a single day made us aware of the problems faced by both authors and editors in their efforts to produce good papers and good journals. For authors it meant a lot of hard work. This included first spelling out clearly and concisely why the work was done, how it was done, what were the results obtained and what did they mean. Was the paper important enough to influence medical practice in India or even elsewhere? There were discussions on whether Indian authors were being discriminated against by Western editors and reviewers, which might be why few papers from India appeared in journals with high impact factors. (The answer to this was not 'no' but 'maybe', and the reasons they said were complex—it was true the papers from India were not always put together well, but the subjects they dealt with also did not always have a wider relevance.)

Stephen Lock suggested that we publish more in, and concentrate on improving, our own journals, and that is where the idea of starting *The National Medical Journal of India (NMJI)* was born (the present editor of *NMJI* is involved in this book's creation). The team also discussed the nitty-gritty of writing clearly and concisely, stressing that simple writing involved a lot of hard work with many, many revisions of the text. All of this would become easier, they said, if would-be writers had proper guidance from experts in the field either through personal contact or from their articles. I, for one, was introduced to many new ideas such as agreeing early on who a paper's authors should be and their order of appearance, asking friends who were not involved in the work for help (colleague treatment), leaving the written piece alone for a week or so to 'mature' before returning to it and being realistic about choosing which journal to send it to and reading its 'instructions to authors' carefully.

We recorded the proceedings and published a small booklet, also called *Better Medical Writing*, which sold out quickly. There was obviously a demand for such guidance relevant to the Indian situation. A year later, Subhash R. Naik held a similar workshop at King Edward Memorial (KEM) Hospital in Mumbai and brought out a book called *Better Medical Communication*. Subhash and his like-minded colleagues in medical writing and editing then organized a series of writing seminars all over India, which provided a tremendous impetus to both the quality and quantity of medical writing from India. Sadly, Subhash died early but not before he had edited another multi-author book called *Communication for Biomedical Scientists*. Now, two of his friends, Peush Sahni and Rakesh Aggarwal, have updated his original effort and are presenting another book here.

I really am very impressed by the result. Peush and Rakesh have brought together a team of 29 authors from 7 countries who have discussed not only how to write a paper but almost every other aspect of biomedical communication that there is. Here you will find detailed guidance not only on writing articles from the introduction to the references but also chapters on electronic publishing, podium and poster presentations and, of course, scientific fraud. A minor omission, and a suggestion for the next edition, is how to speak on a medical subject on television and how to create a short programme for the now ubiquitous and hugely influential 'idiot box' where health matters, I am told, are very popular with viewers.

I enjoyed reading the book and wished it had come out earlier. It would have saved much time and effort on improving my own papers, talks and posters as well as those of my residents. All I would need to do would be to tell them to go and buy this book, consult it over and over again and look after it with great care. It contains everything one needs to know about scientific communication in India and is an updated, modern, worthy and more comprehensive successor to the previous attempt.

So if you are in any way involved in biomedical communication, as I believe all of us will or should be sooner or later, this is the book for you to treasure as the all-purpose reference to me. It is also a major advance, I am proud to say, on *Better Medical Writing* of 29 years ago.

New Delhi, India   Samiran Nundy

Tribute to Professor S.R. Naik: A Scientist and Communicator

Professor Subhash R. Naik was head of the Department of Gastroenterology, Sanjay Gandhi Postgraduate Institute of Medical Sciences (SGPGI), Lucknow, when he passed away more than a decade ago. It seems like yesterday. He was 59.

I first came in close contact with Professor Naik when, in 1982, he joined the Department of Medicine at the King Edward Memorial (KEM) Hospital, Mumbai, and established an academic Department of Gastroenterology. Five years later, he left to join the newly established SGPGI to set up and head the Department of Gastroenterology.

Five years seems a brief period for anyone to start and establish a new department. But Professor Naik was not just anyone. I have no hesitation in saying that he changed the face of academic gastroenterology at KEM. Eager students and the budding faculty were infused with new blood, boundless energy, lively teaching, fervent pursuit of research, encouragement to chase ideas and, most importantly, the refusal to take no for an answer. His students, including me, will always carry that stamp on them. Every successful teaching module in Mumbai in gastroenterology is modelled on what Professor Naik started. He replicated the model at SGPGI over the next 15 years and established that department as among the best in India.

His association with scientific endeavours and publications worldwide was well known. As editor for 6 years and active member of the board in different capacities for another 14 years, he helped establish the *Indian Journal of Gastroenterology* as the premier publication in the field from India. He remained till his last day a respected scientific voice in Indian gastroenterology.

As if that legacy was not enough, Professor Naik also held in Mumbai, in 1987, the first workshop on scientific communication. I had the privilege of working with him on this venture and went on to hold many similar workshops later. It is encouraging to see that since those beginnings, scores of similar workshops have been held in Mumbai and other parts of India. He, along with Dr. Rakesh Aggarwal, published what was probably the first Indian book in this field (*Communication for Biomedical Scientists*). Every endeavour on scientific communication in India brings back memories of Professor Naik, and I see this present effort as a renewed tribute to him.

Those of us who enjoyed the privilege of his company remember him as a counsellor, guide, teacher and inspiration. I could say much more but wish to conclude by voicing my belief that Professor Naik was not only a fine ambassador for Indian science but a very fine human being.

Mumbai, India   Philip Abraham

Contents

About the Editors

Peush Sahni is a gastrointestinal surgeon at the All India Institute of Medical Sciences, New Delhi. He has been involved in journal editing for the past three decades and is presently Editor of The National Medical Journal of India. He is also the President of the Indian Association of Medical Journal Editors and is actively associated with the World Association of Medical Editors. He has been teaching at workshops on writing of scientific papers, peer review, and journal editing for many years.

Rakesh Aggarwal is a gastroenterologist-hepatologist at the Sanjay Gandhi Postgraduate Institute of Medical Sciences, Lucknow, India. He is an active researcher who has published several research papers, review articles, editorials, and book chapters. He has been involved in journal editing for more than two decades and is currently the editor of a major journal in his specialty. In addition, he has been involved in teaching at workshops on research methodology, writing of scientific papers, peer review, and journal editing for several years.

Contributors

Philip Abraham P.D. Hinduja Hospital, Mumbai, India

Amita Aggarwal Department of Clinical Immunology, Sanjay Gandhi Postgraduate Institute of Medical Sciences, Lucknow, India

Rakesh Aggarwal Journal of Gastroenterology and Hepatology and Department of Gastroenterology, Sanjay Gandhi Postgraduate Institute of Medical Sciences, Lucknow, India

Gitanjali Batmanabane Jawaharlal Institute of Postgraduate Medical Education and Research, Puducherry, India

Shobna J. Bhatia Department of Gastroenterology, Seth GS Medical College and KEM Hospital, Mumbai, India

Gourdas Choudhuri Department of Gastroenterology and Hepatobiliary Sciences, Fortis Memorial Research Institute, Gurgaon, India

Lorraine Ferris World Association of Medical Editors (WAME), Toronto, ON, Canada

Research Oversight and Compliance, University of Toronto, Toronto, ON, Canada

Robert H. Fletcher Department of Population Medicine, Harvard Medical School, Boston, MA, USA

Department of Epidemiology, University of North Carolina Gillings School of Global Public Health, Chapel Hill, NC, USA

Department of Social Medicine, School of Medicine, University of North Carolina at Chapel Hill, Chapel Hill, NC, USA

Suzanne W. Fletcher Department of Population Medicine, Harvard Medical School, Boston, MA, USA

Department of Epidemiology, University of North Carolina Gillings School of Global Public Health, Chapel Hill, NC, USA

Department of Social Medicine, School of Medicine, University of North Carolina at Chapel Hill, Chapel Hill, NC, USA

Uday C. Ghoshal Journal of Neurogastroenterology and Motility and Department of Gastroenterology, Sanjay Gandhi Postgraduate Institute of Medical Sciences, Lucknow, India

Nithya Gogtay Department of Clinical Pharmacology, Seth GS Medical College and KEM Hospital, Mumbai, India

Trish Groves BMJ and BMJ Open, London, UK

Farrokh Habibzadeh The International Journal of Occupational and Environmental Medicine Research and Development Headquarters, Petroleum Industry Health Organization, Tehran, Iran

Yvan J. Hutin European Centre for Disease Control (ECDC), Stockholm, Sweden

V. K. Kapoor Department of Surgical Gastroenterology, Sanjay Gandhi Postgraduate Institute of Medical Sciences, Lucknow, India

Rajeev Kumar Indian Journal of Urology and Department of Urology, All India Institute of Medical Sciences, New Delhi, India

Christine Laine Annals of Internal Medicine and American College of Physicians, Philadelphia, PA, USA

Rakesh Lodha Indian Pediatrics and Department of Paediatrics, All India Institute of Medical Sciences, New Delhi, India

John Mackrell Oxford University Press, Oxford, UK

Bandana Malhotra Freelance Medical Editor, New Delhi, India

Ana Marušić Journal of Global Health and Department of Research in Biomedicine and Health, University of Split School of Medicine, Split, Croatia,

University of Edinburgh, Edinburgh, Scotland, UK

David Moher Clinical Epidemiology Program, Ottawa Hospital Research Institute, Ottawa, ON, Canada

School of Epidemiology, Public Health and Preventative Medicine, University of Ottawa, Ottawa, ON, Canada

Sita Naik Apollo Hospitals Educational Foundation, Hyderabad, India

Sanjay A. Pai Department of Pathology, Columbia Asia Referral Hospital, Bengaluru, India

Usha Raman Department of Communication, University of Hyderabad, Hyderabad, India

Peush Sahni The National Medical Journal of India and Department of Gastrointestinal Surgery and Liver Transplantation, All India Institute of Medical Sciences, New Delhi, India

Larissa Shamseer Clinical Epidemiology Program, Ottawa Hospital Research Institute, Ottawa, ON, Canada

School of Epidemiology, Public Health and Preventative Medicine, University of Ottawa, Ottawa, ON, Canada

Dinesh Sinha Byword Editorial Consultants, Delhi, India

Margaret Winker World Association of Medical Editors, Winnetka, IL, USA

The IMRAD Structure

Gitanjali Batmanabane

IMRAD refers to the format in which most biomedical journals publish an original research paper. This framework for a scientific paper spells out how a manuscript should be presented. The letter I stands for Introduction, the M for Methods, the R for Results, the A for And and the D for Discussion. The origin of this format is somewhat hazy; however, Louis Pasteur is said to be the first person who published his work in this format. (1) The format was later made more popular by the famous British statistician Sir Austin Bradford Hill, (2) who worked with the Medical Research Council of the UK and was also a statistical consultant for the *British Medical Journal*.

1.1 Is There a Need for a Format?

In the eighteenth and nineteenth centuries, biomedical scientists published their work mainly in the form of essays or treatises. Those voluminous descriptions were not clearly demarcated into sections. This was acceptable at a time when the number of scientists, the amount of published work and the prospective readership were limited. But as the scientific enterprise expanded, the print runs for journals increased and their distribution became global. Editors became conscious of the high costs of publication and postage, and this prevented potential readers from having access to journals. The need for brevity in scientific writing was recognized as a means of increasing the number of papers published while containing the size of the journals. It is likely that the scientific community also felt the need for a more efficient format of writing and reading, so that they could quickly imbibe the ever-increasing body of knowledge. The IMRAD format was thus introduced to contain

G. Batmanabane
Jawaharlal Institute of Postgraduate Medical Education and Research, Puducherry, India

© The National Medical Journal of India 2018
P. Sahni, R. Aggarwal (eds.), *Reporting and Publishing Research in the Biomedical Sciences*, https://doi.org/10.1007/978-981-10-7062-4_1

costs and make manuscripts more reader-friendly. It is now followed by almost all biomedical journals and is the format recommended by the International Committee of Medical Journal Editors (ICMJE).

1.2 Components of IMRAD

This format represents a sequence of writing components of a paper, which makes for logical presentation of a scientific work. It serves to make information in a paper more easily understandable. This ease of comprehension allows the readers to make quicker decisions about and based on the research paper they have read.

Bradford Hill said that four questions must be addressed in any original research paper (Box 1.1). The first 'why did you start (the study)?' can be tackled in the Introduction. The second question 'what did you do?' can be handled in the section on Methods. The third section, the Results, should contain the answer to 'what did you find?' and the fourth section, the Discussion, should debate the implications of the study and answer the question 'what does it mean?' [2].

The Introduction section (*see also* Chap. 2) provides the background to the study leading up to statement of the problem or limitation in the existing body of knowledge, the justification for the study and the objectives. The Methods section (*see also* Chap. 3) details the methodology followed, so that another researcher may be able to replicate the work, if necessary. The Results section (*see also* Chap. 4) provides the findings of the study, which are summarized as text, tables, figures or a combination of these, and the Discussion section (*see also* Chap. 5) ties all these components together and allows the researcher to state the implications of the work and argue their thesis in the light of what is already known (or not known). The conclusion drawn from the study also forms a part of the Discussion.

Box 1.1 Components of the IMRAD Formats and Question That Each Component Answers [1]

I	Introduction	Why did you start (the study)?
M	Methods	What did you do?
R	Results	What did you find?
A	And	
D	Discussion	What does it mean?

1.3 Advantages of IMRAD

The IMRAD structure provides a simple framework or template for scientists to write their scientific papers. It prevents unnecessary repetition, thus saving print space and readers' time. Since the format follows the sequence in which scientific thought and work progresses, its use makes the contents of a paper easier to understand. It also helps the reader find specific pieces of information. For example, details of a particular laboratory technique would be found in the Methods section.

1.4   Limitations of IMRAD

Not all types of biomedical writing can be fitted in the IMRAD structure. Case reports and reviews (except systematic reviews) are difficult to fit into this framework. Some believe that adherence to a rigid format takes away the author's prerogative to improvise and innovate in presenting their research. The Nobel laureate Peter Medawar criticized this structure for not providing a realistic representation of the thought process of the researcher [3]. For instance, this format may not be appropriate for qualitative research. Also, when the results of some initial procedures in a study determine the subsequent steps performed (e.g. when the results of an epidemiological investigation into an outbreak determine the nature of laboratory tests and follow-up studies undertaken), adherence to the IMRAD sequence may not represent the actual sequence in which various tasks were undertaken. It may appear inappropriate and artificial to describe subsequent experiments in the Methods section, *before* the results of initial work have been revealed.

1.5   Which Journals Do Not Follow This Style?

Some broad-based science journals such as *Science* and *Nature* do not strictly follow the IMRAD structure. These journals publish the Methods section at the end of the paper, and in a smaller font. However, even for such journals, it may help the authors to write the paper in the IMRAD format and then move the Methods section to a later position. Similarly, some journals combine the Results and Discussion sections. This innovation is often a necessity for journals that publish research papers with a large number of sequential experiments, as it is important to first explain the implications of initial experiments for the readers to understand the results of subsequent experiments.

1.6   Other Sections

A research paper also has other sections such as Title and Keywords, as also References—a listing of the published works consulted while preparing the manuscript (*see also* Chaps. 8 and 9). An additional section of the paper is the Abstract, which is a condensed description of the study (*see also* Chap. 7). In fact, because the IMRAD format is so successful in making a piece of research understandable, the Abstract should follow the IMRAD framework.

In conclusion, the IMRAD structure for reporting scientific work has stood the test of time. The fact that most journals use either IMRAD or a minor modification of it implies that it may well outlive the lifetime of the current crop of researchers and scientific writers.

References

1. Day RA. The origins of the scientific paper: the IMRAD format. AMWA J. 1989;4:16–8.
2. Bradford Hill A. The reasons for writing. Br Med J. 1965;2:870–1.
3. Medawar PB. Is the scientific paper fraudulent? Saturday Review; 1 Aug 1964. p. 42–3.

The Introduction Section

2

Uday C. Ghoshal

Most biomedical journals require authors to follow the IMRAD format (*see also* Chap. 1) while writing original research papers. The Introduction is the first section of the body of the paper. The different sections of a paper vary in length, with the Introduction section usually being shorter than the Methods and the Results sections.

The Introduction section should answer the first of the four questions posed by Sir Austin Bradford Hill: 'Why was the study done?' [1]. It should, in brief, familiarize readers with the latest knowledge on the subject so that they do not need to read any previously published papers. It introduces the subject of research, provides the context of the study and encourages those who are interested in the field to read the paper in its entirety. This section should also inform the reader about what motivated the authors to conduct the research.

The Introduction section of a biomedical paper should cover the following points: (1) the importance and magnitude of the particular problem (its prevalence or frequency, disease burden, etc.), (2) the lacunae in the existing literature, (3) the hypothesis underlying the study and (4) the aims of the study. While doing this, one must neither be too brief nor too detailed, and a middle path must be found. A ground rule could be to provide a brief description so that the reader can get an idea of the established facts mentioned in the literature, the gaps in knowledge in the light of which the new study was carried out and the original question addressed in the study. It is important to refer to original research reports and not just review articles. The Introduction section often ends with the hypothesis and the aim of the study.

U. C. Ghoshal
Journal of Neurogastroenterology and Motility and Department of Gastroenterology,
Sanjay Gandhi Postgraduate Institute of Medical Sciences, Lucknow, India

© The National Medical Journal of India 2018
P. Sahni, R. Aggarwal (eds.), *Reporting and Publishing Research in the Biomedical Sciences*, https://doi.org/10.1007/978-981-10-7062-4_2

Box 2.1 provides an example of the Introduction section of a paper. In this example, the first sentence provides information on the frequency of the condition studied in the paper. The next few lines highlight the controversy in the literature available, citing data from a few studies. This part is an attempt to prepare the ground for the new study in the mind of the reader. It culminates in the fourth sentence of the second paragraph ('Hence, there is a need …'), which points to a specific lacuna in the current information and stresses the need for further information. The next sentence further clarifies how the new information would be useful. The final sentence of the introduction lists the study's various aims, as numbered points.

Box 2.1 Sample Introduction

Malabsorption syndrome (MAS) is a common condition in the tropics, including India. The aetiology of MAS in tropical areas differs from that in temperate countries[1] and may be expected to vary over a time period of several years.[2] In the past, tropical malabsorption (TM), popularly known as tropical sprue, was a common cause of MAS in India, and epidemics of TM were described from rural southern India.[3] Sporadic cases of TM have been reported from other tropical countries such as Pakistan, Thailand and Malaysia, and even from temperate countries such as Britain. It is believed that in recent years, with the improvement in the socioeconomic status of the population and in sanitary conditions, as well as the increasing use of antibiotics, the frequency of TM may have declined even in tropical countries.[4] Moreover, there may be a considerable overlap between post-infectious MAS, which is a subgroup of TM, and post-infectious irritable bowel syndrome (IBS), a common condition in temperate countries. Coeliac disease (CD), once thought to be uncommon in tropical countries, including India, is being reported frequently as a cause of MAS among children and adults.[5] However, data on the spectrum of MAS in Indian adults are scanty and contradictory.

It is difficult to differentiate between CD and TM. The response to antibiotics, a criterion used to diagnose TM, may be misleading as patients with CD may have secondary small intestinal bacterial overgrowth (SIBO) which, at least temporarily, may respond clinically to treatment with antibiotics.[6] Thus, it has been proposed that the diagnosis of CD should not be made entirely on the basis of conventional criteria, but should also include a serological test.[7] Hence, there is a need to determine demographic, clinical and laboratory characteristics that may help to differentiate TM from CD in adults with MAS in tropical countries. This may help clinicians to assess the likelihood of CD in a patient through the use of serological tests and the empirical institution of a gluten-free diet in patients with a high probability of the disease even in tropical countries. This study assessed (1) the spectrum of MAS among Indian adults, and (2) features that may help to differentiate TM and CD among them.

Adapted from Ghoshal *et al. Indian J Med Res* 2012;136:451–9

As a thumb rule, the Introduction section should not exceed 1–2 pages of double-spaced, A4 size paper. Too long an introduction may discourage the reader from going through the full paper. It is interesting to note that the Introduction of the Nobel prize-winning paper on the structure of DNA by Watson and Crick was barely two sentences long (Box 2.2). Despite its brevity, it clearly conveyed the originality of the authors' idea.

Box 2.2

'We wish to suggest a structure for the salt of deoxyribose nucleic acid (D.N.A.). This structure has novel features which are of considerable biological importance.'

Watson JD, Crick FHC. A structure for deoxyribose nucleic acid. *Nature* 1953;**171**:737–8

The Introduction should be written in the present tense. It should clearly define the problem that is being studied. It also needs to convey why the authors chose the particular subject and its importance. If the authors or their group have done any related work in the past, it may be mentioned in this section. Research workers in various fields often try to improve upon their previous work, whether by using a better study design or methods or a larger sample size. If this applies to their study, it should be mentioned in the Introduction section. This helps to establish the research group's credentials.

Important statements in the Introduction should be supported with appropriate references. However, this does not mean that a large number of papers should be cited to support each fact in this section. Only the main references that are relevant to the study hypothesis should be cited. Also, the specialized terms used in the paper should be clarified, and the full form of acronyms or abbreviations that are used repeatedly should be provided.

Sometimes, it is important to briefly present the principal method(s) used in the study, including any variation in the standard methodology, particularly if the main aim of the paper relates to the method used or if the authors have tried to make a variation in the method to improve its performance. Some authors, and even some journals, prefer to present the principal conclusion or new observations of the study in the Introduction. For most papers, however, this is not the case, and one should follow the style of the journal to which one wishes to submit the paper.

2.1 How to Write the Introduction

Some general rules of writing apply to all sections of a paper, including the Introduction section. For example, one should avoid writing in the passive voice. Similarly, it is best not to use complex and verbose sentences. It is useful to divide the text into paragraphs, and each paragraph should contain only one idea. The first sentence of a paragraph should introduce that idea and the last should be something of a concluding sentence. For example, the first paragraph could present the magnitude of the problem, the second paragraph could present the controversy in the existing literature and the final paragraph, the aims of the study. The Introduction section of an original research paper must not be written like a mini-review of the subject. For example, one must avoid the temptation of starting with a historical background of the subject.

Since the Introduction section may be written first, it is important to review and edit it after the whole paper is ready. This helps the authors to verify whether it relates to the final results presented and discussed by them. At this stage, it may be useful to run through a checklist of dos and don'ts to verify whether all the important points have been covered and the usual pitfalls avoided (Box 2.3).

Box 2.3 Dos and Don'ts of Writing an Introduction

Dos

1. Does it sufficiently review the relevant literature to familiarize the reader on the subject?
2. Does it state the limitations of the existing literature, or gaps in the current knowledge?
3. Does it state the controversy that the study planned to address?
4. Does it clearly state the study's hypothesis and list the aims of the study?

Don'ts

1. Does it include unnecessary details, such as the history of the disease being studied (except in the case of papers dealing with the history of a disease)?
2. Is the text long and written in a verbose style, in the passive voice and past tense?
3. Are the sentences complex and do they not follow a logical sequence?

Finally, one must remember that it is only through practice that one masters the skill of writing biomedical papers. The words of the Greek philosopher, Aristotle, are relevant in this context: 'For the things we have to learn before we can do them, we learn by doing them.'

Reference

1. Bradford Hill A. The reasons for writing. Br Med J. 1965;2:870–1.

The Methods Section

3

Amita Aggarwal

The key to a successful Methods section is to include the right amount of detail—too much, and it begins to sound like a laboratory manual; too little, and no one can repeat what was done.

Successful Scientific Writing, 2nd ed. [1]

The Methods section of a paper describes how a research study was done. This section is perhaps the most important part of a scientific paper as it describes the strategy and procedures used to answer the research question. Since the validity of the results obtained in a study depends on the approach and techniques used to generate data, a well-written Methods section helps the reader to place the study's conclusions in a context and understand its conclusion better. Further, all good science should be replicable. Thus, this section should describe the study procedures in sufficient detail so that another researcher who wants to replicate the work can do so easily.

A. Aggarwal
Department of Clinical Immunology, Sanjay Gandhi Postgraduate Institute of Medical Sciences, Lucknow, India

© The National Medical Journal of India 2018
P. Sahni, R. Aggarwal (eds.), *Reporting and Publishing Research in the Biomedical Sciences*, https://doi.org/10.1007/978-981-10-7062-4_3

3.1   Contents and Organization

A Methods section should answer the following questions.

1. What was done in the study?
2. How was each of these steps done?
3. How were the data analysed?
4. Did the researcher have ethical clearance and the consent of the study subjects to carry out the research?

This section should present the procedures that were carried out in chronological order. Alternatively, this could be done in the sequence in which you propose to present the results. These days, several studies have a complex design, which involves several interventions, procedures and measurements. To make the Methods sections of papers for such studies easy to understand, it is useful to divide the section into several subsections. For instance, the Methods section in a paper on a two-group, controlled drug trial could be structured as shown in Box 3.1. Of course, depending on the nature and complexity of the study, some of these subsections could be divided further into even smaller segments.

Box 3.1 A Suggested Method of Organizing the Methods Section of a Two-Group Controlled Intervention (Drug) Trial
1. Type of study and overall study design
2. Main methods
    (a) Characteristics of study subjects
    (b) Interventions or exposures
       • Method of assignment of subjects to the two groups
       • Interventions in the treatment group
       • Interventions in the control or comparator group
    (c) Measurement of outcomes
       • Types of measurements made
       • Time points for making each measurement
       • Tools used for and accuracy of each measurement
       • Who made the measurements?
3. Statistical analysis
4. Ethical considerations (including consent)

3.2   The Beginning: Overall Study Design

The first subsection or paragraph should summarize the overall nature and the design of the study since the organization of the subsequent details in the Methods section will depend on that. Research studies can be of various kinds, including (1) primary research studies, such as clinical trials, surveys, laboratory experiments and evaluations of a new test, and (2) secondary research studies, such as systematic reviews, meta-analyses and cost-efficacy analyses. Each of these formats can be further subdivided into several sub-types. For instance, clinical trials can be randomized or non-randomized, uncontrolled (single group) or controlled, open or blinded (masked), etc. Further, the control group could receive either a placebo or another previously known active drug. More complex studies, such as those with a crossover study design and factorial design, would require further subdivisions. Similarly, observational studies may be cross-sectional, case-control or cohort and either prospective or retrospective [2]. Two examples of how one could phrase the first sentence on the overall study design are shown in Box 3.2.

> **Box 3.2 Two Ways to Structure a Sentence on the Overall Study Design**
> - A randomized double-blind, placebo-controlled trial was carried out among patients with active rheumatoid arthritis to assess the short-term efficacy of RA2456, a synthetic small molecule.
> - A population survey was done in the coastal areas of district A in state X between January 2011 and December 2011 to assess the prevalence of blindness in the community.

At times, the study design becomes obvious in the Introduction section itself. In such instances, you could start with the main methods.

3.3   The Main Body

3.3.1   Characteristics of Study Subjects

It is customary to begin with the details of the study subjects (patients and controls), animals or cells, etc. used in the study. In the case of a clinical study, mention must be made of the inclusion criteria, such as the criteria used to diagnose the particular disease that the study relates to, and the specific age group or gender(s) covered. If the study included patients with only a particular subset of disease or disease of a particular severity, this information should be provided. For instance, if the study included patients with severe hypertension, it would be important to indicate what was meant by 'severe' hypertension. Similarly, details of the exclusion criteria, such as the presence of comorbid conditions, complications of the disease, prior exposure to certain drugs, pregnancy, lactation, poor performance status or abnormal laboratory tests, need to be described. The method of the recruitment of patients should be described in detail. For instance, it should be clarified whether all consecutive patients were included or only a subset? In the latter case, some explanation of how the subset was chosen should be provided.

Similarly, there should be a detailed description of the control subjects. This may include whether they were healthy volunteers, disease controls, etc.; from where they were recruited—the community, hospitals, from among blood donors, etc.; and details of their age, gender and race.

For animal experiments, the species, genetic background and source need to be mentioned, since different strains can give different results. Mention must also be made of the gender and age.

For cell lines, the source, origin, phenotypic characteristics, culture medium and conditions, number of passages, etc. need to be included.

A few examples of this segment are shown in Box 3.3.

Box 3.3 Examples Related to Characteristics of Study Subjects, Animals or Other Materials (e.g. Cells)

- Patients with rheumatoid arthritis satisfying the 2010 ACR criteria for diagnosis and having symptoms for at least 3 months were included in the study. The exclusion criteria included the presence of diabetes, pregnancy, renal dysfunction (i.e. serum creatinine of >2 mg/dL) or hepatic dysfunction (i.e. elevated serum bilirubin or ALT/AST >3 times normal). Patients taking >10 mg/day of prednisolone or a disease-modifying antirheumatic drug were also excluded.
- BALb/C female mice, 4–8 weeks of age were obtained from Jackson Laboratories, Bar Harbor, ME, USA. They were reared in germ-free conditions and used between 10 and 12 weeks of age.
- K562 cell line was obtained from National Centre for Cell Sciences, Pune, India, and cultured in RPMI medium in 5% CO_2 atmosphere. After a confluent growth was achieved, the cells were harvested and labelled with Cr^{131}. The labelled cells were used as targets for NK cell cytotoxicity (100,000 cells per experiment) after verifying that the labelling efficiency exceeded 80%.

For all chemicals, the source, catalogue number and generic name should be given. Similarly, for buffers, the pH and molarity needs to be mentioned. For instruments, the name of the manufacturer and the precision and technical specifications are to be included; if the equipment has various settings that may influence the results, the settings used could be included [3]. It is useful in this context to read other published papers in the field to know how much detail should be provided.

3.3.2 Interventions or Exposures

The next part should spell out the details of the intervention. If the patients were studied in special circumstances, such as at a particular time of the day or after an overnight fast, it should be mentioned. The model of all equipment used for the intervention, such as short-wave diathermy, and the details of the manufacturer should be included. If the procedure performed was a standard one, such as endoscopy, there is no need to provide the details; however, if it was a novel intervention, sufficient details should be provided so that the readers can understand and repeat the intervention, if necessary.

If different groups underwent different interventions, then each intervention needs to be described. If multiple interventions were done in the same subject, then each of these interventions, as well as their order, must be specified.

If the paper describes a drug trial, the details of the drug and placebo used, including the source, dosage, route and frequency of administration of each, need to be stated. If the eligible subjects were randomized into different groups, the method of randomization should be described in detail. The methods used for randomization, allocation concealment and blinding, if imperfect, may have an important influence on the results of the study. Providing these details will help the reader to assess the credibility of the results. It is equally important to give the details of the frequency of follow-up and the data recorded at each follow-up visit. Any measurement of drug compliance, such as pill count, should be given. Similarly, the drugs permitted and not permitted as rescue remedies, as also the events for which withdrawal from the study was allowed (flare-up of the disease, drug toxicity, etc.—each being clearly defined) should be listed. Box 3.4 shows the description of the randomization into two groups and the treatment administered to each in a particular study.

Box 3.4 Description of Randomization in a Study
Patients with active rheumatoid arthritis were randomized into two groups in 1:1 ratio, using computer-generated random numbers. One group received methotrexate in a dose of 15–25 mg/week (started at 15 mg/week and escalated by 2.5 mg/week every 2 weeks to the maximally tolerated dose or to a maximum of 25 mg/week) and RA2456 100 mg tablet twice daily. The other group received methotrexate as stated above and a matching placebo tablet twice daily. The patients were followed up every 2 weeks. Drug compliance was assessed at each visit using the pill count. No corticosteroids or intra-articular injections were allowed. For pain relief, the patients could use paracetamol as required, up to a maximum of 2 g/day, which was to be recorded in a diary with date and time.

For laboratory experiments, all details should be provided if a new procedure is used. However, if the procedure used has been previously described, a citation can be provided and the procedure described in brief, making special mention of any modifications that may have been made. If relevant, then details about sensitivity of the assay, as well as intra-assay and inter-assay variability, should be included. The source and performance characteristics (e.g. specificity and sensitivity) of all commercial assay kits used should be provided (Box 3.5).

Box 3.5 Describing the Source and Performance of Commercial Assay Kits
IL-6 was measured in serum using ELISA kits (A&B Labs, MI, USA), according to the manufacturer's instructions. The sensitivity of the assay was 3.15 pg/mL. Intra-assay and inter-assay variabilities were assessed using ten replicates each of the same specimen in eight plates and were found to be 4% and 6%, respectively.

3.3.3   Measurement of Outcomes

The measures of the primary and secondary outcomes should be defined. These can be clinical outcomes or laboratory variables. For quantitative variables, the units of measurement must be specified for each outcome, such as milligrams per decilitre for blood glucose and centimetres for height, even though some of these may appear to be obvious. All qualitative outcomes, which may have been used in the manuscript, should be defined unambiguously, e.g. one must define terms such as improvement in symptoms, pain relief, partial response, complete response, relapse, recrudescence and worsening of clinical condition.

If measurements were made repeatedly, the various time points as well as the outcomes measured at each point should be given. Further, one must describe how each measurement was made, e.g. by using telephonic or direct interviews (at home or in the clinic) or by clinical examination. The members of the research team who made the measurements should also be mentioned. It may be pertinent to specify whether all the measurements were made by the same person or different persons, and in the latter situation, whether any attempts were made to ensure uniformity and assess interobserver variability.

If the outcome was a composite measure, then all its components, as well as the procedure used to combine these, should be defined. The text should be written in such a manner that the interpretation of various combinations of components is unambiguous. It may be important to clarify whether and how the composite outcome was calculated if information on one or some of the components was not available. If this composite measure has been previously validated, one should cite the relevant reference.

Box 3.6 contains a couple of examples of how this subsection can be written.

Box 3.6 Examples of Writing About Outcome Measures
- Blood pressure was recorded at 8:00 a.m. at the start of the study and at 4, 8 and 16 weeks of the study period in a sitting position, using a mercury sphygmomanometer. All measurements were taken by the same nurse.
- The proportion of patients achieving a Disease Activity Score 28 (DAS28) of <2.6 at 24 weeks was the primary outcome whereas the number of patients achieving remission at 48 weeks was the secondary outcome. The DAS28 is a composite weighted score of 28-swollen joint count, 28-tender joint count, ESR by Westergren method and general health measured on a visual analogue scale.[a]

The superscript 'a' indicates that it would be appropriate to provide a reference to the method used for computing DAS28 at this location in the manuscript.

3.4 Statistical Methods

Data analysis methods are an important component of the Methods section. One needs to describe the various statistical tools used to summarize, compare and analyse the data and the software used (mentioning the version) for this purpose. It is also necessary to provide the details of any form of preprocessing that the data may have undergone, such as (1) splitting into categories (with cut-offs used for the purpose, e.g. 'the subjects were divided into four equal quartiles on the basis of their serum triglyceride levels'), (2) normalization against a control (e.g. 'the expression of genes of interest was normalized using the expression of the beta-actin gene as a control') and (3) standardization, log or Poisson transformation to ensure normal distribution of the data or calculation of composite scores. Any procedure used for imputation of missing data must be described. Finally, the p value cut-off used to define significant results (alpha error cut-off) must be specified.

For common statistical tests and procedures, providing the name of the test should suffice; otherwise, one should provide the details of the test or a reference to previous publications describing the test procedure. The type of analysis, whether intention-to-treat or per-protocol, should be specified. However, making a mere mention of either phrase will not do; one needs to describe what each analysis means. Box 3.7 shows an example of the statistical methods section of a paper.

Box 3.7 Example of the Statistical Methods Section
- The data on quantitative and categorical variables were compared between the groups receiving active and placebo treatment using Student's t-test or chi-squared test, respectively. Serum interleukin-6 levels were log-transformed before the analysis. The Disease Activity Score 28 (DAS28; range 1.15–10.4) was calculated from the swollen joint count (out of 28 joints; SJC28), tender joint count (TJC28), serum levels of C-reactive protein (CRP) and global health score (GH) as follows[b]: DAS28 (CRP) = 0.56* $\sqrt{(TJC28)}$ + 0.28* $\sqrt{(SJC28)}$ + 0.014*GH + 0.36*ln (CRP + 1) + 0.96. The proportion of patients achieving ACR20, ACR50 and ACR70 response[c] in the active and placebo treatment groups was also compared. The primary analysis was carried out on an intention-to-treat basis and included all subjects who had received at least one dose of the experimental drug or placebo. In addition, we carried out a per-protocol analysis, which included all patients who had completed at least 3 months of the intended treatment.
- The data were analysed by calculating the odds ratio of the allele frequencies (number of copies of a specific allele divided by the total number of alleles in the group) in the patient and control groups. The genotype frequencies were compared using chi-squared test. Haplotype analysis was done using the HAPSTAT software version 3.0 (available at http://www.bios.unc.edu/~dlin/hapstat/).

The superscripts 'b' and 'c' here in the text are similar to 'a' in Box 3.6.

The section on statistical methods should also include information on the assumptions made and procedures used for the calculation of sample size, any correction used for potential drop-outs and the results of this calculation. If one or more interim analyses were planned or done, the details should be included in this segment (Box 3.8).

Box 3.8 Description of Sample Size
The sample size was calculated for comparison of proportions between the two groups using alpha level of 0.05, power of 0.80, patient/control ratio of 1:2 and allele frequency estimates based on previous studies[d] (PS programme; available at http://biostat.mc.vanderbilt.edu/wiki/Main/Power Sample Size). The calculated sample size ranged from 83–98 for patients to 166–196 for different polymorphisms. We, therefore, planned to enrol 100 patients and 200 controls.

The superscript 'd' here in text is similar to 'a' in Box 3.6.

3.5 Ethical Considerations

Information should be provided on the approval of the relevant institutional ethics committee or institutional review board and the details of the consent process (written or verbal). In studies involving animal experiments, the Methods section must mention that approval was obtained from the animal ethics committee (Box 3.9).

Box 3.9 Describing Ethical Considerations
- The study was approved by the institutional ethics committee. Written informed consent was taken from all patients. The study was done in accordance with the guidelines laid down by the Indian Council of Medical Research (ICMR).
- Studies in animals and humans were reviewed, and the study was approved by the ethics committee of the institution. All subjects provided informed consent before their participation in the study.

3.6 Language and Grammar

Since the Methods section describes work that has already been done, it must be written in the past tense. The writing should be direct and precise. Complex sentences and minor details should be avoided. However, there should be enough detail to enable the reader to replicate the methods, if necessary. The following are a few examples.

3.6.1 Example 1

Ten millilitres of blood was drawn after cleaning the site in an EDTA vial containing 1 mg EDTA. The tube was transported to the laboratory, and plasma was separated by centrifuging the tube for 5 min. The plasma was stored in 1 mL aliquots at −80 °C.

A better way of writing this is:

Ten millilitres of blood was drawn in a vial that contained EDTA. Plasma was separated immediately and stored at −80 °C.

3.6.2 Example 2

Monocytes were separated from peripheral blood and used for further analysis.

This is too non-specific and should preferably be written as follows:

Peripheral blood mononuclear cells (PBMCs) were separated using Histopaque (Sigma, USA) and density gradient centrifugation. Ten million PBMCs were used for monocyte isolation using the plate adherence method. The purity of monocytes was verified by staining for CD16 and analysing in FACS Calibure (Becton Dickinson, USA); specimens with 95% purity were used for further analysis.

3.7 Use of Tables and Figures

In the case of a study with a complex design, a flow diagram may explain the procedures much better than a long paragraph (Fig. 3.1). If several similar items have been used in the study, such as primers for a polymerase chain reaction (PCR), restriction enzymes and bacterial species, a table can be a helpful method of listing these (Table 3.1).

3.8 Use of References

Ideally, all methods, except a few that may have been specifically developed for the study, should have a citation. However, these are omitted in the case of techniques or tests that are in routine use (e.g. the technique for measuring blood pressure or blood sugar and Student's t-test). The citations should be from a well-known journal or a book that is in wide use, and not an obscure source that the reader may not be able to locate easily. The latter defeats the very purpose of providing the reference, which is to allow others to replicate the study. If in doubt about whether or not to provide a reference for a method, it is better to err in the direction of providing it.

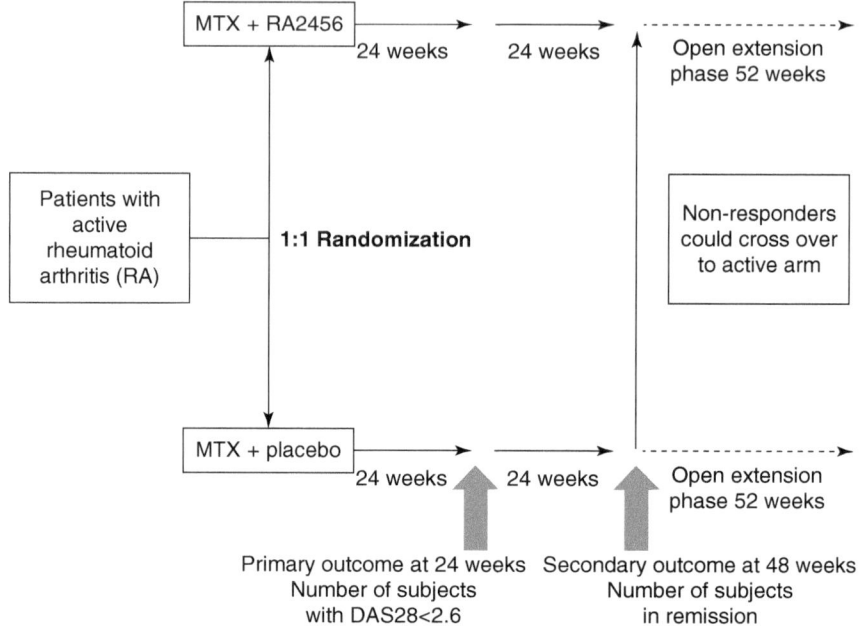

Patients with active rheumatoid arthritis (RA) were randomized 1:1 to receive placebo or the active drug (RA2456) and patients were assessed at 24 weeks for primary outcome and for secondary outcome at 48 weeks. After 48 weeks patients entered open extension phase for next 52 weeks. The non-responders could cross over to active arm after 48 weeks.

Fig. 3.1 Use of a diagram to depict methods of a drug trial

Table 3.1 Example of use of a table in the Methods section of a paper
Table I Primers used for amplification of DNA for various genes using real-time polymerase chain reaction

TLR1	CAGTGTCTGGTACACGCATG	TTTCAAAAACCGTGTCTGTTAA	105
TLR2	GGCCAGCAAATTACCTGTGT	AGGCGGACATCCTGAACCT	67
TLR3	CCTGGTTTGTTAATTGGATTA	TGAGGTGGAGTGTTGCAAAGG	82
TLR4	CAGAGTTTCCTGCAATGGATC	GCTTATCTGAAGGTGTTGCACA	85
18S[a]	CATGGTGACCACGGGTGAC	TTCCTTGGATGTGGTAGCCG	79

[a]18S ribosomal RNA gene was used as a housekeeping control gene

3.9   Special Situations

The principles described above are generalizations that apply to most situations. However, research studies can have differing designs, and certain specific items may need to be described in manuscripts for studies for some particular research designs. Some of these are as follows.

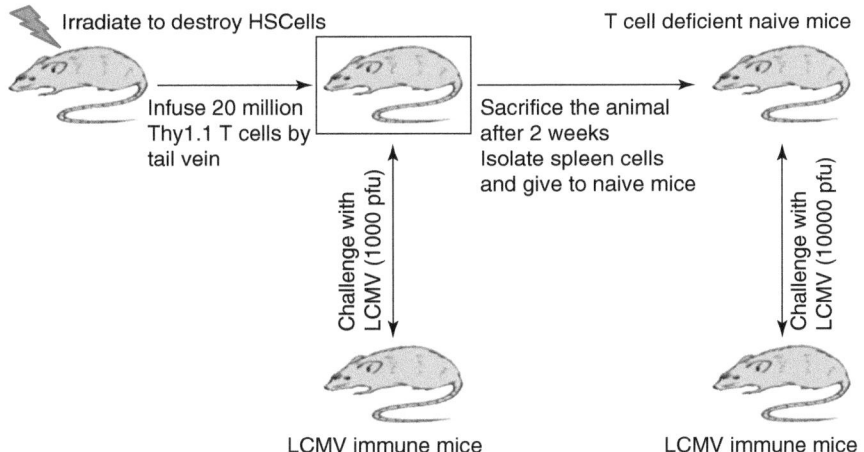

Thy1.2 C57BL6 mice were given 200 Gy irradiation to destroy the haematopoetic stem cells (HSCells). The mice were then reconstituted with 20 million Th1.1 T cells. After 2 weeks the reconstituted and control mice (LCMV immune mice) were challenged with 1000 plaque forming units (pfu) of LCMV. The course of LCMV was studied in both mice. Later the reconstituted mice were sacrificed and spleen cells were isolated from them. Ten million spleen cells were infused into T cell deficient naïve mice. After 2 weeks the mice were challenged with LCMV 10000 pfu and observed for disease.

Fig. 3.2   Use of a picture to depict methods of an animal experiment

3.9.1   Laboratory Studies

For laboratory studies, besides providing the details of the animals and cells as mentioned above, it is also necessary to mention the chemicals used (their source, the vehicle or solvent used to dissolve them), buffers (molarity, pH) and temperature at which the experiment was carried out, as all of these can affect the results of an assay. Since the experimental designs in laboratory studies are complex, it may be useful to provide a simple line diagram explaining the procedure that was carried out (Fig. 3.2).

3.9.2   Randomized Clinical Studies

Of the over 20 items listed in the Consolidated Guidelines for Reporting of Randomized Clinical Trials (CONSORT), several relate to the Methods section (*see also* Chap. 18 on 'Reporting guidelines') [4]. These include the trial design, any changes made to the trial after the study has started, the participants (inclusion and exclusion criteria, setting of the study patients), details of the intervention(s), outcomes (primary and secondary outcomes, the points in time at which these were assessed), sample size, randomization procedure, allocation concealment, blinding, how all these were chosen/conducted and, finally, the statistical analysis. These guidelines are now followed by major clinical journals and are intended to ensure that reports on clinical trials contain sufficient detail to enable readers to understand the impact and applicability of the study to their clinical practices.

3.9.3 Meta-Analysis and Systematic Reviews

The Methods section should include details on the search strategy, criteria used to select (inclusion and exclusion criteria) studies for use in the meta-analysis, procedures used for data abstraction (efficacy and safety data), whether the authors were contacted to obtain supplementary data, and statistical analysis.

3.10 Summary

The Methods section should describe what you have done to answer your scientific question in a simple, clear, systematic way, so that the reader can understand the study design, protocol used and statistical analysis. One should use the past tense and provide enough details to allow for replication of the study.

References

1. Matthews JR, Bowen JM, Matthews RW. Successful scientific writing. 2nd ed. Cambridge: Cambridge University Press; 2000. p. 64. http://eugene.yakovis.com/doc/Matthews%20 Bowen%20Matthews%202000%20(raw%20OCR).pdf.
2. Knight KL. Study/experimental/research design: Much more than statistics. J Athl Train. 2010;45:98–100.
3. Kallet RH. How to write the methods section of a research paper. Respir Care. 2004;49:1229–32.
4. Schulz KF, Altman DG, Moher D, CONSORT Group. CONSORT 2010 statement: updated guidelines for reporting parallel group randomised trials. BMC Med. 2010;8:18.

The Results Section

4

Rakesh Aggarwal and Peush Sahni

4.1 Introduction

The Results section is the part of a research paper that answers the third of the four questions of Sir Austin Bradford Hill, namely, 'What did you find' [1]. It follows the Methods section, which has already answered the question 'What did you do?' [1]. It is therefore logical that results of all the steps enumerated in the Methods must be provided, preferably in the same sequence as their description in the Methods. Also, it is expected that all results would have corresponding methods described and that no new data would suddenly appear in the Results section.

A cardinal rule while writing this section is that it is better to err on the side of excess. It is better to provide your results in more detail than ending up with a Results section that leaves the reviewer or a reader feeling that he needs further data to fully understand your findings. This has become even more important in recent years, with meta-analyses becoming common—it is at times impossible to include in such analyses those papers whose Results sections provide inadequate details. Thus, the emphasis is on providing more data; the issue of consequent increase in the size of manuscripts has been resolved through the use of supplementary data section (*see below*).

R. Aggarwal (✉)
Journal of Gastroenterology and Hepatology and Department of Gastroenterology, Sanjay Gandhi Postgraduate Institute of Medical Sciences, Lucknow, India

P. Sahni
The National Medical Journal of India and Department of Gastrointestinal Surgery and Liver Transplantation, All India Institute of Medical Sciences, New Delhi, India

© The National Medical Journal of India 2018
P. Sahni, R. Aggarwal (eds.), *Reporting and Publishing Research in the Biomedical Sciences*, https://doi.org/10.1007/978-981-10-7062-4_4

4.2 Three Components of Results

Results are usually provided in three components: text, tables and figures (or graphics). These three components should be used synergistically, taking care to avoid repetition of the same information in text and in accompanying tables and figures. However, this advice should not be used as a justification for statements in text such as: 'The results are presented in Tables I to V and Figures 1 to 3'. Such statements are a nightmare for editors and reviewers and hinder effective communication of the findings to the readers. Instead, important messages derived from data in tables and figures should be briefly spelt out in the text and possibly without actual numbers. Such text serves to complement the data shown in the tables and figures, which though should be understandable even without referring to the text.

In contrast to oral presentations, tables are preferred over figures in written presentations. This is because numerical data in a table are more accurate and detailed than those in the graphic format and because a journal reader has more time available to understand a complex table than an audience listening to a talk. Also, numerical data in tables are more amenable to use in subsequent meta-analyses. However, some data are more amenable to graphical representation (e.g. a scatter diagram showing relationship of two variables or a line showing temporal trend of a variable) since the latter conveys the message at a glance.

4.3 Contents

4.3.1 Study Subjects and Groups

The Results section generally begins with a description of the study subjects (patients in clinical studies, clusters in cluster-randomized community trials, animals in experimental studies, etc.) and study groups (e.g. placebo and treatment groups in a drug trial). It helps to provide full details as the readers can then assess whether all the study subjects fulfilled all the inclusion criteria, how they compared with those that the readers encounter in their practice, etc. This is particularly important when data have been generated at a tertiary referral centre, whereas the inference of the study will be applied at the primary or community care level, where the patients may differ from those seen in the referral setting. It helps to provide a table with the salient features of the study subjects; however, if this is done, the same information must not be repeated in the text.

In a study where the subjects are classified into two or more groups that are treated or followed-up differently (for instance, in a drug trial), information on the number and condition of subjects included in each group should be provided. This is often best done using a table containing a column for each study group. This allows the readers to compare the groups quickly. Whether p values for statistical comparison of various characteristics between study groups should be shown is a matter of debate; however, it is increasingly being considered inappropriate when a process of randomization has been used to assign subjects to two groups.

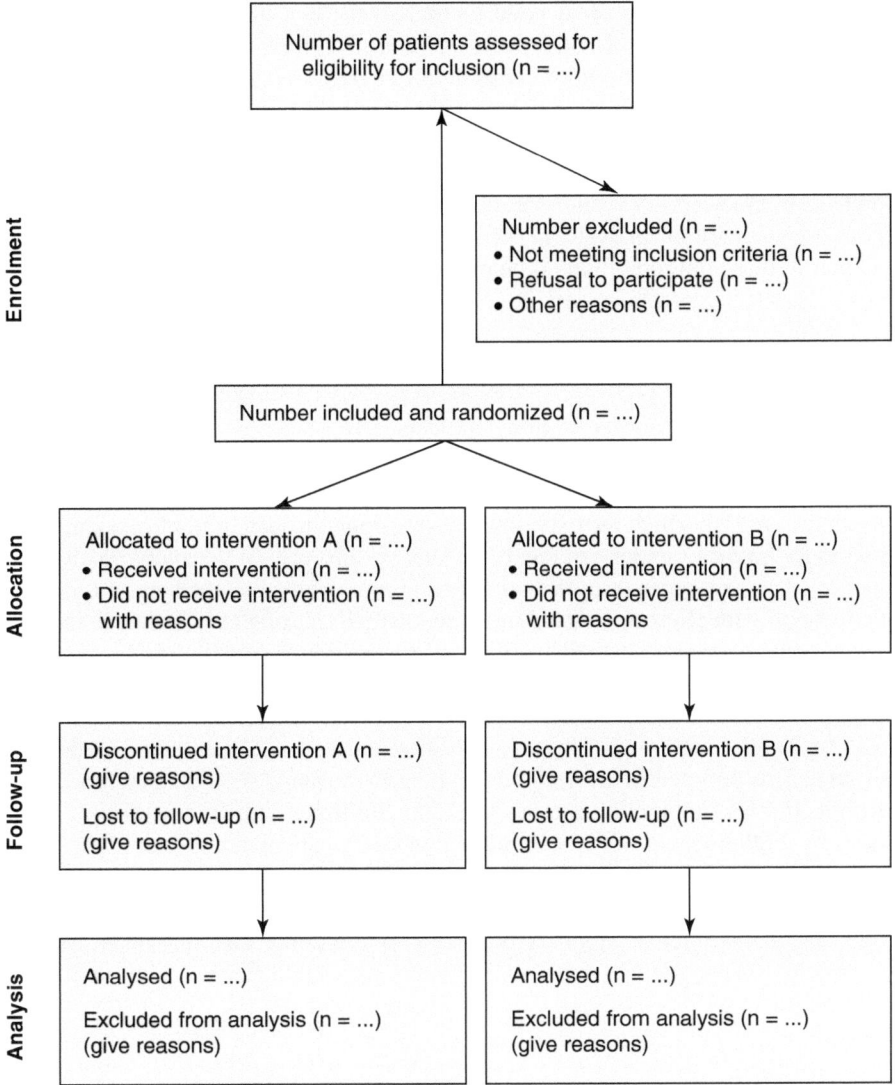

Fig. 4.1 Diagrammatic representation of the flow of patients in a drug trial

4.3.2   Flowchart for Study Subjects

For interventional studies, it is almost mandatory (*see* Chap. 18 on 'Reporting guidelines') to show the flow of patients through various phases (i.e. enrolment, intervention allocation, follow-up and data analysis) of the trial [2]. Such a graphic, known as the CONSORT flowchart (Fig. 4.1), helps the readers know the proportion of patients who fulfilled the eligibility criteria, agreed to participate in the study, completed the treatment, etc. It is also important to mention the proportion that dropped out and the reasons thereof, and the cause of death if any subject died during the study period. Most good journals insist that the CONSORT statement, including providing a checklist and flowchart, is followed, because this helps improve the reporting of randomized controlled trials. This, in turn, enables readers to better understand a trial's conduct and to assess the validity of its results. In a graphic of this type, the numbers must add up correctly so that all subjects who were screened or included in the study are accounted for. Any discrepancies may be interpreted by reviewers (or readers) either as representing carelessness in data collection, organization or analysis on the part of authors or as an attempt to hide data; neither of these interpretations is charitable to the authors.

4.3.3 Results of Various Measurements

The section on description of study subjects is followed by the results of various experiments. It helps to present these in the form of a story; this is possible only if the results are presented in a chronological or a natural order. It does not necessarily mean the order in which the experiments were done; instead, it implies an order that makes for an easier understanding of results. For instance, if the study involves collection of several types of information in a group of subjects, the natural order may be to begin with clinical data and move sequentially through biochemical and serological data to genetic data. The aim is to progress from simple to more complex information. If the Methods were grouped and ordered in several subsections, the Results should follow the same order.

The Results section should have the information on all the variables that were evaluated, as outlined in the Methods section. No variable should be included in the Results if it was not included in the Methods. Similarly, if the assessment of a comparison or relationship was not mentioned in the statistical methods section, there is no place for it in the Results section.

If one is not sure of the sequence in which various results should be presented, a look at some similar papers may be useful. While doing this, one must avoid the temptation to use the text from such a paper as a template, lest one be guilty of plagiarism.

4.3.4 Numerical Data

For numerical data, actual values are preferred over percentages; the latter may be included in parenthesis after the actual numerical values. The only exception perhaps is large cohort studies with several thousand subjects, where percent values alone may be provided. Though frequently used, percent values are misleading if the number of observations is fewer than a hundred. Their use for observations sets of fewer than 50–70 should be discouraged.

Computer software programs automatically calculate means and ratios to several decimal points beyond that in individual observations. Authors often reproduce these as such in their results. The increased number of digits is misleading. One must remember that the values of mean and standard deviation cannot have a degree of accuracy higher than those of the original observations, and hence the use of any additional digits must be avoided. However, others believe that one extra digit beyond that in the original data after the decimal point is acceptable.

Results must be specific and unambiguous. Adjectives such as 'most', 'some' and 'often' should be avoided, as these might convey different meanings to different people.

4.3.5   Statistical Aspects

Data should be summarized using appropriate measures of central tendency and dispersion (or variability). Mean and standard deviation (SD) are the most frequently used measures for this purpose; however, if the data are not normally distributed, median and interquartile range (or range) should be preferred. Authors often confuse SD with standard error (SE) and provide a measure of variability of data without specifying whether it is SD or SE; this must be avoided. Most journals today require authors to also provide confidence intervals around the estimate, since these provide additional useful information.

Probability values may be given as actual p values, or as being above or below a cut-off (e.g. $p < 0.05$ or $p = $ ns, depending on whether or not the test result was statistically significant). However, when using the former option, any p values below 0.001 are usually rounded off to $p < 0.001$; also, one must know that p values can never be zero. One must avoid adding adjectives to the interpretation of the p value ('highly' significant, 'very highly' significant, etc.). Similarly, statistically speaking, differences that are non-significant do not exist. For instance, it is wrong to say 'Increase in weight of animals receiving the dietary supplement was higher than that of animals receiving the conventional diet, even though the difference did not reach statistical significance'. Similarly, it is better to avoid phrases such as 'trend towards significance', 'just short of significance', etc.

4.4   Tables

Tables are frequently used for presentation of data in the Results section. In fact, their use is often indispensable. They allow for a large amount of information to be presented in an organized manner within a small space. They also make for easy retrieval of the required information even though the entire table may appear quite intimidating. For instance, let us consider either the log tables that we used in school or the railway schedule. These are examples of large tables which are referred to only when required. We use these since there is a lot of information placed in a few pages.

A table is an appropriate method of presenting data in a research paper when the aim is to (1) summarize the research findings from a set of experiments done in several study subjects, (2) allow comparison of specific data from two or more groups, (3) relate one set of data to another making their relationship clear (e.g. the relation of weight of animals with their age) and (4) provide raw data to enable readers to make calculations for themselves. When large amount of data are generated, as in epidemiological studies or hypothesis-free laboratory experiments (e.g. microarray or proteomics experiments), the number and size of tables may far exceed the space limit set by a given journal for a printed paper. Most journals today ask authors to submit even such raw data with their manuscripts as an addendum. Journals place such data in electronic format on their website (using labels such as supplementary data, web extra material, additional data, etc.) while printing only the most important tables. Interested readers can then download these supplementary data for viewing or reanalysis. However, such data are usually made available on an 'as-submitted-by-the-authors' basis—without a close examination or formatting. Hence, one must be particularly careful, as any errors in these data are unlikely to be picked up during the peer-review and publication process.

A good table must be compact and complete, i.e. it must be understandable without any detailed reference to the text of the paper. The data in a table must be accurate, important and related to each other; it is not a good idea to include several types of disparate (say clinical, biochemical and radiological) data in one table; in such cases, it may be preferable to create two or more tables, each dealing with data on one aspect. The format of the table must be clear and simple. This can be done by using logical groups for rows and columns and removing any unnecessary ones. A consistent style and terminology should be used throughout the table. The groups to be compared should be so placed that for comparison, the eyes move from left to right, and not from top to bottom.

A table consists of the following parts: (1) a title, (2) rows and columns, (3) row descriptors and column headings, (4) stub (heading for the first column that contains row descriptors), (5) the data in various cells (intersection of each row and column) and (6) footnotes and explanatory notes, if required (Fig. 4.2). Omission of any of these may render the table difficult to understand. Each table must have a short title, which should preferably be self-explanatory and not contain abbreviations. Explanations for all abbreviations and symbols used in a table should be included as footnotes. Symbols for footnotes vary from journal to journal, and the instructions for authors need to be consulted. Some journals use alphabets, others numerals and

Title: Parts of a table

Stub	Column A heading	Column B heading	Column C heading	
			Column C1 subheading	Column C2 subheading
Row 1 descriptor	Cell	Cell	Cell	Cell
Row 2 descriptor	Cell	Cell	Cell	Cell
Row 3 descriptor	Cell	Cell	Cell	Cell

Footnote and explanatory notes

Fig. 4.2 Various parts of a table. Each of these components must be present in a table, except footnote and explanatory notes which are optional

still others symbols, such as *, †, ‡, §, ¶, **, ††, etc. Units of measurement for each variable and the nature of the summary measures used (mean or median, SD or SE, confidence intervals) should be given; where statistical comparisons have been done, p values should be included in the table, either as a separate column or in a footnote.

Each table should be double spaced and placed on a separate page. Tables should be numbered consecutively in the order of their first citation in the text. Vertical rules should not be used within the table since these interfere with reading. Most journals use computer software to convert the electronic files submitted by authors into print files; complex formats and internal rules can interfere with this conversion process. Most journals thus prefer tables to be submitted as separate spreadsheet files or in a generic format (.txt or .csv files).

Some journals may limit the number of tables and figures for a particular type of article. Others may want authors to reduce the number of words in the text to accommodate an extra table or figure. It is therefore wise to check the 'instructions to authors' of the journal to which one plans to submit the manuscript and familiarize oneself with the type of tables and figures in recent issues.

4.5 Figures (Graphics)

The eyes and brain are better at picking up visual clues from pictures than from a set of numbers. Thus, it is easier to convey a message through illustrations than by using tables.

Graphics used in the Results section can be of several types [3], namely, (1) photographic pictures (including radiology images, nuclear scans, pathology images, etc.); (2) line diagrams of surgical findings, surgical technique or other data; (3) graphs or data charts (including pie diagrams, bar diagrams, line diagrams, scatter plots, etc.); and (4) graphics showing molecular data (nucleotide sequences for DNA or amino acid sequences for proteins) which consist primarily of text matter. Each of these types of graphics needs special attention (*see below*). All figures must be professionally drawn, using a computer program. Handwritten or typewritten labels on figures are not acceptable.

4.5.1 Photographic Images

Photographs are used to document observations. These include photographs of patients, radiological data (including CT scans, ultrasound, magnetic resonance imaging, nuclear scans), intraoperative findings, surgically resected specimens, histology slides, electrophoresis gel pictures, fluorescence microscopy images, etc. Such pictures often contain colours or a wide range of greys (known as continuous tone, grey-tone or half-tone pictures). Photographic prints are also frequently used for reporting of physiological data (e.g. electrocardiographic recording of an arrhythmia, electroencephalography recordings, pressure recordings in an animal experiment, oesophageal manometry recordings, etc.) though in such settings, only two (black-and-white) or a few shades of grey may suffice.

A good photograph must be (1) true to the original, (2) clear and have good resolution, (3) of an appropriate size (appropriate reduction or enlargement), (4) of full tonal range for continuous-tone images and a sharp contrast for black-and-white images and (5) accompanied by a legend which explains the features included in the picture. To ensure good-quality reproduction, one needs to pay attention beginning with the initial data acquisition itself. Newer imaging devices allow images to be exported directly to a computer file in a digital format; the quality of such exported images is much better than that of photographs made from printouts or X-ray films. It is helpful to read the manual or consult the manufacturer in case of a specialized imaging device (e.g. radiology equipment) to obtain better-quality images. The images must be acquired at the highest resolution possible—one can always downgrade the resolution later if needed; the converse is not possible.

The area or object of interest must be placed near the centre of the picture. Unnecessary details should be trimmed. It helps to use as few intermediate steps as possible to go from the original picture to the final version because each step is associated with a loss in quality. The size of the final version submitted should be such that the journal does not need to either magnify or reduce its size; thus, it helps to make its width equal to either one column or two columns of the journal's printed page. It is helpful to look at a recent issue of the journal to which the paper is planned for submission to find out whether the journal prefers figures in column width or page width.

For photomicrographs, it is sometimes useful to combine more than one related photographs in one picture (e.g. showing different stages of a disease). The component images should be of similar brightness and contrast. The space between the components of such a composite figure should be just adequate to allow the components to be seen as separate. If images at two different magnifications are to be shown, it may be useful to include the more magnified image as a small inset (preferably in the right lower corner), taking care that important features of the larger picture are not obscured. It is also important to provide an internal scale within the picture or provide a measure of magnification in the figure legend; the former is preferable since the magnification factor may be altered by enlargement or reduction during the printing process.

Important features on the picture may need labelling. The labels should be short and unobtrusive, preferably in the form of single letters whose meaning can be explained in the figure legend. The labels should have an appropriate and uniform font size. Sans serif fonts, such as Helvetica or Arial (which lack thin horizontal extensions), are preferable. Labels should have a colour that contrasts with the background (black when the background is light coloured, and white when the background is dark); if a good contrast cannot be obtained, it may be useful to add a black or coloured square over the picture and place the letter over it in a contrasting colour or shade. Labels must not obscure important features of the underlying picture; use of arrows and lines may allow the labels to be placed away from the object being labelled. Also, arrows of different shapes and sizes can be used to mark different elements within an image and each arrow explained in the legend, to

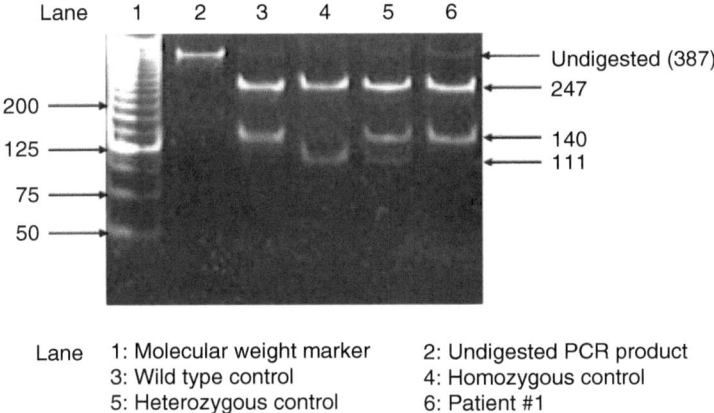

Lane   1: Molecular weight marker   2: Undigested PCR product
       3: Wild type control   4: Homozygous control
       5: Heterozygous control   6: Patient #1

Fig. 4.3 An example of a well-labelled electrophoresis gel picture. The lanes have been numbered and description of each lane is included. Selected molecular weight marker bands are marked on the left and bands of interest in various specimens are marked on the right. Use of thin arrows helps accurate localization of the bands of interest. The labels used are unobtrusive and do not interfere with the picture

eliminate the need to place text labels within the picture. One may try several possible methods of labelling and decide on the best one, possibly in consultation with one of the co-authors or another colleague. An alternative to labelling is to prepare an accompanying line diagram corresponding to the picture and label various structures in it.

Different areas of work and type of images may have their specific requirements. For instance, for gel images, it is important to label each lane and to label the bands of molecular weight markers (Fig. 4.3). It may be worth marking individual bands of interest.

It has become easier to modify/manipulate computer-based images by introducing changes in brightness and contrast, using colour filters or touching-up of details. It is unethical to change the image characteristics to such an extent that the message is altered.

For patient photographs, it is important to obtain the patient's written permission for publication and to use masking to maintain the patient's privacy and anonymity. Also, for radiographic images, care must be taken to remove patient identification information.

Photographs of physiological data (pressure tracings and graphs) can be either continuous tone or black-and-white, the latter being preferable. If these data have been recorded on a graph paper or a paper with grid lines, the background grid interferes with understanding. Therefore, for publication, it is better to record such tracings on a plain paper without a grid. Alternatively, if the grid and tracing are in different colours, it is possible to eliminate the grid by using a colour filter on the camera. Scales for both the variables (along the X- and Y-axes) must be included (Fig. 4.4).

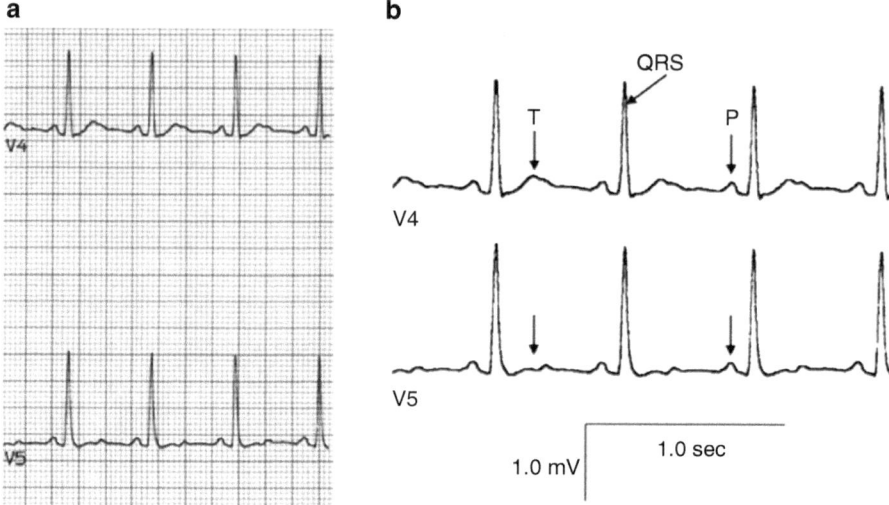

Fig. 4.4 A poor and a good picture for the same data. Section (**a**) shows a black and white picture of electrocardiography recording in which the background grid interfaces with the graph, the two graphs are widely separated leading to wastage of space. In (**b**) grid lines have been removed, the two tracings have been brought closer to each other to save space, and the relevant features have been marked using labels and arrows. Note that scale for both the X-axis and the Y-axis have been added

4.5.2 Line Diagrams

In biomedical science papers, line drawings are sometimes used for reporting data, depicting surgical findings, profiling family trees in inheritance studies, etc. These should be prepared using either a computer program or a drawing by a professional using a black ink pen to produce lines of uniform thickness. In the latter case, labelling should be done using a stencil to ensure a uniform font and letter size. Alternatively, the manual drawing can be scanned and typeset labels added. It should be made clear what each line represents. If the lines intersect, care must be taken to ensure that there is no ambiguity about how each line travels.

4.5.3 Graphs or Data Charts (Pie and Bar Charts, Line Graphs, Scatter Plots and Maps)

Graphs are a powerful medium to summarize and communicate numerical data. However, as discussed above, data tables are preferred over graphs for publication purposes. There are several forms of graphs, each with its specific uses.

Pie diagrams. A pie chart consists of a circle with several wedge-shaped pieces. It is used to indicate the components of a whole group. Each sector (or wedge)

stands for one component, and the area (and hence angle) of each sector is proportional to the size of the component it represents. Pie charts are easy to understand and have a strong visual impact. In a good pie chart, each sector is labelled and filled with a colour or pattern that is easily distinguishable from that of other sectors. The number of sectors should not exceed ten and no sector should be so small as to be virtually indistinguishable. Each sector should represent the number of observations or percentages. Many software programs allow for 3D pie charts, but one must avoid the temptation of using them as in these, the eye cannot easily make out the relative size of each sector (Fig. 4.5). Pie charts have limited use in research papers. These may be used when large amount of data are available, e.g. in an epidemiological study, for small data, a table or a text sentence may be preferred.

At times, two pie charts may be combined to illustrate the differences in distribution of various components between two groups.

Bar charts. These compare one or more sets of measurements using bars (usually vertical) whose heights represent the magnitude of measurement (Fig. 4.6a). Occasionally, horizontal bars are used; this allows long labels for each bar (Fig. 4.6b). Bar charts should be used to compare values of one variable across two or more groups (Fig. 4.6c), and at different time points. More complex bar charts compare the values of several variables. Stacked bars can show a comparison of the total value of a variable and that of its components across different groups (Fig. 4.6d).

Histograms. These are similar to bar charts, except that the bars are placed touching each other and only their tops are shown (Fig. 4.7a). They convey the time course of an outbreak of a disease or the age distribution of a group, etc. Sometimes, a line is used to connect the midpoints at the top of each 'bar' in a histogram to generate a 'frequency polygon' (Fig. 4.7b).

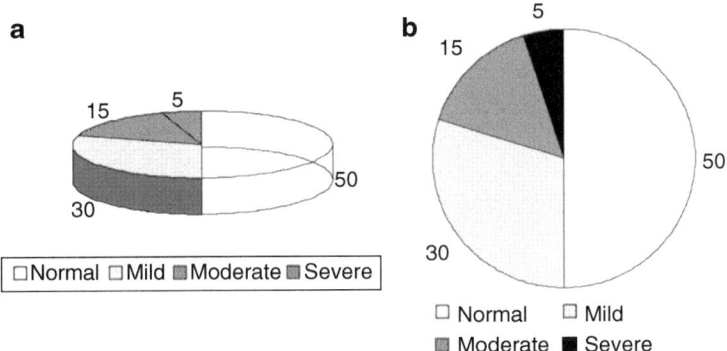

Fig. 4.5 A poor and a good pie chart; In (**a**), the 3-dimensional format interferes with understanding of the graph, the data labels are too small, the filling patterns of the two smallest sectors are indistinct from each other, and the legend has a small font and an unnecessary box around it. In the improved version (**b**), the 2-dimensional format makes for easy understanding, the data labels and legend are larger, and the box around the legend has been removed, and the legends and data labels now use the same font type and size

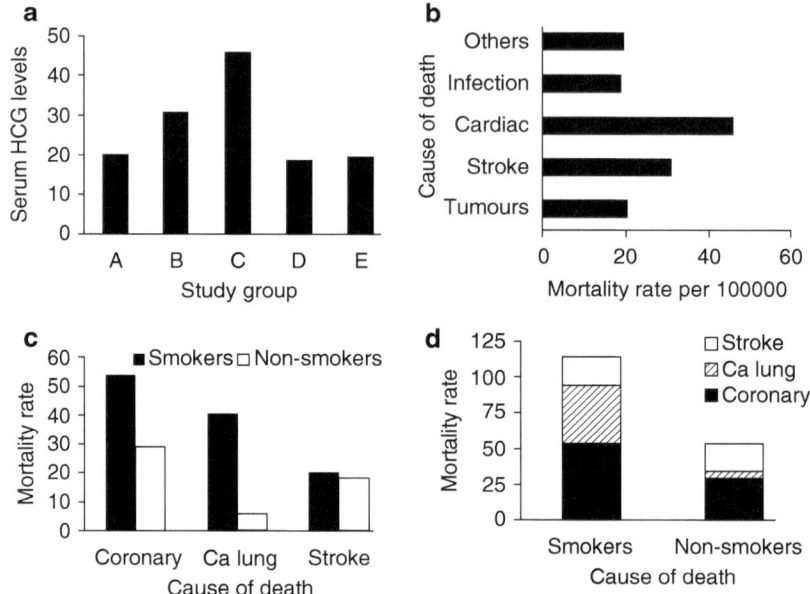

Fig. 4.6 Types of bar charts. Panel (**a**) shows a simple bar chart. Panel (**b**) shows a horizontal bar chart that is useful when the group names are long. Panel (**c**) shows a multiple bar chart; this format arrows comparison of several variables in two or more groups; in these charts, care must be taken to ensure that the bars to be compared with each other (smokers and non-smokers) are placed next to each other. Panel (**d**) shows a stacked bar chart; this format allows comparison of totals as well as various components (here, total mortality and mortality due to various causes)

Line graphs. A line graph can be thought of as a bar diagram where the midpoints of the tops of each bar have been joined by a line. These graphs emphasize the change in a variable rather than the absolute values. Thus, this form of data representation is used where change is important, for instance, to show the change in serum concentration of a drug over time or change in a measurement with age (Fig. 4.8).

Scattergrams. These charts show the relationship between two numerical variables. The value of one variable (usually an independent variable) is shown along the X-axis and that of the other (usually a dependent variable) is shown along the Y-axis (Fig. 4.9). Each study unit (e.g. each patient) is represented by a dot (or a data point). Thus, the chart has as many data points as the number of study units. These charts provide a strong visual impression of the relationship of change in one variable with that in the other. Thus, placement of data points along a line from the left lower corner to the right upper corner indicates an increase in the value of the dependent variable with an increase in the value of the independent variable. Also, data points placed closely together suggest a strong relationship, whereas widely scattered data points indicate a weak relationship. Computer programs allow a trend line to be drawn across the scatter diagram along with the statistical calculation showing any correlation between the two variables; however, the use of such a line should be a deliberate decision, with no scope for misinterpretation.

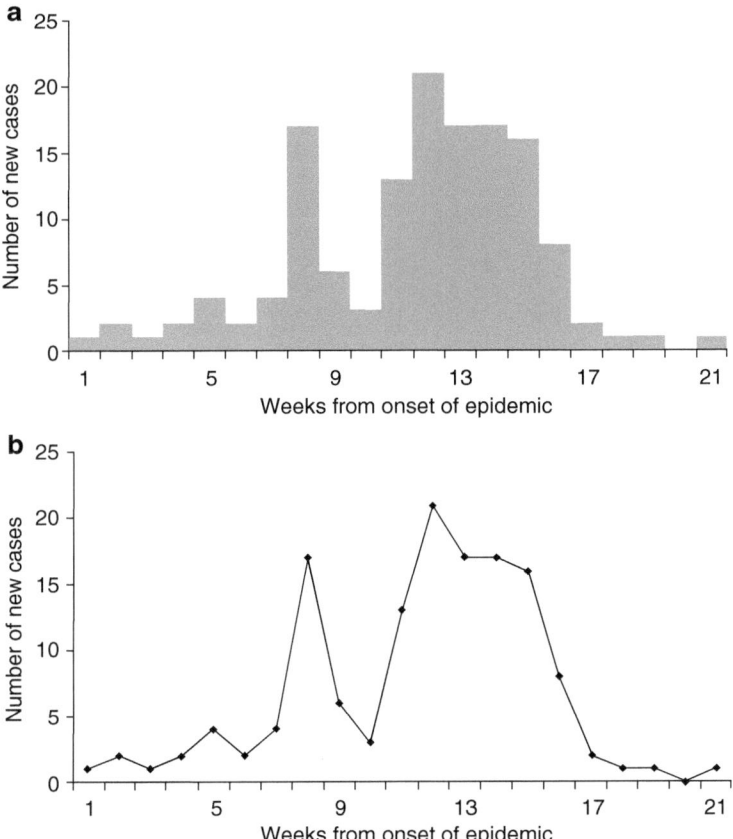

Fig. 4.7 (**a**) An example of a histogram. Such charts are useful for showing age distribution of a population, time course of an outbreak, etc. (**b**) Frequency polygon. This figure shows exactly the same data as shown in (**a**) but in a different format

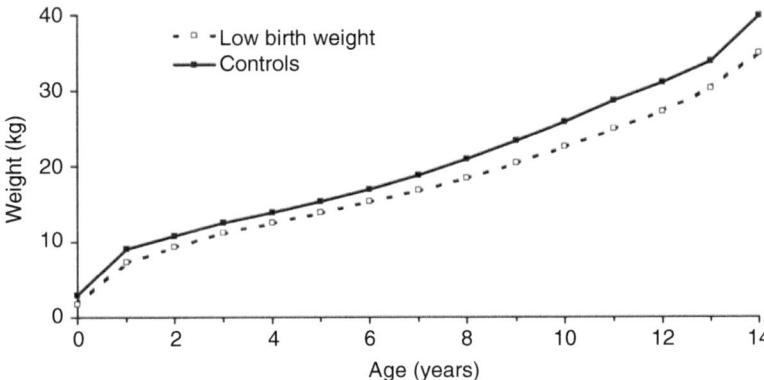

Fig. 4.8 Line diagrams. These show change with time or time trends much batter then bar graphs. Different lines must be drawn in different styles and a legend describing each line must be included

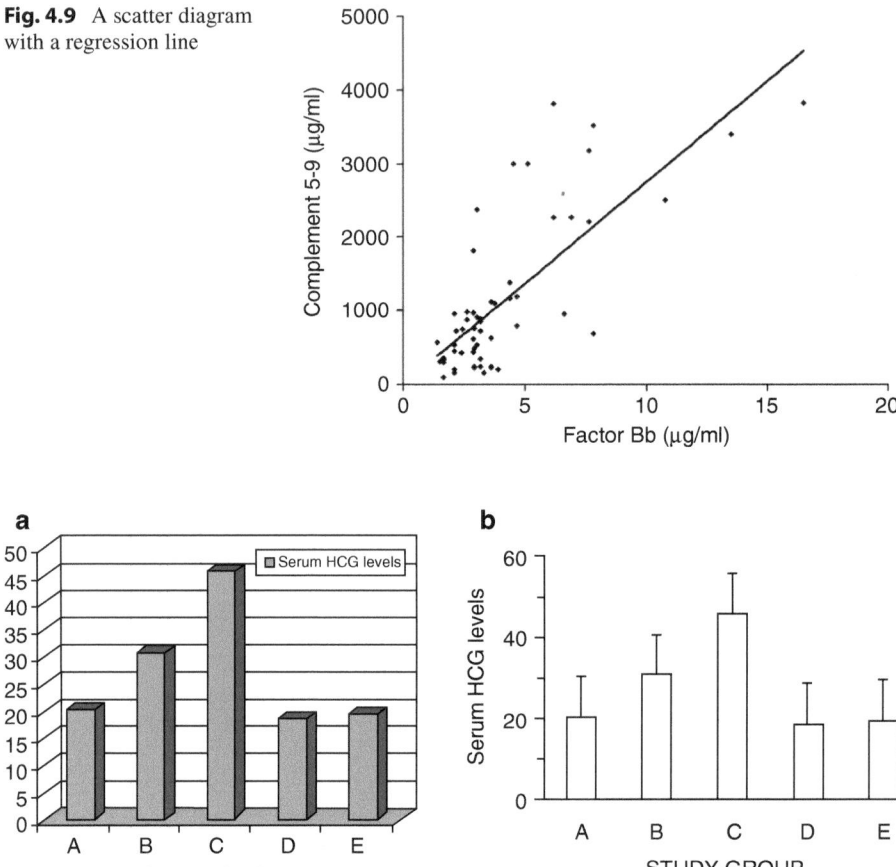

Fig. 4.9 A scatter diagram with a regression line

Fig. 4.10 A poor bar diagram (**a**) and its improved version (**b**). The poor diagram has 3-dimensional bars (the third dimension adds to clutter and makes it difficult to read the value corresponding to each bar on the Y-axis), grid lines (add to clutter), has too many labels on the Y-axis (add to clutter) in a small font (unreadable), and has no label to indicate what it represents (serum HCG levels). The X-axis has a thick line where none is necessary (there is no continuum along X-axis). The X-axis legend is in all capitals (difficult to read) and uses italics font (reduces readability). A legend box included in the right upper corner is not needed (necessary only if the chart has bars of two or more types which need to be distinguished from each other). The improved version (**b**) is much less cluttered, has few unnecessary lines and provides some additional information (error bars added)

4.5.4 Preparation of Graphs

All graphs should be drawn professionally. Use of computer programs has made their preparation easy. However, automatic settings of these programs often produce cluttered graphs. To prepare a good-quality graph, one needs to pay attention to each component by using as little 'non-data' ink as possible (Fig. 4.10). The axis lines must not be too heavy or should not extend far beyond the last group or observation. The two axes should intersect at zero. Starting one or both axes at a non-zero value can be misleading and falsely exaggerate differences; if this is done, then it should be clearly indicated. The nature of scale—whether arithmetic or logarithmic—must be clear. If any of the axes has a discontinuous scale, the change must be indicated by a scale break. Each axis must carry a label indicating the variable it represents. The labels should be large enough to be legible but should not be too large and must not be in capital letters; sans serif fonts are usually preferred. The label for the Y-axis can be placed either vertically along the axis line or horizontally above the Y-axis line. The number of tick marks and labels indicating their values on each axis should generally be limited to 4–6.

The symbols used for different groups (say circles, triangles, diamonds, squares—each filled or unfilled) should be distinct and of appropriate size. Similarly, the patterns used in various bars should be well defined. If a paper has several figures, the pattern used for each group must be consistent for all. In bar and pie charts, a legend should clearly indicate what each pattern (filled, hatched, not filled, etc.) stands for. Variability in data can be shown using vertical lines equal in length to the SD extending above or below (or both) from the mean (i.e. from tops of bars in bar graph or the markers in a line graph). Use of three-dimensional bars, bold fonts and shadowing for text character and grid lines should be avoided.

4.5.5 Use of Geographical Maps

Geographical maps portray selected information and knowledge derived from scientific observation. They occasionally accompany papers on epidemiological studies and show the areas affected by a disease.

Maps may contain several different types of information, such as the distribution of a disease-causing agent (such as a vector or animal), or a timeline if a disease is spreading outward from a smaller area. If directed at health agencies planning a response, health centres and transport links might be shown.

Maps should be uncluttered. Do not name too many towns or physical features but try and show a few locations that are necessary to convey the key message. It is useful to show physical features close to the margins of the map so that a reader can quickly locate the area that he is looking for.

Maps should have a clear title, a clear legend, and an internal line scale. Do not use a scale expressed as a ratio (e.g. 1 cm = 5 km) unless the journal editors request you to do so; this is because the image may be enlarged or reduced during the printing process.

Symbols and gradations of tint should be legible after printing and not just look nice on-screen. Tints above 50% can often be difficult for the eye to separate. Most people can easily identify printed tints below 50% at 15% intervals (e.g. 5, 20, 35 and 50%) (*see* the pie chart on page 41).

A number of cartographic drawing packages are marketed, but advice from a colleague or cartographer can be sought for those who are less acquainted with maps.

CAT TGC CCA TAG GAA AGA TCT AGA
CCC TTC CTT CCT AGT TTT ATC GCT   Times New Roman
AAG GAG GCT TGC ATG GTC ATC ATT

CAT TGC CCA TAG GAA AGA TCT AGA
CCC TTC CTT CCT AGT TTT ATC GCT   Arial
AAG GAG GCT TGC ATG GTC ATC ATT

CAT TGC CCA TAG GAA AGA TCT AGA
CCC TTC CTT CCT AGT TTT ATC GCT   Courier
AAG GAG GCT TGC ATG GTC ATC ATT

Fig. 4.11 DNA sequence data written using three different fonts. The letters align well when written in a non-proportional font (Courier) but not when written in proportional fonts (Times Roman or Arial). Hence, for such figures, a non-proportional font should be used

4.5.6 Graphics Containing Molecular Data

Figures are often used to provide sequences of nucleotides in DNA or RNA and of amino acids in proteins. In addition to providing information on the primary structure of a molecule, such figures try to (1) find homology between different sequences; (2) provide a consensus sequence by aligning various related sequences; (3) locate particular patterns (motifs); (4) display information on folding of protein or mRNA, etc.; and (5) show sites at which these sequences can be cut using specific enzymes. Such graphics have their own particular set of rules to make these simpler to understand.

The first point to consider is whether the entire sequence needs to be included in the manuscript. It is usually adequate to deposit the full sequence data with a central database (say GenBank) and provide the database accession number in the manuscript. Using this information, a reader can access the entire sequence easily on the internet. Thus, the figures to be printed with the paper can then include only the region(s) of particular interest.

Sequence data must be shown using fixed-width or non-proportional fonts (e.g. Courier) in which each letter takes up the same amount of space, allowing proper alignment of letters one above the other (Fig. 4.11); alignment of sequence data is impossible to maintain with the use of proportional or variable-width fonts such as Times New Roman, Helvetica or Arial. Nucleotides usually need to be numbered—this can be done either at the beginning and the end of lines, or above the line showing the sequence. One may need to try various combinations to find the arrangement with the most aesthetic and uncluttered look. It helps to provide a space after every ten nucleotides (or three, if the aim is to indicate different 3-nucleotide long codons) to allow for easier reading of sequences. The regions needing particular emphasis (e.g. regions of homology or non-identity) and specific nucleotides or amino acids (representing sites of action of restriction enzymes, crucial mutations, etc.) can be underlined (using single or multiple lines of varying thickness, if required), overlining, boxes, arrows, bold letters or a stippled background (Fig. 4.12). If several sequences have been aligned, the first sequence can be shown in full and only variations shown for the others; this makes viewing easier. It is helpful to see how data are represented in similar papers.

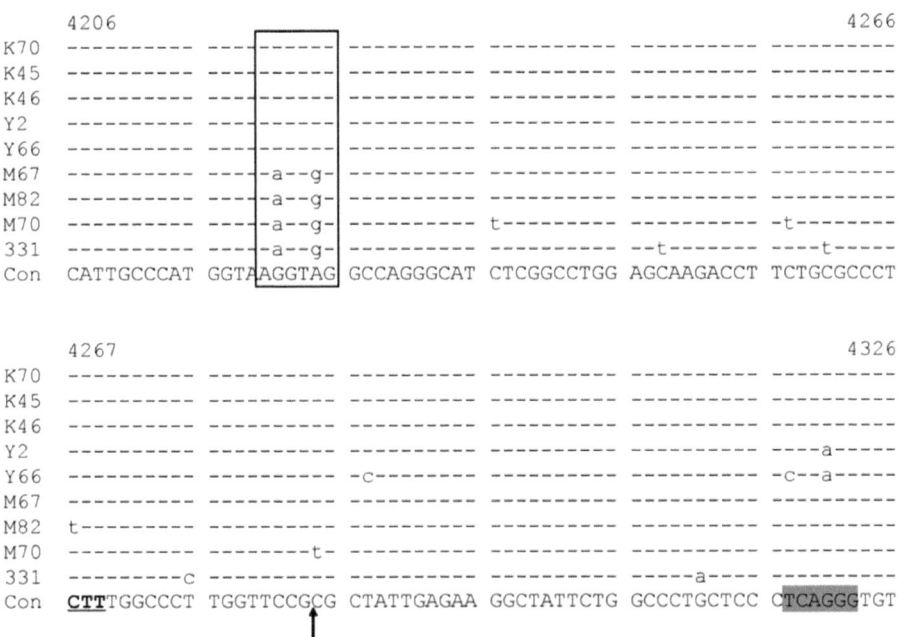

Fig. 4.12 Different methods used to represent various features in figures containing molecular data. The aim is to reduce clutter as much as possible. Only a selected region (nucleotide 4206–4326) of a long DNA molecule is shown. The full DNA sequence is not shown for each of the nine specimens studied (K70, K45, K46, Y2, Y66, M67, M82, M70, 331); instead, only differences from a consensus sequence (Con) are shown. This emphasizes the differences between different sequences, which is the point of interest in the paper. Use of a non-proportional font and spaces after each set of 10 nucleotides give a neat appearance. Nucleotide numbers are indicated at the top of each set of 60 nucleotides and not in each row. Regions or nucleotides of interest can be shown using box, boldface letters, underlining, or a grey background for selected nucleotides, and arrows, etc.

4.5.7 Figure Legends

Each figure must be accompanied by a legend that describes its salient features. The legend should explain any labels used on photographs and define the abbreviation and symbols used. These should also have the explanation for the measure of dispersion used (SD or SE) and any marks that indicate statistical significance. For photomicrographs, the stain used and magnification must be mentioned. In the case of graphs (e.g. pie, bar and line diagrams), the legend should explain the axes, various patterns used for bars or pies and results of any statistical comparisons (*p* values). The figure along with its legend must be fully and independently comprehensible. Legends for all the figures can be printed on a separate sheet.

4.5.8   Precautions While Submitting Figures

These days, most figures are submitted as computer files. The manuscript handling systems in different journals vary in the types of files they can process. Hence, it is important to look up the specifications for a particular journal. These could relate to file format, resolution, file size, depth of colour, permitted compression techniques, etc.

If you plan to submit illustrations in colour, you should ascertain whether or not the journal prints colour images. Some journals publish illustrations in colour only if the author pays the additional cost; this is often difficult if your research is not funded. However, if the authors request, the journals would often agree to include colour images in the online PDF version, even though the print version includes only a greyscale or black-and-white image.

4.6   Pitfalls to Avoid

Common mistakes in the Results section include (1) mismatch of numbers in text and tables; (2) failure to account for all study subjects; (3) inclusion of results for variables that were not mentioned in the Methods section; (4) omission of results for one or more variables (for one or more groups); (5) repetition of data in text, tables and figures; and (6) inclusion of some interpretation, conclusions and speculations. One must make an effort to avoid these common pitfalls. As for the rest of the manuscript, it helps to ask your co-authors and one of your colleagues to read through your results and review your figures and tables. The latter, not being too familiar with the data, are more likely to point out ambiguities and discrepancies. Their feedback should go a long way towards improving this section of your paper.

References

1. Bradford Hill A. The reasons for writing. Br Med J. 1965;2:870–1.
2. CONSORT. http://www.consort-statement.org. Accessed 24 Apr 2015.
3. Briscoe MH. Preparing scientific illustrations: a guide to better posters, presentations and publications. 2nd ed. San Francisco: Springer; 1995.

Suggested Reading

Moher D, Schulz KF, Altman DG. The CONSORT statement: revised recommendations for improving the quality of reports of parallel-group randomised trials. Lancet. 2001;357:1191–4.

The Discussion Section

5

Robert H. Fletcher and Suzanne W. Fletcher

This chapter is about manuscripts describing original clinical research and organized in the traditional (IMRAD) way into Introduction, Methods, Results, and Discussion sections. It also applies to manuscripts in closely related disciplines such as health services research and epidemiology. The laboratory sciences have their own traditions, and our comments bear less directly on that kind of science. Manuscripts not reporting original research are organized in very different ways.

The Discussion is often considered the least structured part of a research manuscript. The Introduction must impart basic information about the importance of the research question, the extent to which it has not yet been answered and how the present study addresses the unanswered question (*see also* Chap. 2). The Methods section reflects the basic elements of the scientific method—research design, population and sample, comparison groups, interventions or exposures, outcomes, measurement methods, statistical analyses and the like (*see also* Chap. 3). The results progress from description of the sample through effects on primary and secondary outcomes, results of subgroup analyses and perhaps sensitivity analyses (*see also* Chap. 4). But in the Discussion, the author might hope to finally be free of all this structure and in a position to speak her or his own mind.

However, the Discussion section of a research manuscript has its own specific purposes too. As stated by the International Committee of Medical Journal Editors (ICMJE), this section should 'emphasize the new and important aspects of the study and the conclusions that follow from them in the context of the totality of the best

R. H. Fletcher (✉) • S. W. Fletcher
Department of Population Medicine, Harvard Medical School, Boston, MA, USA

Department of Epidemiology, University of North Carolina Gillings School of Global Public Health, Chapel Hill, NC, USA

Department of Social Medicine, School of Medicine, University of North Carolina at Chapel Hill, Chapel Hill, NC, USA
e-mail: Robert_Fletcher@hms.harvard.edu; suzanne_fletcher@hms.harvard.edu

© The National Medical Journal of India 2018
P. Sahni, R. Aggarwal (eds.), *Reporting and Publishing Research in the Biomedical Sciences*, https://doi.org/10.1007/978-981-10-7062-4_5

available evidence' and should 'not repeat in detail data or other information given in the Introduction or the Results sections' [1]. A textbook also implies a specific content and order [2].

Having an expected structure makes it easier for authors, who need not cast around for what to say and where to say it; rather, they can follow a simple, basic plan. If they have difficulty finding uninterrupted time to write, they can draft one or another part of the Discussion when they do have the time and inclination, without fear that it will be out of context with the rest. An expected structure also makes it easier for readers to find the information they want.

As with the other sections of a research manuscript, the structure of a Discussion has evolved over time, without a great deal of explicit attention being paid to it in the medical literature or in formal journal policies. To date, relatively little has been published about the craft of writing a Discussion section of a research manuscript. A book, *How to write and publish papers in the medical sciences*, by Edward Huth, former editor of *Annals of Internal Medicine*, includes a page on basics of a Discussion section [2]. Some journals include guidance for writing a Discussion in their Information for Authors [3]. Most books on medical writing are about how to say things and not what should be said. Nevertheless, efforts to define the quality of a research report affirm the importance of the Discussion. Widely used guidelines (such as CONSORT) for the expected contents of research reports include items— interpretation, generalizability and overall evidence—that are ordinarily located in the Discussion [4]. Similarly, a research instrument used to assess the quality of a manuscript included several items that belong in the Discussion: contribution, external evidence, limitations, generalizability and conclusions [5].

For the most part, the skill of writing a compelling, complete and informative Discussion is part of an oral tradition, passed on from senior to junior investigators and from experienced to inexperienced peer reviewers. Little of this art has been recorded for wider dissemination. Despite the lack of explicit, formal attention to the structure of the Discussion section, experienced authors and editors have a clear view of what should be in a Discussion, and readers need to find information in a familiar order.

5.1 Length

The Discussion section should be in proportion to the rest of the manuscript, and it should not be much longer than any of the other sections (Fig. 5.1). For a 3000-word manuscript, Discussion would be approximately 900 words or 3–4 double-spaced A4-size pages. Because of space limits and all that must be included in this section, the Discussion must be tightly constructed, with little room for extra words or ideas.

If the Discussion is much longer, it gives the impression that authors have taken the manuscript as an opportunity to present their ideas about the field, rather than a succinct transmission of a new finding in the context of other research. If it is much shorter, it risks leaving out important information that belongs only in that section of the manuscript.

Fig. 5.1 The appropriate size of the Discussion section in relation to other parts of the manuscript

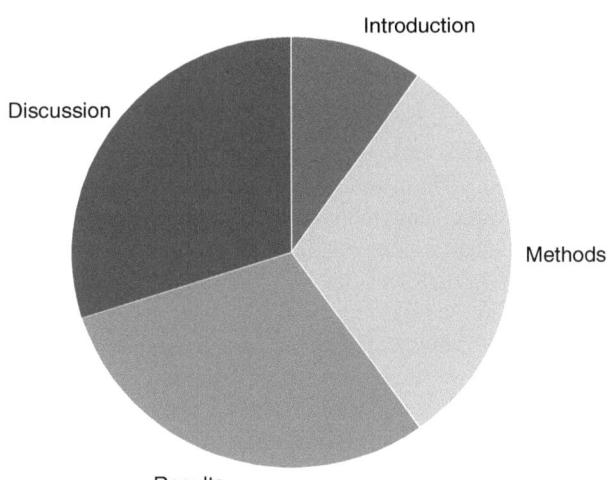

Table 5.1 Components of the Discussion section of a research manuscript

- Summary of main results
- Compare results to earlier studies
- How strong is this study?
- How convincingly has the question been answered?
- Strengths
- Limitations
- Generalizability
- Implications
- Conclusions

5.2   Components

In the following, we discuss the elements of a Discussion section in the usual order in which they appear (Table 5.1). These elements are not ordinarily identified by subheadings but are made clear by topic sentences at the beginning of paragraphs dealing with each issue. There is, of course, some latitude in how this information is presented, especially the order and whether some parts are combined. But authors should not leave any of these elements out of a manuscript unless that is forced on them by severe restrictions to the length of the manuscript.

5.2.1   Summary of Main Results

The Discussion of a research manuscript conventionally begins with a succinct statement of the main research findings. As Huth put it: 'In the first paragraph … you should state concisely the central conclusion, or answer, to be drawn from the data presented in Results' [2]. Has that not been done already in the abstract? Yes, partly, but that part of the abstract is limited to just a few sentences. What about the Results section? Yes, all of the findings worth reporting should be there, but the main results will be in the company of a lot of other (secondary) findings and may not stand out among all the other information. Also, Results should be an account of the facts without interpretation. For example, 'Death rate was 10% in the treated group and 40% in the control group (p<0.05)'. In the Discussion, the author can place a value judgement on the findings. For the example above, it might be 'We found that treatment resulted in a large, clinically important reduction in mortality…'. Whereas Results are described in numerical terms, namely, effect sizes, p-values and confidence intervals, the Discussion also includes briefer, less quantitative, more interpretive and clinically focused descriptions of what was found.

Usually, the main results can be summarized in a paragraph. Using more space for this purpose risks repeating what has already been said in Results rather that providing a summary. However, if the study has a rich array of important findings—for example, intermediate and secondary outcomes, subgroup analyses, and intention-to-treat versus per protocol analyses—this part of the Discussion might require more than one paragraph.

The summary of main results is an opportunity to highlight major strengths of the paper as well. For example, 'This study reports experience with an unusually large cohort with a rich array of data on covariates and long follow-up…'. A word about strengths here might replace the need for a separate mention later in the manuscript, where strengths and limitations are typically discussed (*see below*).

5.2.2   Compare Results to Earlier Studies

The Discussion should place the research findings in the context of previous studies of similar research questions. Some of this might have already been done in the Introduction, where the importance of the research question and the extent to which the answer is already known are established. But in most clinical research articles, the Introduction is just a few paragraphs long and is not the place for an extensive review of the literature. The Discussion is where existing literature is dealt with more completely. Have other studies found similar results? If not, can the differences be explained by differences in patients, interventions, follow-up and outcomes in the previous studies (compared to your study)—that is, because they addressed somewhat different research questions? Or is it more likely that strengths of research methods—reduction in bias and chance—account for the differences?

The Discussion section of a research manuscript is not the place for a definitive review of the literature, comparable to a review paper. The report is mainly about the one study at hand. There are limits to the overall size of the manuscript, and much of the space should be reserved for the study itself. Also, some journals discourage a large number of references. One way to establish the state of the evidence and to save space is to cite the pattern of results found in systematic reviews, or the strongest studies of the question, rather than describing all studies one at a time.

Studies related to the present one should have been identified before the research was undertaken and updated before the research is reported. To take into account all existing information, the effort to find relevant studies should be similar to a systematic review, going beyond electronic searches of databases such as MEDLINE and EMBASE to examine citations in published reviews and textbooks, the articles cited in the articles identified, registries of randomized trials and the recommendations of experts in the content area of the manuscript. However, what is actually reported in Discussion of a research article is less extensive; this requires the authors to choose only the most relevant articles for comparison of each of their findings.

If major studies of a similar research question are in progress, it helps readers to know about them and when results are expected, as long as authors can find some way of citing this information. Similarly, published abstracts (for which papers have not yet been published) can be cited; they do not provide complete enough information to fully judge their validity, but they are information and do help establish a context for the current study.

In this part of the Discussion, authors are subject to a familiar temptation, to selectively cite articles that support their own results. Needless to say, the integrity of the scientific record depends on a fair and balanced account of other studies bearing on the research question. Readers depend on this fairness because it is difficult for them to detect selective citation unless they are familiar with the subject matter of the study.

Authors should also tie their findings to observations from other branches of science. A typical example in a clinical or epidemiological study is to comment on the underlying mechanisms of the disease, as elucidated in laboratory studies of pathogenesis. A report of a randomized controlled trial might discuss reasons why the intervention is promising enough to study in such a costly and labour-intensive way and if its effects differed in subgroups why that might have been expected. For observational studies, the authors should discuss the underlying biological mechanisms that may explain observed associations. For example, a study of antioxidant vitamins and cardiovascular risk might point out how laboratory studies have linked oxidation to atherosclerosis at the molecular level.

It is all too easy to find reasons for observed results after the fact. For example, at a time when observational studies were finding that folic acid intake was associated with lower rates of cancer, it was argued that folic acid protects against cancer by regulating cell growth; later, when an excess number of late-stage cancers was found in patients taking folic acid in a cancer prevention trial, it was suggested that folic acid promotes growth of cancers once they have arisen. To be fair, authors should include all reasonable sides of the story, not just the ones that support their results.

5.2.3   How Strong Is This Study?

Readers expect authors to provide a brief, balanced critique of their work. Often this is done in a 'Strengths and Limitations' section (*see below*). But this might be dealt with in a separate section in which study data are used to establish the credibility of the findings. A common approach is to comment on confidence intervals and the extent to which they identify or rule out a clinically important effect. Another approach is to mention sensitivity analysis—to show how a range of plausible assumptions about missing or uncertain data might have affected the results.

Authors have an opportunity to examine whether their results are internally consistent. Do intermediate outcomes change in the same direction as the end results? Are effects larger in patients who actually received the intervention (per protocol analysis) than in those who did not? Was the effect larger in those who received a larger dose of the intervention? Was the onset of effects consistent with what is known from other studies about the onset of action of the intervention? Answers to these kinds of questions help to establish, apart from research design, how credible the findings are. At best the answers can be obtained from additional analyses of data—that is, studies within the main study.

5.2.4 How Convincingly Has the Question Been Answered?

Authors should address the degree of certainty with which the answer to the question is known, given existing research plus the results of this particular study. There are several approaches. One, proposed by the British statistician Bradford Hill [6], is to see how the pattern of evidence from all studies—size of effect, consistency of results, dose–response relationship, reversibility and so on—supports or refutes study conclusions. Another, formulated by Reverend Thomas Bayes [7], is to ask how the study results change prior belief, built up from all existing evidence before the study results were known. For example, results of a strong study might substantially change belief based on prior weak research, whereas a relatively weak study might have little effect on belief based on many strong studies preceding it. Another approach, called 'falsification', was advocated by the Austrian philosopher Karl Popper [8]. He asserted that science advances by falsification (i.e. when strong research shows that an existing theory cannot be right). Popper thought that knowledge advances by disproving conventional wisdom, not by affirming it.

Whichever approach, or combination of approaches, is taken, authors should make their version of applied epistemology (the basis for knowing what we think we know) explicit. Readers should see an underlying purpose in how authors compare their results with other studies of the research question and not be subjected to an aimless recitation of the results of other studies, with the main metric for scientific validity being that they agree with the study at hand.

Speculations about the reasons for findings, based on previous studies, extrapolation from other diseases or imagination, are common but often excessive. At best, these speculations are hypotheses that need to be tested further by data from the current study, other published studies or even in future studies. At worst, pure speculation can be frivolous and self-serving. For example, an observational study showed that elderly patients with colon cancer experience fewer adverse events after adjuvant cancer chemotherapy [9]. This was consistent with older people who received chemotherapy having been selected for lower risk, receiving less toxic treatment or, actually being, as a group at lower risk of suffering adverse events, everything else being equal. That is, the results were consistent with selection or protection. In this example, several measures of selection—dose, duration and toxicity of drugs—and patients' health before chemotherapy all suggested that the elderly patients in the study had been preselected to be at lower risk and were treated less aggressively. So the Discussion pointed out that at the very least selection was part of the reason treated patients experienced fewer adverse events.

It is helpful to identify the set of possible explanations for study results whether or not they are supported by existing research. That at least helps readers think of the possibilities and how evidence for each might be strengthened or refuted by additional research.

5.2.5 Strengths

Authors should point out the strengths of their study, relying on facts, and not interpretations or opinions. Scientific articles are not the place for persuasion laced with adjectives such as 'strong' or 'rigorous'. Some authors include only limitations, but we believe limitations should be balanced by strengths and, in the spirit of putting one's best foot forward, should be located before limitations.

A new piece of research adds value to the medical literature to the extent that it has examined a question in a somewhat stronger way than studies already published. There is some value in replication of earlier work; however, it is even better if the new research overcomes some of the weaknesses of previous studies. This approach not only advances the state of the science but also is more appealing to peer reviewers and editors, who are looking for new findings. So authors should call attention to aspects of their study that surpass, correct for or overcome defects in previous studies. Is the present study population-based, whereas previous studies were of convenience samples of patients in clinics and hospitals? Is it a randomized controlled trial whereas others are observational studies? Did it have a longer follow-up than that in previous studies? If the study is observational, were the authors able to measure and include in statistical analyses potential confounding variables that were not available to previous investigators?

When the shortcomings of previous studies are noted, stick to the facts and be kind. It serves no good purpose to damage other investigators' feelings or reputations. Authors of those studies may have wanted a stronger study but were unable to do one because of limited resources, insufficient access to data or their research environment. (Sometimes, when the previous study was done, it may not even have been known that a particular variable could be a potential confounder.) Besides, they may be the peer who will review the present manuscript—or your next grant!

While being the first study of an important question is certainly an asset, it is hazardous to claim that unequivocally. There always seems to be someone who has addressed the same research question—perhaps long ago and in an obscure journal—and they might dispute your claim of priority in a letter to the editor. So it is prudent to qualify the claim of priority with 'to our knowledge this is the first…' or 'we could find no other studies…'.

5.2.6   Limitations

Authors may find limitations difficult to write about. Some believe that pointing out faults in their study damages their cause. They might hope that reviewers and editors—and later readers—will not notice weaknesses in the work unless they are pointed out to them. But in fact, a clear, direct summary of limitations, besides being in the best scientific tradition, can be a defence against unfair criticisms. Each limitation mentioned is an opportunity for authors to state what they did to overcome the limitation and why they believe the effect of the limitation does not substantially change the study's main results. (Of course, if they do, that needs to be admitted too and, in the extreme, might be a reason to not write the manuscript at all.) Also, stating limitations is a display of self-confidence and protects against others thinking that the authors are not capable enough to recognize their own shortcomings. Anyway, discerning reviewers will find out the weaknesses in a manuscript whether they have been mentioned or not. Some journal editors, such as the editors of *Annals of Internal Medicine*, believe so strongly in the importance of an explicit statement of limitations that they require that it be part of a structured abstract.

The limitations mentioned should be those that might reasonably be expected to change the results of the study to an important extent. Examples are relatively small sample size (especially in a negative study), low participation rates, short duration of follow-up, lack of data on a potential confounding variable and high drop-out rates. Authors are not expected to include a recitation of all the factors that might affect the internal validity and generalizability of their study regardless of importance.

Authors may have difficulty recognizing limitations in their own work. It is good practice to have a colleague, who is not invested in the study, review the manuscript and suggest what he or she thinks are important limitations.

5.2.7   Generalizability

Generalizability—the extent to which the results can be extrapolated to other patients in other settings—is a value judgement based on a factual description of the study. The study being reported is on a sample of patients who are in a specific setting, met carefully defined inclusion and exclusion criteria and were willing to participate. They may be from the general population, community practice or referral centres. The sample may have been representative of patients in these situations or, because sampling was not random, not representative even of them. Similarly, the study might involve care by exemplary doctors in extraordinary settings or average doctors in ordinary settings. Basic information about sampling and setting should have been reported in the Methods and Results sections but should be summarized in the Discussion, along with the authors' own views about generalizability. It is ultimately up to the reader to decide about generalizability to his or her practice and patients. But that decision will be better informed if the authors not only provide basic information about study patients and setting but also state their own opinions about the generalizability of their study's results and the reasons for their beliefs.

5.2.8 Implications

Clinical research should provide better information to clinicians so that they can make better decisions about the care of patients. Therefore, the 'bottom line' for a research article is how it would affect practice. Do the results suggest that usual care should be abandoned altogether? Do they make us more confident that an alternative to usual care is also reasonable? Do they mainly strengthen our conviction that usual care is the most effective option? Or do they imply that a new treatment is better than the previous conventional treatment or no treatment? For those articles that are about the biology of disease, whether or not they are helpful in the care of patients, how does the new information expand understanding of the disease?

Some authors like to assert that 'more research is needed'. Because this is always the case, it is a 'throw-away' comment. We suggest that authors not use this time-worn cliché phrase unless they point out just what kind of study would advance the field. For example, after consistent findings from randomized trials of highly selected patients, the best way forward may be a practical clinical trial of more ordinary patients and real-world interventions. Another approach is to point out how discrepancies in the existing evidence base could be explained or reconciled.

5.2.9 Conclusions

In recent years, authors and some journals have begun to include a Conclusions section in the Discussion, often set off by a subheading. This is a return to an old practice, before abstracts were a regular part of research manuscripts and conclusions could be readily found in them. We do not favour a separate Conclusions section. It seems to us that there have already been ample opportunities to state the conclusions—in the Abstract and beginning of the Discussion. But to the extent that the conclusions are truly a synthesis of all that has gone before—not only the research results but also their consistency with other evidence, the strength of the research and its generalizability—this section may add value and not just space and so be worthwhile.

Good writers want to end on a high note, a sentence or paragraph that captures the essence of the study at hand and is especially wise about what it means for the care of patients. We suggest that authors try to write such an ending with the understanding that if they come up short, the stakes are not high. The study will still be what it is, and readers rarely read the manuscript from beginning to end, like a novel with an engaging plot. They will remember the main results more than the closing words.

5.3   Final Thoughts

We have described several components of a Discussion section in the order in which they are commonly presented. It often works best to take up these issues one at a time so that readers know just which is being considered at any point in the Discussion. Regarding order, readers have become accustomed to seeing Discussions in a certain way, and it is disconcerting to them if the sequence has been scrambled. However, there is certainly room for variations. For example, some authors place strengths in the first paragraph after they have stated main results. Generalizability may be mentioned where strengths or limitations are addressed.

The main issue is to consider all of the information we have described even if some is left out for good reasons.

References

1. International Committee of Medical Journal Editors. Uniform requirements for manuscripts submitted to biomedical journals. http://www.icmje.org/recommendations/browse/manuscript-preparation/preparing-for-submission.html#f. Accessed 11 July 2015.
2. Huth EJ. How to write and publish papers in the medical sciences. Philadelphia: ISI Press; 1982.
3. Information for Authors, Annals of Internal Medicine. http://annals.org/public/authorsinfo.aspx. Accessed 11 Jul 2015.
4. CONSORT Statement. http://www.consort-statement.org. Accessed 11 Jul 2015.
5. Goodman SN, Berlin J, Fletcher SW, Fletcher RH. Manuscript quality before and after peer review and editing in Annals of Internal Medicine. Ann Intern Med. 1994;121:11–21.
6. Hill AB. The environment and disease: association or causation? Proc R Soc Med. 1965;58:295–300.
7. Goodman SN. Toward evidence-based medical statistics. 2: the Bayes factor. Ann Intern Med. 1999;130:1005–13.
8. Popper KR. Conjectures and refutations. London: Routledge and Kegan Paul; 1969.
9. Kahn KL, Adams JL, Weeks JC, Chrischilles EA, Schrag D, Ayanian JZ, et al. Adjuvant chemotherapy use and adverse events among older patients with stage III colon cancer. JAMA. 2010;303:1037–45.

The 'Argument Matrix': A Structured Method to Write and Organize a Manuscript

6

Yvan J. Hutin

6.1 Rationale

Writing or editing a paper can be a challenging task, particularly for young authors who have limited experience. Often, such authors worry about editorial issues, whereas the key pieces that determine the scientific quality of a paper are different—namely, ideas and argumentation. We propose here a practical method that may be used to organize ideas and argumentation of a paper upfront so that the process of writing the paper becomes easier and more organized. This so-called argument matrix organizes ideas and arguments using a two-way table that keeps track of (1) linear development of ideas (with each horizontal row tracking one idea) and (2) the sections of the manuscript (vertical columns).

6.2 Preliminary Work Before Getting Started on a Paper

6.2.1 Tables and Figures

Analysis transforms data into information that is easily understandable. This information is usually presented in the form of tables and figures, which form the core of a scientific manuscript. Hence, the process of writing starts after the tables and figures have been prepared. The following three steps may be followed to begin writing a manuscript once the tables and figures have been prepared:

Select three to five tables/figures. First, the data analysis results should be reviewed to select the tables and figures that make the most important points, i.e. those that

Y. J. Hutin
European Centre for Disease Control (ECDC), Stockholm, Sweden
e-mail: hutiny@les3voltas.org

© Yvan J. Hutin 2018
P. Sahni, R. Aggarwal (eds.), *Reporting and Publishing Research in the Biomedical Sciences*, https://doi.org/10.1007/978-981-10-7062-4_6

are essential to the arguments of the manuscript. The traditional IMRAD format limits the number of tables or figures to a maximum of five. Aiming for fewer tables and figures is always better. Exceptionally, for large studies, a larger number of tables may be acceptable.

Describing results through short captions. Once the key tables and figures have been selected, writing a short caption for each may help the author step back from the numbers in the table and to see the bigger picture and express it in words or sentences. One approach consists of writing three to five lines to describe the main patterns in each table or figure and any major exceptions to these patterns. These sentences can be used later as part of the Results section.

Formulating a conclusion in view of the initial objectives of the study. Examining the results from the tables and figures expressed in sentences usually helps the author to formulate conclusions. These must be articulated in light of (1) the original study objectives, (2) background information and (3) other elements of information that were known before the study began. In most cases, the conclusion points should answer the study questions or fulfil the study objectives. These elements of conclusions are also useful in formulating future steps, in terms of generating more information or action.

6.2.2   Preparing for an Oral Presentation

Following data analysis and identification of the main conclusions, many authors decide to give a presentation, first for an in-house audience (e.g. colleagues from the department, lunchtime seminar) and later at a scientific conference. A small (fewer than 12) slide-set allows integration of all key aspects of the study in the IMRAD sequence. This lays the foundation for the manuscript. An oral presentation typically includes (1) introduction, (2) methods, (3) results, (4) limitations, (5) conclusions and (6) recommendations. In most cases, such presentations do not allow for a formal Discussion section and the presenter goes directly from results to conclusions in the absence of an explicit description of the mechanisms of interpretation. A useful way to prepare a presentation is to start from the conclusions identified (*see above*). Then, the next steps/recommendations can be formulated working forwards as a logical consequence of the conclusions. Results, Methods and Introduction can then be prepared by working backwards while taking care that these sections contain only the minimum of information needed to understand how the conclusions were generated. If a presentation at a conference is envisaged, the preparation of an abstract also forces the author to prepare a focused line of communication, which may help clarify ideas and provide a rough shape to the proposed manuscript.

6.2.3   Feedback on Preliminary Presentations

Preparation of a slide-set and presentation at internal or external meetings allows feedback from peers. This feedback will help improve the content of the future manuscript and build a full discussion, including limitations. Such feedback on a presentation also provides a preview of what the peer-review process may bring. It may also suggest previous studies on the subject that the authors may not have been aware of and may help in interpreting the findings. Thus, taking notes and keeping track of the comments will help shape the future manuscript.

6.3   Preparing the Argument Matrix

6.3.1   Framing the General Message

In the field of communication for behaviour change, specialists identify a target audience and an expected behavioural outcome. These elements determine the key messages and the type of media to be used. A similar approach may be applied to scientific communication. Authors can ask themselves a number of questions (Box 6.1). First, a review of the current knowledge provides a backdrop. Second, the identification of the new pieces of information delineates the contribution of the current work. Third, the understanding of the implications in terms of action focuses the practical relevance of the information. Fourth, identification of the target audience for the recommendations (e.g. subject matter experts, specialists in a narrow field, primary physicians, general public health practitioners, policy-makers) clarifies the general approach that will be used. Fifth, mapping the readerships of the likely target journals will shortlist categories of audience that could be aimed for. Overall, answers to these questions will frame the key messages (usually two or three, occasionally four) and the way these will be disseminated, including the length of the manuscript (e.g. full paper, short report).

Box 6.1 Planning a Mini-communication Strategy for a Scientific Manuscript
1. What is already known on the subject?
2. What does the study add?
3. What do the findings imply in terms of action?
4. Who needs to know the information to act?
5. Where can this target audience be reached?
6. How should the information be presented?

6.3.2   The Life Cycle of Scientific Investigations

Scientific investigations can be seen as going through a life cycle (Fig. 6.1). Researchers try to identify information needs, such as missing information that would allow better action (e.g. why do diphtheria cases remain high in our region [Step 1]). On the basis of various information needs, they frame a more formal

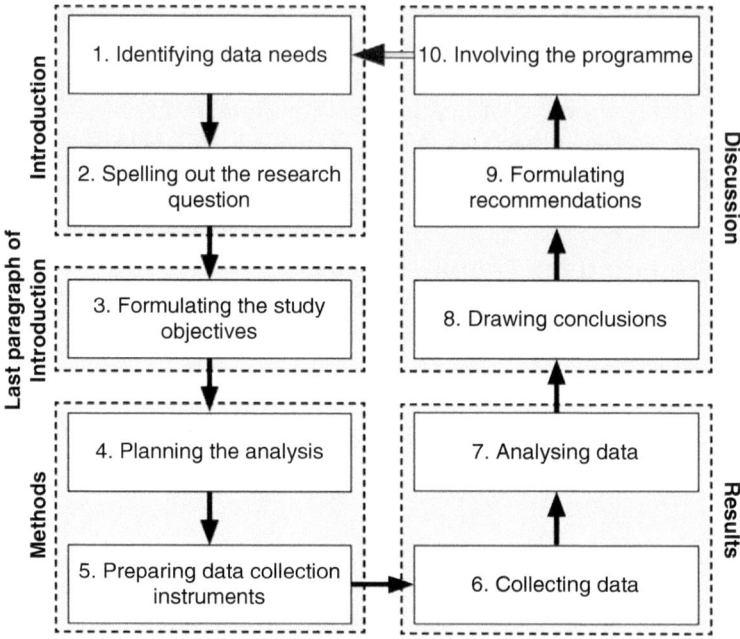

Fig. 6.1 The life cycle of an investigation and its relation to the various sections of a scientific manuscript

research question (e.g. we need to know whether diphtheria persists because of failure to vaccinate sufficient number of children or because of failure of the vaccine to protect against infection [Step 2]). They then convert the research questions in epidemiological terms that explicitly refer to testing a hypothesis or measuring a quantity (e.g. we want to estimate vaccine coverage and vaccine efficacy [Step 3]). Thereafter, they project an analysis plan that will address the study's objective (e.g. compare cases and controls in terms of vaccination coverage or estimate the vaccination coverage in the population [Step 4]). In the next step, they prepare the data collection instrument that will be used to gather the evidence (e.g. questionnaire and forms to abstract data from vaccination certificates [Step 5]). They then collect data (Step 6) using the data collection instruments prepared in Step 5, analyse these (Step 7) using the plan prepared in Step 4 and formulate conclusions (Step 8) that provide answers to the study objectives formulated during Step 3. This is followed by identification of the next steps (Step 9) in terms of action or gathering of more evidence, in line with the research question defined in Step 2. Finally, they engage the stakeholders (Step 10) in the implementation of the next steps. At that stage, new information needs may appear, thereby beginning the Step 1 of a new cycle and launch of a new investigation. Overall, these cycles repeat themselves in a process akin to peeling of onions, with each investigation providing an increased understanding and allowing more effective actions.

6.3.3   The IMRAD Structure

This structure proposes that manuscripts have four sections: Introduction, Methods, Results and Discussion (Table 6.1). This structure facilitates accelerated reading as it arranges all pieces of information in specific places. For instance, a reader already

Table 6.1   The various sections of the manuscript, including content and objectives

Sections	Subsections	Content	Objective	Practical remarks
Introduction	First paragraph	General (global) background information on the subject, while remaining focused on what is relevant to the research question	Provide a global perspective on what makes the question important to study: burden of disease, what is known and what is unknown	Good to write in third place after the methods and results
	Second paragraph	Regional or national perspective on the background information	Zoom in: explain how the general points apply to the regional/ national context	Does not constitute a complete literature review (cannot be too long)
	Third paragraph	Emergence of the research question in the local context, leading to the study objectives	Justify the local research question by making it a logical sequence to the global and regional perspective	Must be limited to what is necessary to make the rest of the paper appear natural and be understandable
Methods		Methods used to answer the research question	Provide the necessary information to judge the quality of what was done to obtain the results	Easy to write first as it constitutes a summarized, edited version of the protocol
Results		Data obtained using the methods	Describe the results of the analysis (i.e. information rather than data) in the absence of interpretation	Good to write in second place on the basis of the tables and figures

(continued)

Table 6.1 (continued)

Sections	Subsections	Content	Objective	Practical remarks
Discussion	First paragraph	Summary of the results (without interpretation): this paragraph may be omitted to save space	Summarize the information generated Introduce the key points that will be interpreted in the paragraphs of the discussion	• Write in fourth place • Put results in big picture terms • Step away from most raw numbers • Introduce the discussion
	Points of discussion (one to four different ones) in separate paragraphs	Organization of an argument around key results to place in perspective/ context and reach an interpretation	Interpret the results to make a point *State what can be said on the basis of the study*	• Write in sixth place • Start from the data • Build a case on the basis of the data and additional sources of information
	Limitations	Enumeration and discussion of the points of limitations	Propose ways to deal with limitations through a good understanding of them *State what cannot be said on the basis of the study*	• Write last • Focus on key limitations • Analyse each limitation fully
Last paragraph of discussion	Conclusions	Summary of the conclusions points reached on the basis of (1) results and (2) a layer of justified, documented interpretation	Bring answer(s) to the research question(s), as much as the study can	• Write in fifth place • Conclusions must bring an answer to the objectives that were announced in the third paragraph of the introduction
	Recommendations	Formulation of the recommendations/ next steps that the conclusions can support	Propose what needs to be done in terms of (1) action and (2) further research	

familiar with the subject can quickly read the abstract, clarify a point of methodology, review the tables and check how the authors made a specific point in the discussion, without reading the full manuscript. A disorganized manuscript will not allow such a quick review. Bradford Hill's proposed four questions guide the writer in understanding the IMRAD format (*see also* Chap. 1). First, the Introduction section answers the question: 'Why did you start?' It contains key background information that sets the stage for the study question or purpose of the study. It highlights specific issues about the problem that may not be known or that may simply not be available (i.e. not yet published or not clear). It progressively zooms in towards a last paragraph that introduces the need of the study and spells out its objectives. Alternatively, the study objectives may be placed in the first paragraph of the Methods section, which is logically equivalent as the end of the introduction and the beginning of the methods are adjacent to each other and only separated by the word 'Methods'.

Second, the Methods section answers the question: 'What did you do?' It reports the information necessary to judge the quality of what was done to obtain the results. Third, the Results section answers the question: 'What did you find?' This section presents the information obtained from analysis of the data obtained during the study. Finally, the Discussion section answers the question: 'What does it all mean?' This discussion is structured and purposive: the facts, numbers, estimates and parameters produced in the results need to be integrated with each other and with external information sources regarding what was known before the study (references) to yield a conclusion that leads to recommendation. Overall, the discussion serves as a bridge that connects the results with the conclusion through interpretations in light of what was already known. This process (what was known, what was done, what was found and what it means) is replicated for the two to three main messages of the papers. Then, the discussion raises what remains unknown (the limitations) before a last paragraph with the conclusions and next steps.

6.3.4 Mapping the Life Cycle of Scientific Investigations to the IMRAD Structure

Overall, the IMRAD structure of the manuscript reflects the life cycle of an investigation (Fig. 6.1), comprising identification of the information needs, research question and study objectives (reflected in the Introduction, Chap. 2), analysis plan and data collection instruments (described in the Methods, Chap. 3), data collection and analysis (summarized in the Results, Chap. 4) as well as conclusions, recommendations and programme involvement (detailed in the Discussion, Chap. 5).

6.3.5 Building the Argument Matrix

The next step in the construction of the backbone of the manuscript is the identification of two to three ideas that will run through the manuscript (Fig. 6.2). Each of these threads will be followed in a linear way through the Introduction (i.e. what was known before this study began? what was the local context?), the Methods (i.e. what methods were used to generate the findings?), the Results (i.e. what are the observations—the facts, the figures?) and the Discussion that can be broken down further into the interpretation (i.e. what can we say on the basis of the findings?), the

a Direction used to construct each idea

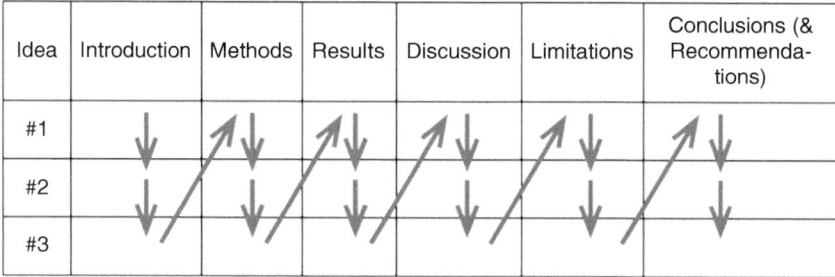

b Direction of placement of text in manuscript

Fig. 6.2 Using an argument matrix to prepare a manuscript. Panel (**a**) shows the linear flow of thoughts for each of the ideas in the manuscript. Panel (**b**) shows the sequence in which various components are assembled in a manuscript

limitations (i.e. what can we not say?), the conclusion (what is the take-home message once all things, including limitations, have been considered?) and the recommendations (what do these conclusions call for in terms of taking action and generating more evidence?). This approach prevents missing links in the development of an idea (e.g. a recommendation that is not backed up by data or a point of interpretation that does not connect what was known before and what was found in the study). It also prevents improper placement of an argument in the wrong section of the manuscript.

The IMRAD structure helps prevent some common mistakes such as providing results in the methods or beginning the interpretation in the Results section itself. Similarly, the argument matrix may help prevent more subtle mistakes in placement of text, which are not real errors in a strict sense. For example, some authors provide some specific background elements only when these are required in the discussion so that they can interpret a finding. However, this may not be the best placement for an element that was known before the study. Placement of these elements in the introduction may help set the stage for the study more effectively. They can help the reader obtain a better understanding of the research question and interpretation of the procedures done and data as these appear in the Methods and Results sections, respectively.

The 'argument matrix' (*see* example in Table 6.2, referring to the study summarized in Appendix 1 [1]) captures the two dimensions in which the manuscript must be thought of—the sequence of arguments in the development of each of the main

Table 6.2 Example of an argument matrix: organizing the content of the various sections of the manuscript in a linear, consistent way for a case–control study on the risk factors for typhoid in Darjeeling district, West Bengal, India

Topics	Introduction	Methods	Results	Discussion	Conclusions	Recommendations
Raw fruits/ vegetables and typhoid	Raw fruits and vegetables previously reported as risk factors for typhoid	Information collected on consumption of (1) raw fruits and vegetables and (2) milk products Data analysis	Association between consumption of selected raw fruits and vegetables and typhoid	Past studies that reported an association between typhoid and raw fruits and vegetables and local information about production of fruits and vegetables and hygienic practices	Consumption of selected raw fruits and vegetables is a source of typhoid	Thoroughly wash raw fruits and vegetables before consumption
Milk products	Milk products previously reported as risk factors for typhoid		Association between use of milk products and typhoid Stronger association among poorer people	Milk not a source of pathogen for typhoid but excellent growth media Contamination through dirty water (adulteration?) Richer people buy industrial products; poorer people buy local products	Local milk products may be unsafe	Promote hygienic practices in local preparation of milk products
Water supply	Reported risk factors for typhoid (including unsafe sources of water supply) Local information, including the fact that water supply is not chlorinated in Darjeeling and that water is scarce and sold by street vendors	Information collected on provision, treatment, handling and consumption of water Data analysis	Absence of clear association between source of water supply and typhoid Association between unsafe water handling practices (open container, etc.) and typhoid	Other studies reporting similar results Impossible to change the water supply in Darjeeling Experience with safe water system with chlorination of water at the point of use (Mention absence of a reference group of people who used treated water in limitations)	Unsafe water handling at the point of use is a source of typhoid in Darjeeling	Promote safe water system with chlorination of drinking at the point of use in safe, narrow-mouth containers

messages (with two to three rows, one for each main message), presented according to the sections of the manuscript (in columns). Rows show the natural linear development of each idea, ensuring that there are no omissions. Columns make a strategic use of the various sections of the manuscript by sections in the way that the reader will ultimately experience the text. Each box of the argument matrix may contain only a few keywords, preferably in nonsentence, 'bullet point' format, which function as placeholders or reminders of the way the logical thought ought to proceed. There is no need to write extensively in the argument matrix table. One could look at it as, the smaller the dots, the easier they connect.

Two sections may particularly benefit from the use of the argument matrix. First, the Introduction may gain through an upfront identification of the information elements that are necessary and sufficient to set the scene. This is to convince the audience that the study needed to be done and plant selected facts in the mind of the reader to prepare a personal process of interpretation. Second, the Discussion benefits through a better planning of how the section will build a bridge between (1) the facts and figures from the study's Results section and (2) the conclusion points. This bridge is built through connecting the results with prior knowledge by means of a process of interpretation so that the results find their meaning in a broader context. Elements of the results presented in the matrix should focus on those that will be the key starting points of the interpretation. The methods are usually straightforward and can sometimes be written on a column that merges cells across from top to bottom to prevent repetition. However, the matrix may work as a useful reminder for the author to specify some of the critical details that would be required to convince the reader that the key results are valid (e.g. use of a validated data collection instrument, use of highly specific reagent to confirm a diagnosis).

6.4   The High-Level Outline

Once the argument matrix has been constructed, it may be used to develop a high-level outline of the manuscript in one to two pages (*see* example in Appendix 2 [1]). The 'outline mode' of word processors allows building the structure of the document in the high-level outline. This high-level outline builds on the points of the argument matrix, by expanding each of these slightly and replacing these in text format in the sequence that the manuscript will follow. In practice, one can cut and paste the elements within the boxes of the argument matrix in a structure made up of the headings and subheadings of the manuscript. The completed high-level outline contains the headings, the subheadings and a short text point under each subheading. Each subheading will serve as a nidus for a paragraph in the final manuscript.

The high-level outline does allow the authors to reorder some of the elements of the matrix so that these follow each other logically and sequentially. For example, the elements of the introduction that were in the first column of the argument matrix may need reordering so that the introduction provides a gradual three-paragraph progression from the general to the specific and from the global to the local. One way to write these short points is to think of these as what the reader will have to remember when he begins reading the next paragraph. The high-level outline can also expand the discussion elements to locate and connect the main information points that will bridge the information presented in the results with the conclusions. Overall, the finished high-level outline represents a blueprint of the final manuscript. If the five tables and figures prepared earlier are added to the end of the document, the product obtained is draft zero of the manuscript that just requires expansion. Once this is done, the work of preparing the complete manuscript appears easier.

6.5   Different Ways to Use the Argument Matrix Approach

There are two ways to use an argument matrix to draft a manuscript. Ideally, a 'primary argument matrix' may be prepared as the first step in the drafting of a manuscript, as has been described above. This is the easier method, since it helps organize ideas ahead of the actual task of writing. However, there are times when a manuscript has already been drafted, but it lacks organization. In such a situation, a 'secondary argument matrix' may be used, to help organize various components of a manuscript better.

Working with a secondary argument matrix to reorganize a manuscript involves a series of steps. First, you need to read the entire draft manuscript and identify the two to three main messages of the manuscript. This may be difficult if there are some missing links in the development of ideas (e.g. an element of background is omitted; the data are not connected with prior knowledge to construct an interpretation). At times, some discussion is needed among the authors to identify these central ideas and extract these from the disorganized manuscript. Second, a 'secondary' argument matrix is prepared that develops the main messages the way these should have been presented in the first place in the paper (closing the gaps that may have been observed in the draft and restoring the natural sequence in the development of the ideas). Third, a second reading of the manuscript is done using two to three highlighters (either physically on paper using highlighter pens or electronically on a computer using 'text highlighting' function) to colour-code the places in the manuscript where elements related to each idea occur, using separate colours for each idea. These allow the mapping of the key elements for each idea in the different IMRAD sections of the manuscript. This review also flags separately the elements that are unnecessary (those that remain uncoloured); these can then be deleted in the next version of the draft. Fourth, the secondary element matrix makes use of the highlighted draft and uses a graphic code to explain if the elements mentioned in the matrix were (1) already present in the manuscript and at the right place (e.g. use of bold to present the bullet point in the matrix), (2) present in the matrix but misplaced in a different section (e.g. use of italics) or (3) absent from the manuscript (e.g. use of underlined). Using a secondary argument matrix prepared in this way along with the draft highlighted with the colour coding is usually an effective way to reorganize a paper. A next draft can then eliminate the unnecessary points, keep the points marked as being at the right place, move the misplaced points to locations where they belong and add the ones that were missing.

6.6   Summary

The argument matrix and high-level outline are simple tools that can help break down the manuscript writing process into elementary tasks that result in intermediate, shareable products. These products can serve as useful discussion points among co-authors so that a consensus on the main ideas can be developed ahead of and during the writing process. The main authors can construct the primary or secondary argument matrix and the high-level outline as a team during a short, 1-day retreat. Technology now allows newer and possibly more effective methods of organizing meetings (e.g. chat room on the Internet, Internet-based phone conference). This allows an in-depth review of the study, its findings and implications to determine whether the objectives were reached and whether the conclusions indeed bring an answer to the research question. This builds consensus among all the co-authors and facilitates the next steps for the preparation of the manuscript.

Acknowledgements The author is thankful to Marta Valenciano and Johan Giesecke who provided critical comments on earlier drafts.

Appendix 1: Abstract
Risk Factors for Typhoid in Darjeeling, West Bengal, India: Evidence for Practical Action

Sharma PK, Ramakrishnan R, Hutin Y, Manickam P, Gupte MD

Objective: To identify risk factors for typhoid and propose prevention measures.

Methods: Case–control study; we compared hospital-based typhoid cases defined as fever >38 °C for > or = 3 days with fourfold rise in 'O' antibodies on paired sera (Widal test) with community-, age- and neighbourhood-matched controls. We obtained information on drinking water, fruits, vegetables, milk products and sanitation and calculated matched odds ratios (MOR) and attributable fractions in the population (AFP) for the risk factors or failure to use prevention measures.

Results: The 123 typhoid cases (median age, 25 years; 47% female) and 123 controls had similar baseline characteristics. Cases were less likely to store drinking water in narrow-mouthed containers (MOR 0.4; 95% CI 0.2–0.7; AFP 29%), tip containers to draw water (MOR 0.4; 95% CI 0.2–0.7; AFP 33%) and have home latrines (MOR 0.5; 95% CI 0.3–0.8; AFP 23%). Cases were more likely to consume butter (OR 2.3; 95% CI 1.3–4.1; AFP 28%), yoghurt (OR 2.3; 95% CI 1.4–3.7; AFP 34%) and raw fruits and vegetables, including onions (MOR 2.1; 95% CI 1.2–3.9; AFP 34%), cabbages (OR 2.8; 95% CI 1.7–4.8; AFP 44%) and unwashed guavas (OR 1.9; 95% CI 1.2–3.0; AFP 25%).

Conclusion: Typhoid was associated with unsafe water and sanitation practices as well as with consumption of milk products, fruits and vegetables. We propose to chlorinate drinking water at the point of use, wash/cook raw fruits and vegetables and ensure safer preparation/storage of local milk products.

Appendix 2: High-Level Outline
Risk Factors for Typhoid in Darjeeling, West Bengal, India, 2005–2006: Evidence for Practical Action

Introduction
- Typhoid remains common and kills. It is transmitted through the faecal–oral route, and humans are the sole reservoir of its pathogen.
- Asia accounts for a high proportion of the global typhoid burden. The local epidemiology of the disease has been studied but is incompletely understood.
- The Darjeeling district of the West Bengal state of India has high typhoid rates in a context of poor water and sanitation. In this situation, understanding the risk factors for infections is the key to prevention.

Methods
- Case–control study in Kurseong subdivision of Darjeeling with matched community controls

Cases and Controls
- Typhoid: fever of at least 38 °C for 3 or more days with a positive Widal test between January 2005 and October 2006. Matched, population-based control group matched for neighbourhood and age.

Data Collection
- Standardized questionnaire for demographic characteristics and risk factors by field workers in Nepali. Referent exposure period: 14 days before onset/recruitment.
- Widal test.

Sample Size
- Assuming a prevalence of exposure of 10% among controls, for odds ratios of at least 3, 95% confidence interval and 80% power: 112 cases and 112 controls (+10% for non-responses = 123/123).

Data Analysis
- Time, place and person analysis for 2005. Matched odds ratio for the neighbourhood control group. Adjustment for multiple comparisons. Attributable fractions, stratification and dose–response relationship.

Human Subjects
- Protection.
- Ethical committee clearance.

Results
Descriptive Epidemiology
- 123 cases. No deaths. 2005 incidence from 3 to 14 per 100,000 (peak in September during rainy season). Even distribution. Persons under 30 years of age had higher incidence.
- Median acute phase antibody titre in 123 typhoid cases was 1:160 (range 1:80 to 1:320).

Characteristics of Cases and Controls
- 123 cases and 123 healthy neighbours. Cases were more likely to be Hindu, upper caste, monthly income <Indian Rupees 1500 and live in wood houses.
- Cases were less likely to have piped water than matched controls. Cases were less likely to store drinking water in narrow-mouthed containers, to take out water by tilting the container and more likely to scoop out water with a cup (attributable fractions).
- Cases more likely to consume selected raw unwashed fruits and vegetables (with some dose–response and attributable fraction data).
- Cases were more likely to eat butter and yoghurt (dose–response, attributable fraction, stronger association among poorer people).
- Cases less likely to have latrines at home (attributable fraction).

Discussion
- Two areas of risk factors: (1) fruits and vegetables and (2) milk/milk products. People with safer patterns of water use were at lower risk of illness.
- Fruits and vegetable reported elsewhere. Many opportunities for contamination through water. Likely to be causal. Possible explanations.
- Milk cannot be a source of typhoid (animals do not have typhoid infection), but milk products could be contaminated because of poor handling/adulteration, and milk is a good culture medium for typhoid. Stronger association suggests that local cheaper products are more likely to be sources of disease.
- Water use data suggest some contamination takes place at the point of use, pointing to possible relevance of safe water systems. Latrine use decreases incidence of typhoid.
- Limitations: (1) unable to confirm diagnosis with blood cultures, and (2) no capacity to examine the impact of water treatment as there was none taking place locally.
- Opportunities to prevent typhoid in a number of areas. Recommendations: (1) safe water systems/latrines/sewerage, (2) washing/cooking of raw fruits and vegetables and (3) hygienic practices in the preparation and storage of local milk and milk products. Further studies to characterize the quality of drinking water. Surveillance to evaluate the effectiveness of the proposed prevention measures.

Tables/Figures

- Table I: Incidence of typhoid cases by age and sex, Kurseong sub-division, Darjeeling, West Bengal, India, 2005
- Table II: General characteristics of typhoid cases and controls in Kurseong, Darjeeling district, West Bengal, India, 2005–2006
- Table III: Selected exposures among typhoid cases and controls, Kurseong, Darjeeling district, West Bengal, India, 2005–2006
- Table IV: Odds of typhoid according to increasing gradients of exposure, Kurseong, Darjeeling district, West Bengal, India, 2005–2006

Reference

1. Sharma PK, Ramakrishnan R, Hutin Y, Manickam P, Gupte MD. Risk factors for typhoid in Darjeeling, West Bengal, India: evidence for practical action. Tropical Med Int Health. 2009;14:696–702.

Writing an Abstract

7

Nithya Gogtay and Shobna J. Bhatia

The Merriam–Webster dictionary defines an abstract as 'a brief written statement of the main points or facts in a longer report …' [1]. In a research paper, the abstract is a concise, selective summary of the entire contents of a study.

Medical researchers need to write abstracts not only for publication in journals but also for presentation to conference organizers, conference delegates and, occasionally, to those who provide funds. The abstract should be carefully tailored to its audience and structured as advised by the journal or committee to which it is being submitted.

7.1 Need for a Good Abstract

The abstract for a journal is usually the first part of the text that is read. It is usually placed at the very beginning—after the title and before the Introduction. One cannot understate the importance of the impression it can create.

Editors frequently judge whether or not a submitted article falls within the scope of their journal from a reading of the abstract—and a poorly written abstract may not see an otherwise acceptable paper advance to the peer-review stage.

A good abstract has always been considered important. However, in recent years, with the advent of the Internet, online abstracting services and online

N. Gogtay (✉)
Department of Clinical Pharmacology, Seth GS Medical College and KEM Hospital, Mumbai, India
e-mail: nithyagogtay@kem.edu

S. J. Bhatia
Department of Gastroenterology, Seth GS Medical College and KEM Hospital, Mumbai, India
e-mail: sjb@kem.edu

© The National Medical Journal of India 2018
P. Sahni, R. Aggarwal (eds.), *Reporting and Publishing Research in the Biomedical Sciences*, https://doi.org/10.1007/978-981-10-7062-4_7

65

journals, the abstracts have become more widely available to prospective readers. This has further accentuated the importance of composing a succinct, stand-alone version of one's paper which encapsulates the highlights of the research. Journal websites, electronic literature databases and search engines often include a paper's abstract. The inclusion of certain keywords and phrases relevant to the main elements of a subject enhances an abstract's 'searchability'. This, in turn, improves the chances of the abstract (and the whole paper) being brought to the attention of an interested audience. For similar reasons, book chapters sometimes open with an abstract.

Another reason for preparing an abstract is to submit one's work for presentation at a conference (either as an oral or poster paper). Scientific committees use the abstract to decide who should be invited to present their research work at the meeting (or at an award session). The quality of an abstract may thus influence decisions about acceptance of a paper for presentation at a conference, approval or selection for a travel grant and choice for a best paper award.

Preparing an abstract for a conference or a presentation can also help focus thoughts on starting the actual process of writing and so shape the subsequent paper.

7.2 Qualities of a Good Abstract

An effective abstract should contain only material that is relevant to a paper, that is, the key elements that convey its essence. It should be clear and concise, should have a logical structure and should follow the chronology of the main manuscript.

It should adhere to the length and structure specified by the journal or conference organizers and is written in a style so engaging that the reader is disposed to find out more.

Similarly, abstracts in conference proceedings should entice the reader to visit the poster display or to attend the author's oral presentation in preference to others—particularly where there are competing parallel sessions.

7.3 Classification of Abstracts

7.3.1 Descriptive Versus Informational

Descriptive abstracts are somewhat in contradistinction to some of the qualities of a good abstract that have been indicated above—they simply provide a flavour of what the paper contains and do not lay out its findings or conclusions. These abstracts are shorter, 100–150 words in length, and provide an outline of the work than a summary of the work done. The reader has to go through the entire paper to find out what it contains. They occur mainly in reports from the social sciences and humanities but also in some basic science journals and textbooks. Some journals prescribe short descriptive abstracts for review articles and for case reports, but fortunately these now appear less frequently than before.

Informational abstracts, on the other hand, communicate the entire report—albeit in brief. Such abstracts usually have a prescribed length in the range of 250–300 words, but this can vary depending on the purpose for which these are written (*see below* under 'Structured Versus Unstructured' abstracts, and 'Conference Abstracts'). These include sections on the purpose (rationale), methods, results and conclusions, i.e. they follow the classical IMRAD format. Because these abstracts provide the findings and conclusion, some readers may be content with this information and decide not to read the entire paper.

7.3.2 Structured Versus Unstructured

Abstracts can also be classified as unstructured and structured. The former are free flowing, whereas the latter are divided into sections that conform to the structure of the main manuscript. Medical journals introduced structured abstracts in the 1980s, and most now favour their use for original research papers. However, both forms have their advantages and disadvantages.

Depending on the journal, a structured abstract could have a few or several subheadings and subsections. For example, it could use a minimum of four headings—background (and rationale), methods, results and conclusions, with each broadly corresponding to the four components of the IMRAD format. However, it might also contain a larger number of subheadings—objective, design, setting, participants, intervention, primary outcome measures, results and conclusions. This is particularly common with interventional studies such as randomized controlled trials or systematic reviews. This expanded format ensures that key aspects of the research method are presented in the abstract for readers to understand quickly what was done or what was not done.

Research on these two types of abstracts has shown that readers generally prefer structured abstracts. They perceive abstracts in this format to be more informative, to be easier to read and recall and to facilitate the peer-review process.

In a study that examined the quality of abstracts published in three general medical journals using 33 objective criteria in eight categories (purpose, research design, setting, subjects, intervention, measurement of variables, results and conclusions), the scores for mean overall quality were significantly higher for structured than for unstructured abstracts (0.74 vs. 0.57; $p < 0.001$) [2].

However, structured abstracts do take up more space in print journals. Hence, often journals also allow a larger allowance of words for such abstracts.

On the other hand, some data suggest that structured abstracts are just as likely to omit important pieces of information as the more traditional (unstructured) abstracts. In addition, there are authors who feel that the structured abstract straightjackets their presentation, and they prefer to write in the more free-flowing form of the unstructured abstract.

7.3.3 Conference Abstracts

A conference abstract is much like a manuscript abstract, but it is 'sold' to two sets of people—first the conference organizers and then the conference delegates.

In general, conference organizers prefer completed work so, as far as possible, do not write in the future tense. For example: It is much better to write 'Our study shows that administration of ABC for six weeks led to a 30% increase in XYZ' than 'I will present the results on effect of administration of ABC on XYZ' or 'the results will be discussed'. It is important to check the conference website for instructions and deadlines and follow these to the letter! (*See also* Chap. 25 on 'Podium presentation'.)

Some conferences will allow the author to submit a longer abstract than those normally written for a journal manuscript (up to 400 words or so), and they may even accept the occasional figure, table and reference. However, usually there are restrictions on the number and size.

7.4 Writing an Abstract

An abstract is best written after the entire manuscript has been completed. The structure follows the IMRAD pattern (Introduction, Methods, Results and Discussion). What was the purpose of the study? What was the methodology used? What were the findings? And what does it mean anyway?

As the abstract is written for the same audience as the entire manuscript, the same technical expression and level of language should be used throughout.

All abbreviations, acronyms, mathematical expressions and special symbols should be defined.

Standard nomenclature and notations should be used. In general, no figures, tables or references should appear, except in conference abstracts (*see above*).

It is always useful to consult the instructions to authors before beginning to write the abstract and to look at abstracts of papers already published on the journal's website.

The first step is to read through the entire paper and decide what needs to go into the abstract. The key points from the IMRAD can be highlighted and then extracted. Sentences should be specific and quantitative.

The word limit often makes writing of the abstract difficult as a large volume of information has to be condensed and conveyed in a very small space. It is preferable to use the active voice although the use of an occasional sentence in the passive voice may help shorten the text.

The introduction or background should be the shortest subsection and just give an outline of what is known, the gaps in the knowledge and why the study was carried out.

The Methods section is longer and should contain sufficient information for the reader to understand exactly what was done. Important facts such as randomization, sample size, number of cases versus the controls, drug dosages, duration of the study and measures of the primary and secondary outcomes must be clearly stated.

The Results section is usually the longest and the one most readers are interested in. It is important to present as much detail and as clearly as possible. Measures of effect (odds ratios, relative risk, risk difference, etc.) and p values should be included where appropriate. The data and statistical values must be to the same level of accuracy and decimals as in the main manuscript.

The Discussion section is omitted from the abstract so the next section is the Conclusions. This contains the primary take-home message, the importance of the findings and how they might be generalized. The key conclusions should be presented in two to three lines. As these will be taken at face value, they need to be presented carefully and truthfully. Any hype or unjustified extrapolations from the results must be avoided.

Once a first draft is written, it is useful to edit redundancies and substitute concise phrases for verbose passages. Brevity is of essence here. Editing is vital and the abstract must conform to the guidelines regarding length. It always helps if a co-author or interested person reads through the abstract. In fact, someone who has never been involved with the report can often identify text that is confusing, verbose, ambiguous or redundant.

7.5 Manuscript Revision and the Abstract

When a paper is revised, the abstract must also be revised. Authors need to check the following: (1) Does the abstract match the revised paper? (2) Do any new data added to the paper also need to be added to the abstract? (3) Have figures and values changed? (4) Have the conclusions changed in any way? Each of these points needs to be addressed.

The CONsolidated Standards for Reporting Trials (CONSORT) and their extensions offer clear, unambiguous instructions on how to write an abstract for manuscripts that report the results of randomized clinical trials. The items outlined by CONSORT for an abstract that reports a parallel group randomized study include details of the trial objectives, trial design (method of allocation, blinding, etc.), participants in the trial (description, numbers randomized and analysed), interventions intended for each randomized group and their effect on primary efficacy outcomes and harms, the trial's conclusions, the trial's registration name and number and the source of its funding.

Extensions of the CONSORT statement provide additional information on specific requirements for abstracts of non-inferiority trials and cluster randomized trials. Similarly, guidelines of the Preferred Reporting Items for Systematic Reviews and Meta-analyses (PRISMA) provide instructions for writing abstracts for systematic reviews and meta-analyses. The broad headings are title, background, methods, results, discussion and others. Some aspects of this information differ from that required for interventional studies. These include identifying the study as a systematic review or meta-analyses (or both), the key databases searched, the search strategy, methods used for assessing risk of bias, relevant characteristics of studies, direction of effect (which treatment or group does the study favour) and how relevant the study is to clinicians and patients.

References

1. Merriam–Webster Dictionary. www.merriam-webster.com/dictionary/abstract. Accessed 9 Nov 2015.
2. Taddio A, Pain T, Fassos FF, Boon H, Ilersich AL, Einarson TR. Quality of nonstructured and structured abstracts of original research articles in the British Medical Journal, the Canadian Medical Association Journal and the Journal of the American Medical Association. CMAJ. 1994;150:1611–5.

Suggested Reading

Andrade C. How to write a good abstract for a scientific paper or a conference presentation. Indian J Psychiatry. 2011;53:172–5.
Ferrero F. Writing a scientific paper abstract. Arch Argent Pediatr. 2015;113:104–5.
Hopewell S, Clarke M, Moher D, Wager E, Middleton P, Altman DG, et al. the CONSORT Group. CONSORT for reporting randomised trials in journal and conference abstracts. Lancet. 2008;371:281–3.
Hutton B, Salanti G, Caldwell DM, Chaimani A, Schmid CH, Cameron C, et al. The PRISMA extension statement for reporting of systematic reviews incorporating network meta-analyses of health care interventions: checklist and explanations. Ann Intern Med. 2015;162:777–84.

Title, Keywords and Cover Letter

8

Philip Abraham

After a research paper has been written with due attention paid to the IMRAD format and Abstract and References, a few other requirements must be completed before it is ready for submission to a journal. These include the Title, Keywords and Cover letter—all of which are important.

8.1   Title

A typical reader of biomedical journals is perhaps as busy as the author. The reader is mostly looking for what is interesting and relevant, just as the author is eager to convince the reader that his/her article meets just those criteria.

Several factors influence the reader's decision to read or not to read an article. Arguably, the most important is the title. Most people who read hard-copy versions or online-first versions skim through the titles and read an article only if they find its title interesting or relevant. The purpose of the title, therefore, is to convince readers that it is worthwhile to pause and wade through the text, that they will benefit from reading the whole article. If the reader is unclear about the article at the initial stage, the rest of the article might as well not have been written.

It is obvious that the title should be interesting and eye-catching. Examples abound in our daily newspapers. However, medical writing is a little more complex. While journalists may get away with being flowery or even frivolous, the prime requirement for the title of a medical article is to state the facts. Conjuring up an attractive and appropriate title within the given limits is an art. Several guidelines and approaches have been suggested to help in this task. A few simple steps may make the job easier even for a beginner. These are listed below:

P. Abraham
P.D. Hinduja Hospital, Mumbai, India
e-mail: dr_pabraham@hindujahospital.com

© The National Medical Journal of India 2018   71
P. Sahni, R. Aggarwal (eds.), *Reporting and Publishing Research in the Biomedical Sciences*, https://doi.org/10.1007/978-981-10-7062-4_8

- Begin by putting together a few sentences that describe what happened in the study, e.g. 'I evaluated the effect of a *new beta-adrenergic blocker BAB75 on portal hypertension*. I did this by measuring the *hepatic venous pressure gradient* (HVPG) in *mongrel dogs* in whom *liver cirrhosis* was produced using *carbon tetrachloride*. The HVPG was measured before and after the *administration* of the drug *for 7 days*. I found that the new drug compared well with the standard non-selective beta-blocker *propranolol* in reducing HVPG'.
- The italicized words in this passage hold the message to be conveyed in the title. The trick now is to decide which of these words or phrases need to be selected to convey the message briefly, adequately, but not fully (the bikini principle)—they should tease the reader by revealing just enough to attract his/her attention while arousing his/her interest in knowing what lies hidden in the article. At times, a title that states everything that the article contains may discourage a reader from exploring the full text. Needless to say, what is revealed should be representative of the whole.
- Next, one must string the selected words together—*new beta-adrenergic blocker BAB75, portal hypertension, hepatic venous pressure gradient, mongrels, liver cirrhosis, carbon tetrachloride, administration for 7 days and propranolol*—and rearrange them logically as *new beta-adrenergic blocker BAB75, propranolol, 7 days' administration, hepatic venous pressure gradient, portal hypertension, mongrels, liver cirrhosis and carbon tetrachloride*.
- Some of the words will need to be sacrificed or combined (e.g. *portal hypertension* and *liver cirrhosis* can be combined into *cirrhotic portal hypertension*) for the sake of brevity. What remains is *new beta-adrenergic blocker BAB75, propranolol, 7 days, cirrhotic portal hypertension and mongrels*.
- Hence, a reasonable title would be 'New beta-adrenergic blocker *BAB75* compares favourably with propranolol in reducing cirrhotic portal hypertension: A 7-day study in mongrels'.
- Note that a long title can be made more readable if it is split into a title and subtitle. The subtitle can be used to mention whether the study is a randomized, controlled trial or a retrospective data analysis, or whether an article is a review or meta-analysis, or to mention the study animal species/gender; all this is essential information and contributes to completeness.
- Note also that commonly used introductory phrases such as 'A study of...', 'The use of...', 'The first cooperative study...' or 'Observations on...' are not only wasteful but also irksome.

A few points need to be re-emphasized. The title should relate to the contents of the article and should be informative. One should not mislead the reader. One must not be frivolous in an attempt to avoid being boring. Abbreviations or jargon should be avoided as they could mislead the reader. One should be enthusiastic about thinking of a title.

What does this whole discussion tell us? That, yes, medical journalism is, indeed, drab and boring. But all is not lost: mercifully, we are allowed to take some liberties in this dreary exercise. One can try to make the titles of commentaries, editorials and letters interesting. For these, catchy titles are acceptable, provided they are truthful and representative. However, here, too, one must avoid the temptation of using foreign words or jargon. A short question or a teasing introductory phrase ('Who wins the battle of the bulge?' to comment on an article on gender differences in obesity) may attract the reader without being misleading.

An equally important role of the title is to provide keywords (more on that later) that help to slot the article in indexes (of journals or of indexing agencies), in which an interested browser is likely to find it. Since many journals specify a word limit for titles (usually 80 characters or so), it is important to exclude wasteful words.

8.2   Keywords

Print journals prepare their annual index on the basis of the keywords in the title as well as an additional list of keywords that authors are advised to provide. Specialist journals may compile their index by selecting from their own lists of keywords. Many journals have discontinued the practice of printing an annual index simply because readers rarely refer to these any longer. For this reason and because every author craves for a universal readership authors now use keywords to maximize the chances of their article being featured in the electronic indexing agency listings

In those ancient, precomputer days, when the only worldwide 'search engines' or compilations known to the medical world were voluminous hard copies printed by indexing agencies (e.g. Index Medicus), it was important to choose words that would ensure listing of the article in the right places in these indexes. Index Medicus, for example, had (and still has) its Medical Subject Headings (MeSH). The yearly printed version was discontinued in 2007, and MeSH is now available only online, as part of the electronic MEDLINE/PubMed article database, created and updated by the US National Library of Medicine.

It takes little effort to identify keywords in the title, but what is important is to check whether they match the keywords in listings such as MeSH. This may not always be easy. For example, the concept that a particular article deals with may be too specialized or cutting edge to feature in the indexing agencies' listings of keywords. When faced with a dilemma, the right thing to do, of course, is to stick to a title that is representative of the article's contents rather than going for mass appeal. In situations such as these, it is a relief if journals have a system that allows for the addition of more keywords.

Many journals allow the author to list seven to ten keywords after the Abstract. These are not necessarily words; they may also be short phrases. This facility should be used to list words that do not feature in the title, and preferably not in the abstract, since these two sections will be accessed in the electronic databases in any case. In fact, this list should include descriptive words (especially qualifiers; *see below*) about the article from MeSH that may not even feature in the full text of one's manuscript. This might further increase the chances of the article being accessed.

MeSH contains subject headings, known as descriptors, which are arranged in a hierarchical tree; the same word may feature in different branches of the tree. The list is revised every year. These are followed by standard qualifiers, such as epidemiology, diagnosis and complications, which may accompany various subject headings. It is advisable to peruse the MeSH before selecting the keywords for the article. One way is to use the MeSH Browser facility or to study the hierarchical structure using the 'navigate from tree top' approach (details are available on the website www.ncbi.nlm.nih.gov/MeSH). Another way of finding appropriate headings is to search PubMed for articles on similar topics and review the MeSH headings assigned to those articles.

Since 2014, the National Library of Medicine of the USA has made available an online tool—'MeSH on Demand' (at https://www.nlm.nih.gov/mesh/MeSHonDemand.html)—for selection of keywords. A user can simply paste text from the manuscript (of up to 10,000 characters) as input and run this tool; the latter searches through the text and outputs the likely MeSH keywords. The user can then review these suggestions, retaining those that represent key concepts covered in the paper. This method needs no prior familiarity with the MeSH vocabulary or software download and works very well.

It is easy to scan PubMed for a particular word or phrase in the title and abstract. The flip side of this kind of scanning is that it may turn up useless ('false-positive') articles that are of no interest to the reader, simply because they contain the particular word even though it may be in an unrelated context. One advantage of using the descriptors and qualifiers in MeSH is that they match the drop-down menu on PubMed's search facility, allowing for a more accurate match between the contents of various papers and the readers' expectations.

8.3   Covering Letter

When sending a paper to a scientific journal, the author should also send a brief covering letter introducing the manuscript. This letter will not be the deciding factor, but its contents might help the editor decide whether the article should be sent for peer review (and to whom) or turned back from the internal review process itself.

The primary purpose of the covering letter is to highlight the important findings of the study, i.e. to outline its contribution to the promotion of science, and to impress upon the editor (who cannot be an expert in every aspect of a field) that the article has something worthwhile to say and should thus be given due consideration. One must try not to either go overboard or be overly modest in doing this. One should make sure that the covering letter is short, as one must respect the editor's time—he/she has only limited time to evaluate many papers.

In addition, suggesting the names of a few potential reviewers in the cover letter may be helpful for the editor. This can be done even if the journal does not explicitly ask for names. A precaution that must be taken is to steer clear of suggesting persons who are associated with the authors (conflict of interest) or likely to be biased in favour of the authors. The editor can easily become aware of any such association or bias with the help of a quick search through PubMed or through other means. Equally importantly, the author may discretely state why he/she feels that certain persons may not be appropriate as reviewers because of their known bias or because they have competing interests.

8.4   Summary

The title is the part of the paper that is read most often; thousands of readers will scan the title. Abstracting and indexing services will also use the title. The title should, therefore, succinctly describe the contents of the paper. One should use descriptive words that one would associate with the contents of the article. The title should be short and unambiguous, yet be an adequate description of the work. Paradoxical as it may sound, it should be a good blend of clarity and brevity. Titles should never contain abbreviations and jargon. It should be borne in mind that the majority of readers will find one's paper via electronic database searches, and search engines use keywords found in the title.

In addition, a title should grab attention and lure the reader into reading the text. It must promise some kind of benefit to the reader, as a reward for the valuable time it demands from him/her. Since one's aim is to attract readers, one should make it easier for them to find one's article and tempt them to read it.

Most journals ask for a list of keywords, which they can use to classify and organize their content. As for the title, the list of keywords is important for search engines and readers to easily find one's article if it is related to what they are looking for. One must be careful when choosing keywords and remember that they need not be single words; they can also be short phrases.

Finally, the covering letter should be brief but should clearly put across to the editor one's honest evaluation of the paper and how one feels it contributes to science. To do justice to one's paper, one may also suggest the names of unbiased reviewers who one feels would be competent to evaluate the paper.

References and Bibliographic Software

9

Bandana Malhotra

A reference is a way to present other people's work or ideas, usually in relation to one's own, by acknowledging the original sources of knowledge in a document or presentation. New research is mostly undertaken to validate or negate the findings of others, answer questions that may arise from earlier research or answer a fresh question. Whatever the reason for the research, it will be based on work that has been done earlier. References are cited for the following reasons:

- As credit for the original work
- To direct readers to the original source of the information
- To add credibility to one's own work

9.1   How Does One Write a Reference?

A marker is introduced in a manuscript wherever one wishes to refer to a previous piece of work. This is known as a *citation*. This citation marker refers the readers to details that allow them to identify and obtain the complete original source of the work referred to; these details constitute a *reference*.

In research papers and other journal articles, references are listed together at the end of the document. However, in other documents such as official reports, these may be listed as footnotes at the bottom of each page where citations to these appear. The source may be a journal article, book, chapter in a book, newspaper article, website, CD, video or audio cassette, legal document or any other identifiable and obtainable published source. Unpublished documents and observations do not form

1

B. Malhotra
Freelance Medical Editor, New Delhi, India

© The National Medical Journal of India 2018
P. Sahni, R. Aggarwal (eds.), *Reporting and Publishing Research in the Biomedical Sciences*, https://doi.org/10.1007/978-981-10-7062-4_9

a part of the reference list, but their details are provided in brackets at the place of mention within the text.

9.2   When Should References Be Cited?

References should be limited to those that have a direct bearing on the author's work. In scientific writing, references are most often needed in the Introduction and Discussion sections of an article. The Methods section of a paper may also have references (*see* Chap. 3). In the Introduction (*see* Chap. 2), sufficient background information is needed about the topic under investigation, along with a brief summary of what has already been done in the field. Thus, relevant and important previous work should be appropriately cited in the references. In the Discussion section (*see* Chap. 5), it is important to compare and contrast previous major work in the area. While providing conflicting results from other studies, the possible reasons for the differences should be discussed. Comparison with work that has similar results should be highlighted, along with the additional work done in the present study. It is important for authors to check all original sources of information and ensure their accuracy and relevance by reading each article in full (and not just depending on the abstracts).

9.3   Which References to Cite and List?

References are the author's responsibility. Academic honesty is important, and failure to cite references properly may lead to being accused of inappropriate, incorrect or selective referencing. Authors should also ensure that none of the references cited are retracted articles. PubMed may be used to check for this by using the search term 'retracted publication'.

All references should be easily accessible and retrievable. Some journals prefer the use of references obtained from journal articles listed in PubMed or other bibliographic databases. Abstracts of conference proceedings are not regarded as formal publications, as they have not been peer-reviewed. Citing these should thus be avoided.

References to papers that have been accepted for publication but not yet published may be cited and listed as 'in press'. Authors should have proof of acceptance for publication. Papers that have been submitted but not yet accepted are designated as 'unpublished observations'. However, this should be avoided unless absolutely necessary. If information has been obtained from an unpublished or informal source such as a letter or email, it is identified by the term 'personal communication' followed by the name of the person and the date in parenthesis. The nature of the communication should also be provided, such as letter, email, conversation, etc. in square brackets within parenthesis. An example of this may be data cited by national programme managers before these have been officially published. It is advisable to seek permission from the source before including such information. Personal communication and unpublished observations are given within the body of the article in parentheses and not included in the reference list at the end.

Weblinks are often cited as references. The content on websites may change from time to time, and some weblinks may cease to exist. Therefore, it is important to cite the date of access of uniform resource locators (URLs). One should remember that information on websites may not be peer-reviewed.

9.4   Systems of Referencing

There are two main systems of referencing: the Harvard system and the Vancouver (ICMJE) system. The Harvard system has been in use for longer and is also known as the author–date system, while the Vancouver system is more recent in origin and also called the numbered system. Journals and book publishers may have their own styles, but these are largely slight variations of the two main systems. Most biomedical publications follow the Vancouver system or variations of this. The Harvard system is used more frequently by publishers in the social sciences and literature. Whichever system one uses, it is important to be consistent throughout. Other systems of referencing include the American Psychological Association (APA) style, the Chicago Manual of Style and Modern Language Association (MLA) style.

9.4.1   The Vancouver System

The Vancouver system was so named after a meeting of editors of some leading medical journals, colloquially known as the Vancouver group, held in Vancouver, BC, Canada, in 1978. At this meeting, the International Committee of Medical Journal Editors (ICMJE) was formed. This system of referencing was initially proposed by the ICJME and further developed by the National Library of Medicine in the USA. It is also known as the author–number system (Box 9.1).

Box 9.1 Example of the Vancouver System
WHO estimates that nearly half of all deaths in children under 5 years of age in developing countries could be attributed to undernutrition.[1] In India, a number of studies[2–5] have reported on malnutrition, particularly undernutrition among children under 5 years of age. The Government of India has adopted a number of schemes to address the problem of nutrition among children under 5 years of age and primary school students, the most notable being the Integrated Child Development Scheme (ICDS) and mid-day meal schemes. In comparison, fewer studies have focused on undernutrition among adolescents[6,7] or programmes tackling adolescent nutrition.

References
1. WHO. *Turning the tide of malnutrition: Responding to the challenge of the twenty-first century.* Geneva: WHO; 2000 (WHO/NHD.007).
2. Dutta A, Pant K, Puthia R, Sah A. Prevalence of undernutrition among children in the Garhwal Himalayas. *Food Nutr Bull* 2009; 30:77–81.

3. Arlappa N, Balakrishna N, Laxmaiah A, Brahmam GN. Prevalence of anaemia among rural pre-school children of West Bengal, India. *Ann Hum Biol* 2009;4:1–12.
4. Bhanderi D, Choudhary SK. An epidemiological study of health and nutritional status of under five children in semi-urban community of Gujarat. *Indian J Public Health* 2006;50:213–19.
5. Jones G, Schultink W, Babille M. Child survival in India. *Indian J Pediatr* 2006;73:479–87.
6. Kurz K, Johnson-Welch C. *The nutrition and lives of adolescents in developing countries: Findings from the nutrition of adolescent girls research programme.* Washington, DC: International Centre of Research on Women; 1994.
7. Das DK, Biswas R. Nutritional status of adolescent girls in a rural area of North 24 Parganas district, West Bengal. *Indian J Public Health* 2005;49:18–21.

In the Vancouver system, references are cited as Arabic numerals immediately after a sentence or fact in the manuscript text that requires a citation. The references are numbered consecutively throughout the text, including in tables and figures. These may be written as superscript numerals or aligned with the text in parenthesis or square brackets—or even as superscript numbers in parenthesis or square brackets. The citation may be inserted after the punctuation mark or before, depending on the style followed by the journal.

Examples
- For the general adult population, it was considered that the recommendation for when to start … would possibly remain unchanged until the results of ongoing randomized trials are available.[11, 12]
- For the general adult population, it was considered that the recommendation for when to start … would possibly remain unchanged until the results of ongoing randomized trials are available (11, 12).

The ICMJE Recommendations (previously known as the Uniform Requirements for Manuscripts Submitted to Biomedical Journals; *see* Chap. 20) have been developed by the ICMJE to offer guidance to authors on various aspects of reporting research, including referencing according to the Vancouver system. This system prescribes different formats for citing various types of information sources, such as a journal article, a book, a chapter in a book, a legal document, a website, proceedings of a conference, etc. The US National Library of Medicine maintains a list of such formats (available at http://www.nlm.nih.gov/bsd/uniform_requirements.html). A detailed book entitled *Citing Medicine* has also been published (available free online at http://www.nlm.nih.gov/citingmedicine).

Most biomedical journals have switched to the Vancouver system of referencing, albeit with minor variations in style. It is best to check the style of referencing followed by your target journal, which is generally given in the 'Instructions for authors' section.

Journals often follow a style that lists the first six authors of a publication followed by et al., but some may list only three authors followed by et al. Journal names are often abbreviated to their accepted forms (the National Library of Medicine establishes an abbreviation for a title, available at http://www.ncbi.nlm.nih.gov/nlmcatalog), to save on space. However, journals with a single name such as *Gastroenterology* or *Hypertension* are written in full. Journal names are usually italicized, as are book titles and any other published material. However, most journals have their own style, and this needs to be followed when submitting an article for publication.

Some examples of formats for references of journal articles and other published material are given below. For details, the reader is referred to http://www.ncbi.nlm.nih.gov/books/NBK7256/.

Journal Articles
- Standard journal article
  - The *scheme* of writing a journal article is as follows:
  - Author A surname initials, Author B surname initials, Author C surname initials, …. Title of article. *Journal name* (abbreviated) Year (month); Volume number (issue number): Page spread.
  - If the journal is paginated continuously across a volume (which is frequently the case), the month and issue number may be omitted. If there are more than six authors, list the first six authors followed by et al. If there are six or fewer authors, then list all the authors.
  - *Example:* Jordan MR, La H, Nguyen HD, Sheehan H, Lien TT, Duong DV, et al. Correlates of HIV-1 viral suppression in a cohort of HIV-positive drug users receiving antiretroviral therapy in Hanoi, Vietnam. *Int J STD AIDS* 2009;20:418–22.
- *Organization as an author*
  - Centers for Disease Control and Prevention (CDC). Achievements in public health. Reduction in perinatal transmission of HIV infection – United States, 1985–2005. *MMWR Morb Mortal Wkly Rep* 2006;55:592–7.
- *Both personal authors and an organization as an author*
  - Cohen MS, Chen YQ, McCauley M, Gamble T, Hosseinipour M; the HPTN 052 Protocol Team. Prevention of HIV-1 infection with early antiretroviral therapy. *N Engl J Med* 2012;55:143–8.
- *Volume with supplement*
  - Newell ML, Brahmbhatt H, Ghys PD. Child mortality and HIV infection in Africa: A review. *AIDS* 2004;18 (Suppl 2):S27–34.
  - The 'S' before the page number signifies that these page numbers are of the supplement.
- *Issue with supplement*
  - Brown T, Peerapatanapokin W. The Asian Epidemic Model: A process model for exploring HIV policy and programme alternatives in Asia. *Sex Transm Infect* 2004;80 (5 Suppl 1):i19–24.

- The 'i' before the page number signifies that these page numbers are of an issue.
- *Article published electronically*
  - Granich R, Kahn JG, Bennett R, Holmes CB, Garg N, Serenata C, et al. Expanding ART for treatment and prevention of HIV in South Africa: Estimated cost and cost-effectiveness 2011–2050. *PloS One* 2012;e30216. doi:10.1371/journal.pone.0030216.
  - The 'e' after the year shows that this is an electronically published article.
  - A digital object identifier (DOI) is a unique alphanumeric string assigned by a registration agency (the International DOI Foundation) to identify content and provide a persistent link to its location on the internet. The publisher assigns a DOI when an article is published and made available electronically.
- *Article published electronically ahead of the print version*
  - McNairy ML, El-Sadr WM. The HIV care continuum: No partial credit given. *AIDS* 2012 May 17 [Epub ahead of print]. Available at http://www.ncbi.nlm. nih.gov/pubmed/22614888 (accessed on 23 Jul 2015).
  - Some journals publish an electronic form of the article before the printed version. This is denoted by Epub ahead of print.

Books and Other Monographs
- *Personal author(s)*
  - Poolchareon W, Chantaratat Na Ayuthaya P, Pawanaporn W, Teokul W, Tantinimitkul C. *Development of AIDS prevention and control program in Thailand*. Nonthaburi: Heath System Research Institute; 1999.
- *Editor(s), compiler(s) as authors*
  - Narain JP (ed). *AIDS in Asia*. New Delhi: Sage Publications; 2004.
- *Organization as author*
  - World Health Organization. *Global tuberculosis control 2009: Epidemiology, strategy and financing*. Geneva, Switzerland: World Health Organization; 2009.
- *Chapter in a book*
  - Pongpan S, Poolkaysorn S, Sankote N, Plipat T. Situation of HIV in Thailand. In: Plipat T, Pongpan S, Kladswas K, editors. *Prevalence and incidence of HIV infection in Thailand, 2009*. Nonthaburi: Bureau of Epidemiology, Ministry of Public Health; 2010.
- *Electronic material*
  - CD-ROM
  - Dorland. *Dorland's illustrated medical dictionary* [CD-ROM]. Amsterdam: Elsevier; 2007.
- *Website*
  - National Commission for the Protection of Human Subjects of Biomedical and Behavioral Research. The Belmont Report. Available at http://ohsr.od. nih.gov/guidelines/belmont.html (accessed on 6 Nov 2010).

Advantages. As reference numbers appear as superscripts, they do not intrude on the text, allowing the eye to navigate the text more easily. It is also easy to prepare the complete list of references at the end of the article and not miss any reference as they are numbered.

Disadvantages. The reader has to go to the reference list to identify the reference. If references are added or deleted, the citations throughout the document and the reference list have to be renumbered.

9.4.2 The Harvard System

This gives the author's name and date as a citation marker in the body of the text in parenthesis after a sentence or fact that needs a reference. The full details of the references in the document are arranged alphabetically at the end according to the first author's surname. The names of books, journals and other published material are usually italicized (Box 9.2).

Box 9.2 Example of the Harvard System

Text

Historically in this region, coverage and 'dosage' of harm reduction interventions has been low and continues to be so. It has been argued that coverage is perhaps too low to have the desired epidemiological impact (WHO 2010; Sharma et al. 2009; Mathers et al. 2010). Provision of suboptimal doses of methadone remains an issue in many settings. For example, in China, a recent study by Lin and Detels (2011) showed that in 28 clinics, the methadone dose was 35 mg/person/day. While it is acknowledged that there is likely to be wide variation in dosage, there are too many examples of underdosing in OST interventions. Similar issues have been noted in Nepal and Myanmar (Sharma et al. 2009).

References

Lin, C. and Detels, R. A. (2011). A qualitative study exploring the reason for low dosage of methadone prescribed in the MMT clinics in China. *Drug and Alcohol Dependence*, 117:45–9.

Mathers, B. M., Degenhardt, L., Ali, H., et al. for the 2009 Reference Group to the UN on HIV and Injecting Drug Use. (2010). HIV prevention, treatment, and care services for people who inject drugs: A systematic review of global, regional, and national coverage. *Lancet*, 375:1014–28.

Sharma, M., Oppenheimer, E., Saidel, T., et al. (2009). A situation update on HIV epidemics among people who inject drugs and national responses in the South-East Asia Region. *AIDS*, 23:1405–13.

World Health Organization. (2010). Report on people who inject drugs in the South-East Asia Region. New Delhi: WHO Regional Office for South-East Asia.

Some important points to remember while citing journal articles
- Cite the journal name that was used at the time of publication. For example, the *British Medical Journal* officially changed its name to *BMJ* in 1988. Cite articles from 1987 and earlier as *Br Med J*, not *BMJ*.
- Cite the version you saw. For example, do not cite the print version if you have used the internet one.
- Do not include information on the type of article, such as 'editorial', 'case report', etc. as part of the article title. These may be placed after the article title in square brackets.
- Be consistent in typography, such as the use of bold, italics, etc. to indicate volume number, page spread, etc. It is best to follow the style of the journal you want to send your article to.

General rules for article title
- Enter the title of an article as it appears in the publication.
- Capitalize only the first word of a title, proper nouns and acronyms.
- Use a colon followed by a space to separate a title from a subtitle, unless some other form of punctuation (such as a question mark, period or an exclamation point) is already present.
- Articles in non-English languages may be translated into English; place the translated title in square brackets. The name of the language of the original article is included after the page spread.
- End a title with a period unless a question mark or exclamation point already ends it.

Example
- *In-text citation*
  - Nitrogenase activity was measured by acetylene reduction assay in 2 ml culture aliquots (David et al. 1980).

Reference List
David, K.A.V., Apte, S.K., Banerji, A., and Thomas, J. (1980). Acetylene reduction assay for nitrogenase activity: gas chromatographic determination of ethylene per sample in less than one minute. *Appl Environ Microbiol.* 39:1078–80.
In this example, the authors' names are not directly cited in the text and are placed in parentheses at the end of sentences. The text could instead also be written as follows:
David et al. (1980) measured nitrogenase activity by acetylene reduction assay in 2 ml culture aliquots.
This system follows certain rules

Journal Articles
- If there are *two authors*, they are listed in the text as A and B, followed by the date.

- *Example:* They exhibit exceptional DNA repair capacities and can recover after acute exposure to radiation (Mattimore and Batista 1996).
- If there are *three or more authors*, only the first author's name is written followed by et al. and the date.
  - *Example:* A major limitation of *D. radiodurans* is its heterotrophy and inability to grow in nutrient-limited minimal media (Venkateswaran et al. 2000).
- If the *author's name is part of the sentence*, then the date is provided in parenthesis after the name.
  - *Example:* Shirkey et al. (2003) have questioned the validity of such a hypothesis.
- If *more* than *one article is referred to*, the names of all authors and dates are written chronologically, separated by semicolons.
  - *Example:* Current recommendations for humans are that ARV prophylaxis should be administered within 72 h (Smith et al. 2005; WHO 2008).
- If there is *more than one publication by the same author or group of authors*, these should be listed chronologically, with the older ones listed first.
  - *Example:* Viral load predicts the risk of both sexual transmission and vertical transmission of HIV-1 (Anglemyer et al. 2009, 2011).
- Where the *author or same group of authors has more than one publication in the same year*, consecutive lower case letters starting with 'a' are added after the year.
  - *Example:* Viral load predicts the risk of both sexual transmission and vertical transmission of HIV-1 (Anglemyer et al. 2010a, 2010b).
- When giving *a direct quotation*, the page number(s) must be cited.
  - *Example:* It is claimed that government in the information age will 'work better and cost less' (Bellamy and Taylor 1998, p. 41).
- If you wish to *cite a work given in another article*, acknowledge both sources in the text, but include only the article you have actually read in the reference list.
  - *Example:* The study by Barr-Sinoussi et al. (1983) cited by Quinn et al. (2000) says that lowering the viral load through the use of antiretrovirals lowers the risk of HIV transmission.
  - In this example, give the full reference of Quinn et al. only.

References of journal articles should be in the following general format:
- Author A surname, initials., Author B surname, initials., Author C, initials. (Year). Title of article. *Name of journal* Volume number: Page spread.

Books and Other Monographs
- References to the work of an author that appears as a *chapter in a book* edited by someone else should be cited within the text using the name of the contributing author and not the editor of the whole work.
  - *Example:* In-text citation
  - High resolution ultrasound examination of the neck undertaken with 7.5–15 MHz probes forms the mainstay of thyroid imaging (Gwyther 2012).
  - Reference list

- Gwyther, S.J. (2012). Imaging in thyroid cancer. In: Greene, F.L. and Komorowski, A.L. (eds). Clinical approach to well-differentiated thyroid cancers. Delhi: Byword Books Private Limited.
- If a work is by an organization and has *no personal author*, the work is usually cited by the organization that commissioned the work.
  - *Example:* It has been argued that coverage is perhaps too low to have the desired epidemiological impact (WHO 2010).
- When citing *information found on a website*, the authorship of the website should be identified. This may be a corporate author, an organization or company. The date of publication may be found at the bottom of the page. The date of accessing the website must be given in the reference.
  - *Example:* NHS Evidence. (2003). *National Library of Guidelines* [online]. Available at http://www.library.nhs.uk/guidelinesFinder (accessed 10 October 2011).
- The reference *list for books* should be compiled in the following manner: Author surname, initials., (Year). Title of book. Edition. (only include this if not the first edition) Place of publication (this must be a town or city, not a country): Publisher.

Advantages. As the author's name appears in the citation in the text, the reader can often immediately identify the reference. This is particularly useful for readers who are familiar with the literature in the field, as they will be able to identify the work cited without having to turn to the reference list at the end of the document. The date also tells the reader how recent the work is. A reader can thus follow an argument in a logical manner.

Disadvantages. If many references are cited, the list of authors may break up the text and make it difficult to follow the thread of the argument. Care is needed to ensure consistency between the text and the reference list, especially if any references have been added or deleted.

9.4.3 Differences in Referencing Between Journal Articles and Books

- Journal references omit information on place of publication and publisher, whereas book references carry these details.
- Journal titles are often abbreviated; book titles are not. The brevity in citing journal articles stems from the need to conserve space.

9.5   Common Problems with References

1. *Quoting too many references:* Only a few key references need to be given. It is not necessary to cite all the possible articles that support a particular argument. The only exception may be in papers reporting meta-analyses, where all papers

with particular characteristics may need to be cited at the place such papers are referred to.

2. *Quoting too few references:* Omitting key or relevant references can dilute the strength of an argument. However, universally known and accepted facts need not be referenced, e.g. Water comprises three-fourths of the earth's surface *or* The population of India is increasing.

3. *Inaccurate quoting of references:* It is the author's responsibility to check that each reference is listed accurately and completely.

4. *Not quoting a reference where one is needed:* This implies not giving credit where it is due and could lead to allegations of plagiarism. However, copying and pasting material from an article and providing a reference at the end does not absolve you of that allegation.

5. *Using varying styles for quoting references:* Ensure that all references are in a uniform style, adhering to the style preferred by the journal you wish to send your article to.

6. *Not crediting sources of data:* All data in tables, graphs and figures, other than those obtained in the current study, must be credited.

7. *Quoting inaccessible sources as references:* All references must be easily accessible to the reader. Unpublished reports and informal observations must not be included in the reference list and should instead be given as 'personal communication' or 'unpublished observation' within the body of the article in parenthesis.

8. *Quoting from secondary sources or without reading the full paper:* It is not a good practice to cite references from secondary sources such as review articles. This may lead to inaccurate referencing as the contents of the cited paper may be different from those mentioned in the secondary source. For the same reason, citing a research paper after reading only the abstract is also not an acceptable practice.

9.6 Reference Management Software

If a paper is short, the task of inserting citation markers in the text and preparing the reference list—while ensuring complete concordance between the citations and bibliography—is easy and can be done in a couple of hours. However, if the paper is long and contains several references, including some that are cited at several places in the text, this task can be quite arduous. Further, if for some reason, one moves some text that contains one or more references from one location in the paper to another, the entire process may need to be redone. Also, if one decides to submit the paper to another journal that follows a different style for formatting in-text citations and bibliography, reformatting the citations and references can be a challenging task.

In recent years, the task of inserting citations and preparing a bibliography has been simplified by the development of computer software programmes, known collectively as bibliography management or reference management tools. These tools allow an author to create his/her own database of references related to any topic. Such personal databases can contain a large number of references of different types (e.g. journal articles, books, book chapters, conference proceedings, etc.). New references can be appended to the database either by typing in the material manually or, more conveniently, by downloading these from computerized literature databases, such as PubMed, Embase, Science Citation Index, etc.; the latter process also obviates any typographical errors. In most of these software, the database can also hold full-text files (e.g. PDF files) for each paper, where available. The contents of these databases can be searched easily using queries in one or multiple fields, making it easy to search for a particular paper using some information that one may recall, e.g. the author name, a few words of the title, keywords, journal name, year or even a word or phrase in the full text.

Having prepared a database of references for a particular subject, preparing manuscripts related to it becomes fairly easy. All one needs to do is to simultaneously open two software, a word processor and the bibliographic software, on one's computer. When one reaches a location in the document where a citation is to be placed, one can shift to the bibliographic software, find and choose the relevant papers to be cited and then move back to the word processor and paste the citations. The software places an appropriate citation (either as a number—superscripted or in brackets—in the case of Vancouver style or the first author name and year in the case of Harvard style) at the chosen location and also simultaneously adds the reference to a bibliography at the end of the manuscript.

Once the document is complete, the two software (word processor and bibliographic software) collaborate and insert the citations in the text and prepare a bibliography with references formatted according to the style selected by the author. The manuscript document does not hold the reference as formatted text but merely as a link to the database entry. Thus, the format of references can be changed, for instance, from Vancouver style to the Harvard style, simply by selecting the desired format in the software, and the citations and bibliography are automatically updated.

Several bibliographic software, both commercial (e.g. EndNote, Reference Manager) and free (Zotero, Mendeley, etc.), are available. Their features vary and the commercial software offer somewhat greater flexibility. For an author who intends to write more than a couple of papers a year, it is useful to choose one of these software programmes and then invest the time and energy (and possibly money) in learning how to use them.

9.7   Summary

- Cite references when you refer to previous work on which your work and arguments are based.
- Use a few key references and not several. Sometimes journals lay down the number of references for a particular type of article.
- Ensure that you have read all the references you quote.

- Format all references uniformly according to the style of the journal you wish to submit your article to.
- Do not use abstracts as references as far as possible. Use the full paper as a reference.
- Ensure that all the references cited by you are easily accessible.
- Ideally, cite articles listed in PubMed or other recognized bibliographic databases.

Sources

1. U.S. National Library of Medicine. International Committee of Medical Journal Editors (ICMJE). Uniform requirements for manuscripts submitted to biomedical journals. Med Educ. 1999;33:66–78. https://www.blackwellpublishing.com/products/journals/freepdf/med339.pdf. Accessed on 30 May 2015.
2. Peh WC, Nq KH. Preparing the references. Singapore Med. J 2009;50:659–61; quiz 662.
3. Anglia Ruskin University. Harvard system. http://libweb.anglia.ac.uk/referencing/harvard.htm. Accessed on 30 May 2015.
4. De Montfort University Leicester. The Harvard system of referencing. http://www.library.dmu.ac.uk/Images/Selfstudy/Harvard.pdf. Accessed on 30 May 2015.
5. National Center for Biotechnology Information. Bookshelf. Chapter 1: Journals. 15 September 2011. http://www.ncbi.nlm.nih.gov/books/NBK7282/. Accessed on 30 May 2015.
6. James Lind Institute. Why referencing? Referencing styles in medical writing. http://www.jli.edu.in/blog/why-referencing-referencing-styles-in-medical-writing/. Accessed on 30 May 2015.

Copyright Issues

10

Dinesh Sinha and John Mackrell

10.1   The Principle of Copyright

The online Oxford English Dictionary defines copyright as "The exclusive and assignable legal right, given to the originator for a fixed number of years, to print, publish, perform, film, or record literary, artistic, or musical material" [1]. These legal rights vary from country to country and what may be considered permissible in one country might not be permissible in another.

The concept of copyright, or the *right to copy*, is closely connected with the concept of intellectual property (IP). According to the World Intellectual Property Organization (WIPO), IP refers to "creations of the mind, such as inventions; literary and artistic works; designs; and symbols, names and images used in commerce" [2]. It goes on to state that "copyright (or author's right) is a legal term used to describe the rights that creators have over their literary and artistic works." Works covered by copyright range from "books, music, paintings, sculpture, and films, to computer programs, databases, advertisements, maps, and technical drawings" [3]. It is important to recognize that copyright applies to a creative *work*. There is however no protection for the idea behind a creation; ideas and facts are *not* subject to copyright.

In most countries, writing, music, images, videos, and design are automatically protected. However, creators of such material can do much to prevent their work from being plagiarized. They should claim (or assert) ownership on a certain date and ensure that they can be easily traced. In practice, the creator may assign his or

D. Sinha (✉)
Byword Editorial Consultants, Delhi, India

J. Mackrell
Formerly with Oxford University Press, Oxford, UK

© The National Medical Journal of India 2018   91
P. Sahni, R. Aggarwal (eds.), *Reporting and Publishing Research in the Biomedical Sciences*, https://doi.org/10.1007/978-981-10-7062-4_10

her legal rights to the publisher of the work, who is likely to be more familiar with copyright law and thus be in a better position to pursue any breach or infringement of the right to copy, including through legal proceedings. Thus, the principle of copyright includes the legal means by which a tangible expression of a creative *work* is protected. Besides legal implications, the concept of copyright also has ethical and moral considerations.

There is a limit on the time for which an author, or an author's estate, can benefit from the protection that copyright affords. The term of copyright is *not* eternal and is dependent on the nature of the creative work and the law in the country of publication. Literary creations pass into the "public domain" (i.e., become freely available for all to exploit) at least 50 years or more after the death of the copyright holder (or the last surviving author in the case of multiauthor works). The term of copyright is life of author plus 60 years in India; it is life plus 70 years in the US and UK. It may be longer in the case of corporate authorship (i.e., when the paid employees of a company or institution author a work, or a corporate body pays an agency to create a work).

For other forms of IP (such as trademarks, appearance, names, and invention), protection may not be automatic but needs to be applied for and the work registered (e.g., for trademarks and patents).

This chapter discusses some issues concerning copyright in the context of reporting and publishing research in the biomedical sciences.

10.2   Rationale of Copyright Law

The development of copyright law over time has generally kept in step with the advances in science, technology, and economy. Before the advent of the printing press in the fifteenth century, the methods of making copies were manual and cumbersome. Copies of any written work were made by hand. The invention of printing made it easier and efficient to generate a large number of copies from a single "master." Continual improvements to the basic printing processes made the act of producing replicas both quicker and less expensive. Beginning in the 1960s, the typesetting and prepress processes have undergone digitization. This has enabled text or data to be transferred electronically, usually through a dedicated cable or a small portable device such as a compact disk or memory stick. The simplicity of digitization coupled with the development of the Internet has universalized the act of publishing (uploading) and the act of copying (downloading). This has brought copyright issues center-stage.

10.3   International Conventions and National Laws

The practice and law of copyright evolved in England, France, and the USA during the eighteenth and nineteenth centuries. The Berne Convention of 1886 was the first international effort to codify copyright law to protect intellectual works and the rights of their authors [4] and then updated on nine occasions up to 1979. This was supplemented more recently by the WIPO Copyright Treaty (WCT) of 1996, a special agreement under the Berne Convention, which deals with "the protection of works and the rights of their authors in the digital environment" [5]. Additionally, such digital works are granted certain economic rights.

The Treaty also provides copyright protection for two newer types of work: "(1) computer programs, whatever the mode or form of their expression; and (2) compilations of data or other material ("databases")" [5]. Based on these Conventions, individual countries have enacted and amended their copyright laws from time to time to reflect their socioeconomic realities and technological advancements and challenges. For instance, the US Digital Millennium Copyright Act of 1998 extended copyright provisions to works originating in the digital media [6]. Similarly, the Indian Copyright Act of 1957 has been amended several times. Of these amendments, those made by the Copyright (Amendment) Act 2012 [7] have been the most substantial. Some key amendments of 2012 extend copyright protection to the digital environment; there are now penalties for those who circumvent technological protection measures; and there are definitions of the rights and liabilities of Internet service providers. Other countries have also revised their copyright acts to accommodate the challenges thrown up by rapid technological advances in the digital domain (*see also* Chap. 20 on "Electronic publishing").

10.4 Creative Commons Licenses

Several creators of novel work have altruistic motives, and they may be happy to allow others the right to freely use their work while retaining some ownership. Creative Commons (CC) is a "non-profit organization that enables the sharing and use of creativity and knowledge through free legal tools." [8]. Founded in 2001, CC aims to realize the full potential of the Internet by facilitating "universal access to research and education … to drive a new era of development, growth, and productivity." CC copyright licenses provide authors or creators of work a "standardized way to give the public permission to share and use [their] creative work on conditions of [their] choice." Authors can thus modify their copyright terms from the default position of "all rights reserved" to one of "some rights reserved" [8].

It should be noted that open access of the published material under CC licenses does not imply merely free access but is a much broader concept. It also gives freedom to others to use your work as if it was their own, improve or build upon it, and to disseminate it further (*see also* Chap. 19 on "Open access journals"). Thus, those interested in giving people the right to share, use, and even build upon their work should consider publishing it under a CC license and define the limits of their copyright.

10.5 ICMJE on Copyright

The International Committee of Medical Journal Editors (ICMJE) recommends that "Journals should make clear the type of copyright under which work will be published, and if the journal retains copyright, should detail the journal's position on the transfer of copyright for all types of content, including audio, video, protocols, and data sets. Medical journals may ask authors to transfer copyright to the journal. Some journals require transfer of a publication license. Some journals do not require transfer of copyright and rely on such vehicles as Creative Commons licenses. The copyright status of articles in a given journal can vary: Some content cannot be copyrighted (for example, articles written by employees of some governments in the course of their work). Editors may waive copyright on other content, and some content may be protected under other agreements" [9].

Many publishers ask for an exclusive license to publish, i.e., they want the authors to grant them all the rights in a particular piece of work (including subsidiary rights such as those for any translations, publications in electronic format, and derivative works such as compilations of a series of articles which may include this work), before they would agree to publish the article in a particular journal. Some journal publishers accept the signature from the corresponding author who warrants that all the other authors have consented to assign to the journal the copyright for the article; by contrast, others follow a policy that requires each author to assign copyright individually [10]. (*See also* Box 1 on page 204, Chap. 20 on "Electronic publishing.")

10.6   Copyright Notice: Asserting Ownership

As mentioned above, creators of original works need to claim copyright; this is done by adding a notice to their work. A copyright notice has three elements, namely, (1) the word copyright or the symbol "©", (2) the name of the copyright owner, and (3) the year of the first publication of the work—(e.g., © *The National Medical Journal of India*, 2016). If a journal is owned by a society, an association, or a company, the copyright notice reflects this status. For example, the copyright notice in *The Lancet* states:

Copyright © 2016 Elsevier Limited except certain content provided by third parties

and that in the *New England Journal of Medicine* states

Copyright © 2016 Massachusetts Medical Society.

10.7   Copyright in Book Publishing

In book publishing, the agreement between the owner of the IP (*author*) and the publisher is on mutually agreed terms (including the terms of royalties and marketing territories). Various limits may apply to the use of such work—for instance, time, number of copies disseminated, and reuse of the material in other languages or other media such as ebooks.

The information on copyright is mostly given on a page called "the copyright page," which follows the title page (i.e., the page carrying the title, author[s]/editor[s] name[s], and the name and logo of the publisher). The copyright notice (© name of copyright owner, year) is often accompanied by another notice, indicating the extent of rights claimed, such as:

> All rights reserved. No part of this publication may be reproduced, stored in a retrieval system, or transmitted, in any form or by any means (electronic, mechanical, photocopying, recording, and/or otherwise) without the prior written permission of the publishers.

For books on medical topics, there may be an additional disclaimer such as:

> Dosage schedules are being constantly revised and new side-effects recognized. The reader is thus strongly urged to consult the printed instructions of drug companies before administering any of the drugs recommended in this book. It is possible that errors might have crept in despite our best efforts to check drug dosages.

The UK Copyright, Designs, and Patents Act of 1988 requires that authors assert their moral rights to be identified as authors/creators of a particular work [11]. This means that, even if the copyright is assigned to a publisher, the author asserts his or her moral rights to be identified as a creator. This notice is generally given below the copyright notice as:

> The moral rights of the author have been asserted.

10.8   The Concept of Fair Use (or Fair Dealing)

In the context of research, copyright law permits the limited use of copyrighted text without asking for permission from the IP owner. This use is covered by the phrase "fair use" or "fair dealing," which is a "legal term used to establish whether a use of copyright material is lawful or whether it infringes copyright" [12]. When the copyrighted material is used for noncommercial, research, or educational purposes, the extent of such "fair use" or the length of the text used is determined primarily by the honesty of the user. Usually, only part of a work may be used [13]. Such fair use does not include reproduction of a table, figure, flowchart, or photograph included in a research article; for such use, permission should always be obtained from the copyright holder. Whenever in doubt, it is advisable to err on the side of obtaining permission from the copyright holder rather than ignoring this requirement. However, in certain cases (subject to fair use), tables or flowcharts can be modified and "adapted from" the original—but this must always be done with due acknowledgment.

Thus, copying "to earn recognition" should be done with sufficient acknowledgment to the copyright owner (together with the title and other description that clearly identifies the work that has been copied), and any copying "to earn financial benefit" should only be done with the explicit permission of the IP owner. (For a detailed discussion on plagiarism and copyright, *see* Chap. 24 on "Scientific fraud and other types of misconduct.")

10.9   Obtaining Copyright Permission

All research builds on previous work, and authors often need to "reproduce" previously published material to support their argument (besides citing many other sources as references). It is the responsibility of the author or contributor to seek permission for the copyrighted material used in preparing the manuscript. Publishers expect the relevant written approval and documentation of copyright permission to accompany the final draft of the manuscript. The author must also apply for permission to reproduce his own previously published work.

Most websites on the Internet have "terms of use," which give information regarding the copyright status of their content and the mode of obtaining permission. Publishers' websites often provide authors with guidance on how to seek copyright permission and the mechanism for obtaining it. Some publishers deal directly with copyright requests; others refer requests to the Copyright Clearance Center (CCC) or direct the enquirer to RightsLink®, the licensing arm of the CCC [14].

10.10   Summary

The act of downloading (i.e., copying) any material from the Internet that we feel is relevant has become second nature to us. We must remember that, irrespective of whether an explicit copyright statement is appended to it or not, the principles of copyright also apply to any material on the Internet, because this is as much a medium of publishing as any book or journal or compact disk. Ethical and moral considerations demand that the material we download for research purposes is treated with due diligence and respect for the copyright owner. Open access journals attempt to disseminate knowledge more widely for the common good while still preserving the rights of IP owners. Many such journals publish articles under a CC license. Though it may be permissible to use such material freely for one's work, one must still acknowledge such use by providing full details of the original source and following the conditions laid down by the original authors in their CC license.

Acknowledgments The authors have benefited from correspondence in Listserve managed by the World Association of Medical Editors (WAME) and the Copyright Permission FAQs of Taylor and Francis.

References

1. Oxford   English   Dictionary.   www.oxforddictionaries.com/definition/english/copyright. Accessed 7 Sept 2015.
2. World Intellectual Property Organization, Geneva, Switzerland. www.wipo.int/about-ip/en/. Accessed 29 July 2015.
3. World Intellectual Property Organization, Geneva, Switzerland. www.wipo.int/copyright/en/. Accessed 29 July 2015.
4. Berne   Convention.   1886.   keionline.org/sites/default/files/1886_Berne_Convention.pdf. Accessed 29 July 2015.

 5. Summary of the WIPO Copyright Treaty. 1996. www.wipo.int/treaties/en/ip/wct/summary_ wct.html. Accessed 29 July 2015.
 6. The Digital Millennium Copyright Act of. 1998. www.copyright.gov/legislation/dmca.pdf. Accessed 7 Sept 2015.
 7. Copyright office, Government of India. http://copyright.gov.in/. Accessed 29 July 2015.
 8. Creative Commons. http://creativecommons.org/. Accessed 29 July 2015.
 9. ICMJE. Recommendations for the conduct, reporting, editing, and publication of scholarly work in medical journals updated December 2014. www.icmje.org/recommendations/browse/ publishing-and-editorial-issues/copyright.html. Accessed 11 Sept 2015.
10. http://group.bmj.com/products/journals/instructions-for-authors/licence-forms. Accessed 2 July 2015.
11. The UK Copyright, Designs and Patents Act. 1988. http://www.legislation.gov.uk/ ukpga/1988/48/part/I/chapter/IV. Accessed 11 Sept 2015.
12. www.gov.uk/government/uploads/system/uploads/attachment_data/file/375954/Research.pdf. Accessed 7 Sept 2015.
13. www.law.cornell.edu/uscode/text/17/107. Accessed 7 Sept 2015.
14. RightsLink for permissions. Copyright Clearance Center. www.copyright.com/rightsholders/ rightslink-permissions/. Accessed 14 Oct 2015.

Suggested Reading

AMA manual of style: a guide for authors and editors. 10th ed. New York: Oxford University Press; 2007. p. 186–209.

Lang TA. How to write, publish, and present in the health sciences: a guide for clinicians and laboratory researchers. Philadelphia: American College of Physicians, ACP Press; 2010.

Letters, Editorials and Book Reviews

11

Sanjay A. Pai

Research articles are the *raison d'etre* of most biomedical journals; however, all good journals also have other sections that seek to involve the reader and offer a balance of scientific information and entertainment. These include letters to the editor, editorials and book reviews. Of these, the editorial and the letter section form the 'voice' of the journal.

As with research articles, you should read the instructions to authors before writing for these sections. It is helpful to read some recent issues of the journal to familiarize yourself with the style and contents. This chapter focuses on general medical and science journals. You may need to make modifications for specialist journals. The editors of journals are often flexible, within reasonable limits. You may need to sound them out before you start writing an article for their journal to gauge their interest.

Conflict of interest, either financial or otherwise, is an important issue in biomedical publishing, and you will need to state all such issues in any manuscript that is being submitted. You must also give your complete name, affiliation and contact details for all submissions.

11.1 Letters

The 'letters to the editor' or the 'correspondence' section is the first section of a journal that many people look up. This is because the letters usually offer a mix of science and literature. Besides, this section often covers a wide spectrum of topics.

Letters can be used as a forum to agree—or disagree, as is more often the case—with a paper published recently in the journal or to address an issue of general

S. A. Pai
Department of Pathology, Columbia Asia Referral Hospital, Bengaluru, India

© The National Medical Journal of India 2018
P. Sahni, R. Aggarwal (eds.), *Reporting and Publishing Research in the Biomedical Sciences*, https://doi.org/10.1007/978-981-10-7062-4_11

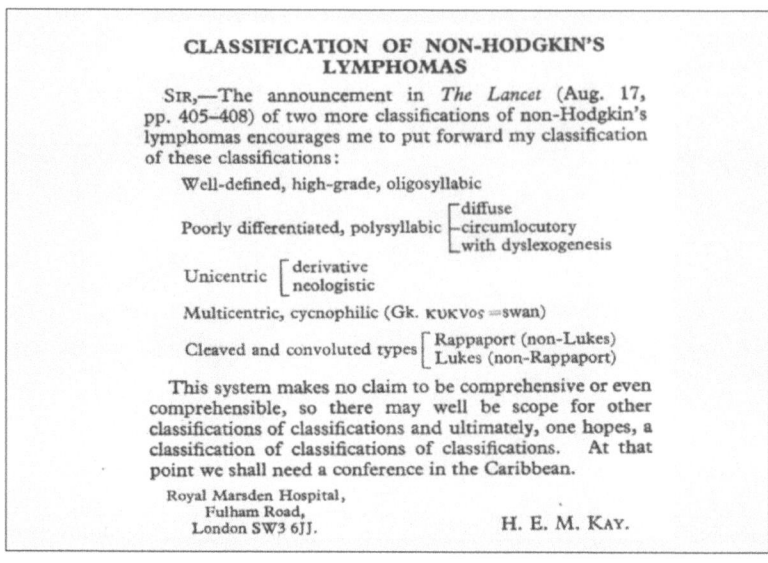

Fig. 11.1 Reproduced with permission from Kay HE. Classification of non-Hodgkin's lymphomas. *Lancet* 1974;2:586

interest, such as an aspect of public health, a social issue related to medicine or teaching methodology. Letters may also sometimes be used to publish primary data or a small case series or, occasionally, a brief case report. Though it is uncommon to find humour in a biomedical journal (the Christmas issues of the *BMJ* and *Canadian Medical Association Journal* are notable exceptions), the letter column offers authors an opportunity to showcase their wit and humour. It is often in this column that many young medical writers make their literary debut, especially now that case reports have become increasingly hard to publish. A letter may be in response to a previously published article, an editorial or even a letter to the editor. It may be a stand-alone letter expressing the viewpoint of the author or may take the form of a query that seeks specific information. Letters can also be used to make a point: Humphrey Kay did this when he used his acerbic wit in a letter in *The Lancet* [1] to protest against the numerous classifications of non-Hodgkin's lymphoma (Fig. 11.1). A letter may serve as a means of criticizing and commenting on the journal's policies. A random thought or hypothesis might also find its way into the letter column of a journal. In short, 'letters' is the most flexible section of a journal.

How does one go about writing a letter? First of all, you must be sure that you have something worthwhile to say. If your letter is in response to an article, it is important to read the original article carefully: you must make sure that your interpretation of the data or the author's discussion is correct. It is not uncommon for letter writers to make mistaken assumptions or jump to conclusions, criticize a paper and then, to their embarrassment, learn from the author's rebuttal that they had not read the paper carefully.

It is perhaps more important and difficult to craft the title of a letter than that of a research paper. Unlike a research paper, a letter has no abstract. Hence, the title must do justice to the subject and serve to attract the reader. It could be provocative or declarative. Since a letter has no abstract and the only words likely to be recognized in a PubMed search are those in the title, it would usually make better sense to choose a scientific phrase over a literary one.

A letter usually has a limited word count, so it is essential to be concise and to the point—and prompt. Letters form an important part of the scientific dialogue between the primary researcher and the readers and, as pointed out by Sahni [2], act as the post-publication debate on the article. Hence, most journals expect the response to be fairly quick.

The time within which a journal expects a letter to be submitted varies widely. For instance, *The Lancet* expects a letter (written or e-mailed, as is now the case) in response to a paper to be submitted within 2 weeks of the publication of the issue that contains the paper; the word limit is 250. However, the word limit for a letter of general interest, which is not related to a paper previously published in the journal, is 400. By contrast, *The National Medical Journal of India* (*Natl Med J India*) accepts letters submitted within 6 months of the publication of a paper (i.e. in the previous three issues) and allows one to use about 300–500 words for you to make your point. This difference in the time limit for the submission of letters is partly related to the frequency of publication of different journals: a weekly journal would require a shorter response time, while a monthly or quarterly journal would accept letters even a few months after the publication of the research paper.

The *BMJ* now requires prospective letter writers to submit their letters as rapid responses on the web. Some of these are used later as formal letters in the print version of the journal. *The New England Journal of Medicine* (*N Engl J Med*) accepts responses within 3 weeks of the publication of a paper. All this, of course, limits opportunities for those who receive their journal by snail mail. The rapid response column of the *BMJ* allows readers to submit letters at any stage—even years after the paper has been published. However, it is extremely unlikely to get published in the paper journal at that stage. Not all e-letters, even if submitted immediately, are published in the paper version of the journal; consequently, only some of those published in the PubMed indexed version of the journal will get indexed.

Unlike with original papers, some journals do not accept letters written by more than a particular number of authors—*The Lancet* limits it to five, while the *N Engl J Med* and *Nature* accept up to three authors. The *Natl Med J India* has no such stated restriction.

It is common practice to begin with a statement referring to that part of the data that you wish to comment on. In a humorous analysis of the letters published in the *Journal of Clinical Pathology*, D.S. O'Briain [3] has pointed out that most letters begin with the phrase 'I (we) read with interest the paper by ...' (Fig. 11.2). Such a statement is superfluous because the letter would never have been written had the author/s not been interested in the topic! However, it does make for a civil beginning to a letter. Readers would do well to read Dennis Wright's [4] equally witty response

Fig. 11.2 Reproduced
with permission from
O'Briain D. I read with
interest the paper by ... *J
Clin Pathol* 1994;**47**:868

I read with interest the paper by . . .

Four of the six letters to the Editor in the
April issue of the Journal begin with the
statement "I (we) read with interest the
paper by . . ." (IRWITPB). One might have
assumed that the preparation of a letter was
sufficient evidence of an interest, stimulated
in turn by reading the relevant paper. So
why are they telling us of their interest?

Clearly many writers have information
which supplements or clarifies an aspect of
a paper or which corrects an error but there
may be some additional factor, some intensity of interest which stimulates the letter,
so, if subjective feelings are to be included,
why stop at the bland "interest"? Why not
indicate the author's true feelings and
begin, for example, with, "We read with
mounting indignation the flawed paper
by . . .," or "We were devastated to see in
print a study almost identical to our soon-
to-be-completed study", or "We were
dumbfounded to find that our paper was
not cited by . . ." The "interest" of other
writers might be a code concealing lyrical,
cynical or even machiavellian approaches.

I looked over the most recent 16 issues of
the Journal and found that almost 40% (22
of 56) of letters began with IRWITPB or its
variants (one writer was *very* interested,
another fascinated; one simply said he very
much enjoyed the paper). A warning to
IRWITPB writers is the response to one letter, [they] may have read our article "with
interest", but clearly they have not read it
with "great care". The prevalence of
IRWITPB indicates that rather than hiding
an undisclosed intensity of interest, it has
become a cliché to introduce a letter and, as
such, should be discouraged . . . or is anyone interested?

DS O'BRIAIN
*Histopathology Department,
St James's Hospital,
Dublin 8
Ireland*

Fig. 11.3 Reproduced with permission from Wright DH. I read with interest the paper by … *J Clin Pathol* 1994;**47**:1058

I read with interest the paper by . . .

In his letter[1] dealing with letters that begin "I read with interest the paper by . . ." (IRWITPB) Dr O'Briain should have addressed the authors' reply that so frequently starts, "We thank Bloggs for his/her interest in our paper" (WTBFHIIOP). What the authors of such letters probably mean is, "Trust Bloggs to point out that he/she published a larger series than ours 10 years ago" or "Damn Bloggs for noticing that our p values are out by a factor of 10".

Over the years, I have noticed that it is uncommon for writers of WTBFHIIOP letters ever to admit honestly their mistakes even when these are pointed out to them in unambiguous terms, preferring to deny, obfuscate, or side-step their errors. Perhaps the problem lies with the fact that letters and authors' replies are not subject to peer review, merely to the perfunctionary scrutiny of an over-worked editor. Perhaps that is how this one got through or am I to expect an ITWFHIIML reply?

D H WRIGHT
*University Department of Pathology,
Southampton General Hospital,
Southampton SO16 6YD*

1 O'Brien DS. I read with interest the paper by . . . [letter]. *J Clin Pathol* 1994;**47**:868.

---

to O'Briain's letter (Fig. 11.3). As stated earlier, a letter itself could prompt another letter.

One must not be rude even if one vehemently disagrees with the paper's conclusions: it is better to disagree politely and get one's point across. It is important to use adequate and proper references to support one's argument.

One should try to end the letter with a statement that emphasizes or encapsulates all that one has said. It must get the message across and clinch the argument.

Some journals have no objection if the letter is accompanied by a table, a figure or an image if it enhances the content. However, these should be kept to a minimum and used only if necessary.

Finally, some information for those enamoured by impact factors: letters are usually not considered while calculating the impact factor of a journal.

11.2   Editorials

An editorial is a commentary or an opinion piece. In the past, editorials were written only by the editors of a journal and were often unsigned. However, this has changed over the past two decades. Now, an editorial may either be written by the editors of the journal or by experts who are not directly associated with the journal, by invitation from the editor. An example of the former is *The Lancet*, the editorials of which are signed '*The Lancet*' as they are written in-house by the editorial team. *The Natl Med J India*, *N Engl J Med* and the *BMJ* fall into the latter category. An advantage of the signed editorial is that it establishes transparency, and the reader is aware of exactly whose views are expressed. Besides, a signed editorial gives one recognition among one's peers.

As with letters, there is a wide range of topics that can form the subject of an editorial. The most common type of editorial is the commentary that accompanies an important research article in the same issue of the journal. An editorial may pertain to an important research paper in another journal. Editorials may comment on a social issue or political decision that might have an impact on health services, a change in the health policy, an advance in medicine or a change in medical thinking. The list is endless.

Usually, an editorial is commissioned by the editor of the journal. A leader in the field, a subject expert or a person who was one of the peer reviewers for a paper is invited to write the editorial. However, most editors welcome suggestions for editorial topics from readers and potential authors. Most editorials are written by experts. Occasionally, an editorial may be co-authored by a junior colleague.

An editorial is a commentary, hence the synonym 'commentary' (or even 'leader'). Unlike the research paper, an editorial does not have a structured IMRAD format. A well-written editorial is characterized by a smooth flow of ideas and coherent argument that is put forth cogently. Unlike a review article, which must contain all the evidence and offer a final, balanced and objective view of the topic on the basis of the data available, editorialists have the right to take a stance and focus on one or a few aspects of the topic. Editorials are often written on controversial topics. For instance, topics such as euthanasia and the death penalty often polarize people. Editorials on such subjects are meant to make the reader ruminate on the topic. On occasion, the editor of the journal may decide to counterbalance one editorial with another that offers the opposing view in the form of a debate. Like the letter to the editor, the editorial offers the author an opportunity to express an out-of-the-box opinion.

On what basis does the editorialist take a stand? In its instructions to authors, the *BMJ* states that it must be made clear whether the editorial is based on expert opinion, personal experience, observational studies, trials or systematic reviews.

The editorialist is expected to write the editorial in such a manner that a person who has no or little knowledge of the subject should be able to learn something about it, while someone with considerable knowledge of the field must also be able to derive something from it—a tough task, indeed, but manageable! This task has to be accomplished within the word limit set by the journal. The *BMJ* has set a word limit of 800 words and allows 12 references, while the *Natl Med J India* allows the author 1000–1200 words and 12 references.

Like letters, editorials do not have abstracts and it is thus imperative for the writer to choose the title with care. The title should be such that it interests the reader and simultaneously may be picked up in relevant online searches.

Editorials rarely undergo formal peer review, in the strict sense of the term. This is because the author is generally an acknowledged expert in the field; the commentary practically never contains primary research data or analysis that requires peer review. Usually, an editorial is reviewed by the editor or members of the editorial board. The editor would expect submissions of a high standard; if the standard is not met, the editorial may be sent back for the writer to improve upon it, or it may even be rejected. One must try to spare a thought for the harassed editor: usually, editorials are commissioned after the original research paper has been accepted for publication and often just before the issue goes to press. Thus, it is important to submit the editorial on time and try to get it as close to perfect as possible. If one fails to do so, one risks never being invited by the editor to write another editorial again.

Being invited to write an editorial is considered prestigious in the academic world. It would be a breach of faith in terms of one's profession and prestige and the editor's trust, if one submitted a poor editorial.

11.3 Book Reviews

Most journals have a section for book reviews. *The Lancet* terms this section 'perspectives' as it also contains reviews of some movies, television programmes, DVDs, etc. The books reviewed may be textbooks, monographs or even general or popular literature, including works of fiction that are related to the world of medicine and science. While some editors do worry that carrying this section means losing precious pages and delaying the publication of important scientific research papers, the general verdict seems to be that some pages should be devoted to book reviews. Book publishers are happy because the review serves to advertise the book (assuming that the review is favourable) for the price of just one book (that sent out to the person who writes the review). In addition, it gives the book wide exposure among readers and potential buyers. The readers are happy because they learn of new books in their field and often gather bits of knowledge of other subjects as well. Those who review the book improve their knowledge, derive pleasure out of reading it, can add another line to their curriculum vitae and get to keep the book!

At the very beginning of a book review, one must state the title of the book, names of the authors or editors, year of publication, edition, name of the publisher, number of pages, price and ISBN number. This gives the reader an idea of the utility and relevance of the book, as well as its availability [5].

Book and media reviews, too, can have only a limited word count, often about 400 words. You must check with the editor if you wish to write a longer review. Some journals discourage this, though the *Natl Med J India* accepts longer reviews. As with letters to the editor, but unlike editorials, students are sometimes welcome to contribute to this column—particularly reviews about textbooks. Though there are no strict rules to be followed, the task of writing a book review is not easy. It is probably easier to explain what not to do than to elaborate on how to write a book review. Many tyros seem to believe that the review must consist of an enumeration of the chapters of the book, with a précis of each chapter. This is entirely undesirable. Since book reviewers are also called critics, some take the opportunity to criticize and quibble over minor errors while losing sight of the larger picture. A book review is not an opportunity to settle old scores. In fact, it is advisable to insert a statement on conflict of interest if you believe that your review may be affected adversely or, otherwise, because of your relationship with the author.

My own practice is to make notes on a piece of paper while reading the book. I specifically make a note of the page number of the material that I intend to quote in my review and often incorporate it in the review. This saves my time later, as well as that of the reader, when it comes to looking up a particular statement. Book reviews are essays in creative writing. A good book review deftly interweaves some of the existing knowledge in the field and the thesis put forward by the author of the book. As an expert who is commenting on a book, you are expected to know about the author's previous works, especially in the same field, as well as other books on the subject. Some aspects that need to be commented on are as follows.

- Does the book fill a long-standing gap in knowledge?
- What is the target audience?
- Is the book likely to serve the purpose of the target audience, or would they be better off giving the book a miss? In either case, one must reason out one's argument.
- Are there factual, scientific errors in the book? If so, are they errors of omission or commission?
- How can the book be improved? Does it have obvious lacunae? Are there specific important issues that have not been touched upon?
- Does the text offer a balanced view or do different chapters contain opposing views? Do different chapters send out contradictory messages which can confuse readers, especially students?
- If the book is a multi-author work, as is the case with most textbooks nowadays, are the chapters consistent? Is there repetition of data?
- Is the language easy to understand or would one constantly have to go scurrying to the dictionary (or the web) to look up words and terms?
- Are the illustrations good? Are they in focus and are they appropriate?
- Is there evidence of plagiarism or other misconduct? (One must be cautious here, as one would not wish to lay oneself open to libel).
- Does the book appear to be written hastily?
- Are there too many printer's devils in the book—a sign of carelessness on the part of the publisher?

- Are the references adequate, correct and up to date? Remember that the book may finally get published only 1–2 years after the authors submit their chapters to the editor. If the latest reference is over 2 years old, it is a cause for worry.
- Does the book offer value for money?
- If the book under review is a textbook, will it replace the book one currently refers to or will it remain a reference book?
- Is the print easy to read?
- Is the binding strong and strong enough to ensure that the book lasts until the next edition? One must remember that all one's comments are likely to be used by the author to improve the next edition, so one needs to do a thorough job. However, as with any scientific communication, it helps to be polite. With practice, one can learn the art of writing a scathing yet diplomatic review!

A good book review is one that arouses the reader's interest sufficiently to motivate him/her to acquire the book at any cost. Book reviews are not indexed, of course, but can be added to one's curriculum vitae.

A few years ago, the *Annals of Internal Medicine* decided to structure even its book reviews. While this makes for a certain uniformity in the reviews (the text must be arranged according to headings provided such as 'field of medicine, format, audience, purpose, content, highlights, limitations and related reading'), in my opinion, it removes the buoyancy that one associates with a creative essay. Now, however, the journal seems to have done away with book reviews altogether.

11.4 Summary

For all forms of manuscripts, one must make it a point to write and rewrite until the article sounds right. It is useful to put aside the final draft and read it again after a week, or at least a couple of days, to see if there are any jarring parts that need to be edited.

As with all manuscripts, it is useful to bounce one's article off a colleague or two as they can offer an unbiased, honest opinion. Often, someone who is not directly connected with the field may be in a good position to decide whether the article—letter, editorial or book review—is readable and likely to be enjoyed or understood by most of the readers of the journal you are writing it for.

References

1. Kay HE. Classification of non-Hodgkin's lymphomas. Lancet. 1974;2:586.
2. Sahni P. Other papers—leaders, reviews, letters, book reviews. In: Naik SR, Aggarwal R, editors. Communication for biomedical scientists. New Delhi: ICMR; 2003.
3. O'Briain D. I read with interest the paper by…. J Clin Pathol. 1994;47:868.
4. Wright DH. I read with interest the paper by…. J Clin Pathol. 1994;47:1058.
5. Peh WC, Ng KH. Writing a book review. Singap Med J. 2010;51:685–8.

Case Reports and Case Series

Rakesh Lodha

In the era of evidence-based medicine, one often questions the utility of case reports and case series. Whereas papers in this category are placed at the bottom of the pyramid of quality of evidence, they often provide useful information that may improve patient care and also provide leads for new research. Several examples in the literature support this role.

Case reports can describe important observations regarding the presentations of various diseases and their diagnosis and also provide new ideas or insights for management. Many aspects described in such reports may not be detectable in clinical trials. Description of aspects of a disease that are different from those of classical cases mentioned in textbooks helps clinicians to improve patient care. However, the rarity of conditions reported in case reports may appeal only to a few and may not add much to everyday clinical practice.

12.1 Role of Case Reports

A case report of Kaposi's sarcoma in a young homosexual man was the seminal observation that led to the identification of acquired immune deficiency syndrome (AIDS) [1]. The use of propranolol in severe capillary haemangiomas of infancy stemmed from the observation of improvement of haemangioma in an infant who was receiving propranolol for obstructive hypertrophic cardiomyopathy; corticosteroids had been ineffective earlier [2]. Observations of novel adverse effects of drugs are often first published as case reports. Case reports also have a role in scientific

R. Lodha
Indian Pediatrics and Department of Paediatrics, All India Institute of Medical Sciences, New Delhi, India

© The National Medical Journal of India 2018   109
P. Sahni, R. Aggarwal (eds.), *Reporting and Publishing Research in the Biomedical Sciences*, https://doi.org/10.1007/978-981-10-7062-4_12

writing as they help authors to get started in scholarly writing. Case reports are often the first publications by a successful scientific writer in her/his early academic career.

12.2   What Cases Are Suitable for Reporting?

Publishable patient case reports include those that:

- Describe uncommon, perplexing or novel diagnostic features of a disease or condition
- Describe a therapeutic challenge, controversy or dilemma
- Describe a new surgical procedure
- Identify a new medical error or medication error or device malfunction that results in patient harm
- Describe a life-threatening adverse event
- Describe a dangerous and predictable adverse effect of a drug that is rarely recognized
- Describe a rare or novel adverse drug reaction
- Describe a therapeutic failure or a lack of therapeutic efficacy
- Describe a rare or novel drug–drug, drug–food or drug–nutrient interaction
- Discover an unlabelled or unapproved use of a medication
- Use a life-saving technique that has not been previously documented
- Discover an interaction between a drug and a laboratory test that yields a false-positive or false-negative result
- Describe the effect of a particular drug in pregnancy and lactation
- Detect novel pharmacokinetic or pharmacodynamic principle
- Use technology to improve patient outcome

12.3   The Structure of a Case Report

The general format of a case report includes an abstract, introduction, case details, discussion and references. The authors should decide upon the journal for submission and follow the instructions for specific segments. The usual word limit for the reports is 1000–1500 words.

12.3.1 Abstract

Most journals carry a short abstract for case reports as well. This may be structured or unstructured. The abstract should highlight the salient features of the case report. It is inappropriate to write 'the details of the case are described in the report'.

12.3.2 Introduction

This section should be concise and interesting enough to draw the reader's attention. It should provide the background information, which will then form the basis for the discussion. It should be supported by an adequate review of the literature. If there are only a few relevant publications, it is appropriate to cite all of these here. If, however, several publications on the issue are available, only the most important and relevant ones should be cited. The Introduction should then provide the justification for reporting the case. It is worthwhile to write a description of the case in a sentence. Typically, the Introduction is limited to one or two paragraphs.

12.3.3 The Case Report

A clear description of the case in chronological order is an essential requirement for the manuscript. The patient should be described in adequate detail to help readers understand the scenario and reach their own conclusions about the diagnosis and management. To maintain brevity and to keep alive the readers' interest in the report, the authors should avoid giving details that are not relevant to the diagnosis.

History and examination: Age, gender and any other relevant demographic details should be included. However, any information that could lead to identification of the patient should be avoided. The patient's chief complaints, history and course of symptoms should be described, followed by a brief account of the present condition, past history and family history. Relevant physical findings should be reported; if required, the relevant negative findings should also be mentioned. At times, clinical photographs are included to highlight the distinctive features; in such cases, care should be taken to hide any features that may allow the person to be identified. It is preferable to take consent from the patient for publishing any clinical photograph as many journals insist on patient consent before publication.

Diagnostic workup: Patients included in case reports often have complex conditions and undergo many investigations. The results of the laboratory tests and other diagnostics that support only a particular diagnosis should be reported. Appropriate units should be presented; the reference range of values should also be reported particularly for the uncommon tests. For detailed textual reports such as histopathology and cytopathology, only the salient features should be presented. It is useful to include relevant photomicrographs, radiographs, endoscopic images, electrocardiographs, etc.

Interventions and clinical course: The management of the patient may be the key reason for reporting the case. In such cases, adequate details have to be provided. On the other hand, in case reports where the clinical features are the highlight, the management may be mentioned only in brief. The course of the condition may be described where necessary, e.g. when assessing the effect of an intervention, describing the natural history of a condition.

12.3.4 Discussion

As for other types of articles, the Discussion section is an important section even for case reports. The Discussion should highlight the uniqueness of the case. It should compare the case reports with the published literature. It should also describe the implications of the case being described for future practice. In this section, the author must discuss features that support the validity of the case particularly when a causal association is being reported; this could require clarification of the temporal relationship of the purported cause and effect. This is applicable for reports that describe novel drug-induced adverse effects; in such cases, it may be important to include details that help exclude other causes of the adverse manifestation. The authors should also list the limitations of the case and should describe its relevance.

The published literature should be summarized, and a summary of the previous cases, with a few citations, should be provided. A table may be useful to highlight the relevant facts of the case being discussed compared with those of previous cases described in the literature; it provides an effective summary of the data and is easy to read and understand.

There should also be a description of how the case(s) compares and contrasts with those reported earlier. The possible explanations for the differences and similarities should be provided. The constraint of limited word count for case reports makes it imperative that the discussion is brief.

Finally, the important features of the case report need to be summarized, highlighting its unique features with conclusions and recommendations.

12.3.5 Conclusion

The author must provide a justified conclusion based on the case report and the literature reviewed in the Discussion section. Speculative statements should be avoided; one should avoid making judgements based on limited and questionable information or on a few case reports. Only justifiable, evidence-based recommendations should be stated.

12.3.6 References

The guidelines of the target journal should be followed. All the references cited should be read and evaluated; transferring an unread reference cited in another article is inappropriate. Such citation, if found to be erroneous, either before or after publication of the case report, has the potential to cause embarrassment to the author.

12.4 Case Series

In this type of paper, several cases with a similar unusual feature or aspect are combined into one report. The approach to writing a case series is similar to that of reporting solitary cases. It is helpful to summarize the key details of the cases objectively in a table. In addition, descriptive statistics may be used, e.g. to report mean/median age. Alternatively, each case may be described individually in one to two paragraphs. It may be important to indicate whether the case series includes consecutive cases or the cases are selected to emphasize one feature. If the former, one should indicate how the cases were identified or if the latter, were they searched for, for instance using certain diagnostic keywords or codes of the International Classification of Diseases (ICD) in a hospital database.

For a case series paper to be effective, it must maintain focus on the shared aspect being reported rather than describe each case in great detail. One should clearly state if any important data are not available in a particular case, which is quite common when the cases are collected retrospectively. If the cases were treated in different institutions, reference ranges for a specific test may need to be mentioned separately for each hospital.

The Discussion section is the key to success for both case reports and case series. This section emphasizes the shared feature of all the cases while trying to rule out any confounders.

References

1. Hymes KB, Cheung T, Greene JB, Prose NS, Marcus A, Ballard H, et al. Kaposi's sarcoma in homosexual men—a report of eight cases. Lancet. 1981;2:598–600.
2. Léauté-Labrèze C, Dumas de la Roque E, Hubiche T, Boralevi F, Thambo JB, Taïeb A. Propranolol for severe hemangiomas of infancy. N Engl J Med. 2008;358:2649–51.

Suggested Reading

Cohen H. How to write a patient case report. Am J Health Syst Pharm. 2006;63:1888–92.
Kooistra B, Dijkman B, Einhorn TA, Bhandari M. How to design a good case series? J Bone Joint Surg Am. 2009;91(Suppl 3):21–6.
McCarthy LH, Reilly KEH. How to write a case report? Fam Med. 2000;32:190–5.

Books and Chapters in Books

13

V. K. Kapoor

Writing a book requires a thorough knowledge of the subject matter. It may not require original research—an essential for a research paper in a journal—and requires few resources. But it does need much commitment and a great deal of time.

13.1 Types of Books in Biomedicine

In library jargon, a book is classified as a monograph to differentiate it from serials and periodicals, such as magazines and journals or newspapers, which come out at regular intervals. However, in common usage, a monograph is an authoritative work focusing on a single topic or theme, e.g. an uncommon disease such as primary sclerosing cholangitis (PSC). Whereas an undergraduate textbook may contain only a few lines on this topic, a monograph may devote hundreds of pages to the subject. The different types of books include:

- A textbook—targeted mainly at students and covering the syllabus for a course of study
- A reference book—covering anything and everything about a specialty or a subject
- An atlas—a collection of pictures, photographs or drawings with some explanatory text (used for medical topics mainly to describe procedures, e.g. surgical operations and endoscopic findings)

V. K. Kapoor
Department of Surgical Gastroenterology, Sanjay Gandhi Postgraduate Institute of Medical Sciences, Lucknow, India

© The National Medical Journal of India 2018
P. Sahni, R. Aggarwal (eds.), *Reporting and Publishing Research in the Biomedical Sciences*, https://doi.org/10.1007/978-981-10-7062-4_13

There are several other types of books. A book may be a collection of review articles on a particular topic (such as *Recent advances in…*, or *Progress in…*). Also, the proceedings of a symposium/conference may be recorded and transcribed to produce a book. This is, however, not an easy task as it is very difficult to convert the spoken word into written text. An oral presentation usually does not cover all aspects of a topic, whereas a written text is expected to do so. Moreover, speakers may not like everything they say to be quoted or appear in print under their name; the transcribed text from a speech must always be sent to the speaker for approval.

In addition, there are books that are written specifically to help students prepare for competitive examinations or revise course material before an examination (such as *Lecture Notes on…*).

13.2   Readership

Before an author starts writing a book, he/she should identify who the prospective readers are. For instance, would it be used by undergraduate, postgraduate or post-doctoral students to cover a certain curriculum and pass their examinations? Or would practising doctors refer to it to better manage their patients? Or would academicians and researchers use the book as a resource for in-depth information? Books on scientific (especially medical) subjects may be written for the lay public as well.

A book may target students or practitioners of a single discipline, e.g. surgery, or for those belonging to several specialties, e.g. those dealing with cancer, including surgeons, medical or radiation oncologists, pathologists, radiologists, palliative care specialists, etc. Therefore, the readership should be kept in mind throughout the process of writing the book.

13.3   Purpose of Writing a Book

Besides providing information, the primary purpose of writing a book is to educate the reader by imparting knowledge, aiding comprehension (understanding of the knowledge, as in practical manuals) and facilitating its application (the use of the knowledge in a given situation). Information is available for free and in plenty on the internet. Knowledge is different: it is processed and relevant information. Finally, wisdom is crystallized knowledge which the author effectively imparts to the reader to achieve good outcomes in a particular situation. A lecture also imparts education, but the published work reaches a larger audience; a book has a longer lifespan than a lecture, and many published works outlive their writers.

Earning name and fame (among one's peers) or satisfying one's ego ('me too!') is often a motivation for writing a book (vanity publishing). Such books fall in the 'print-and-forget' category, i.e. a few, usually self-funded copies are produced and distributed (often as complimentary copies), and there is no serious attempt to promote and distribute them. Their educational value, too, is often suspect.

Monetary benefit is usually not the primary aim of writing books as very few authors make a substantial amount of money from their books. More than 300,000 titles are published in the USA every year, but only a fraction is deemed a financial success.

13.4   Structure of a Book

Most books follow a standard structure. The text is generally divided into three parts—the preliminary pages (prelims), the main text and the end matter (or back matter).

The principal components of the preliminary pages are the title page, containing title and subtitle, author or general editor's name perhaps with degrees and affiliations and name of publisher; title verso, the page following the title page that carries details about the publisher and printer, International Standard Book Number (ISBN), disclaimer, cataloguing information and, most importantly, copyright statement; a table of contents; and a preface (written by the author). Other elements that might be included in the preliminary pages are a dedication page, a foreword (written by an authority on the subject matter of the book), an introduction, acknowledgements, abbreviations and a list of contributors.

The main text is divided into chapters, and these are sometimes clubbed together into parts. Notes and references may be placed at the end of each chapter. The end matter may contain appendices, bibliographies, notes and references (if these are not at the end of chapters) and an index.

There are sometimes pages of plates that are printed separately and bound into the text in sections.

The pages of the book are bound into a printed card cover or a hard case with a printed jacket. The cover includes the title, author or editor's name (with no degrees or affiliations) and perhaps the name of the person who has written the foreword. The cover is the prerogative of the publisher, although author's suggestions are usually welcomed. However, if the book is part of a series, the publisher is very unlikely to change a cover design to accommodate the wishes of the author!

13.5   The Writing Process

The process of writing a book usually starts with an idea, which is captured in the title of the book. It could also start with a perceived demand for a book on the subject, which prompts a publishing house to approach a prospective author to write a book. A plan is then made, both in terms of the time frame (if there is a deadline) and the contents of the book. The latter includes drawing up a list of chapters and even listing the sections, subsections and specific contents of each chapter.

To write a book, one may take time off from routine work, e.g. take a sabbatical specifically or go on a stint abroad, where there may be fewer clinical, teaching, administrative and research (and social) responsibilities. Alternatively, one could find 'free' time during one's routine job, e.g. using waiting time during long journeys.

One could either write the whole chapter (or maybe the entire book!) at one go or keep jotting down points and making notes to put together at a later stage. A perfect draft is rarely written in the first attempt. One needs to write, review and revise, and this may have to be done several times over. Incubating the manuscript for a few weeks before reviewing it makes it easier to find mistakes, lacunae and deficiencies in the 'previous' version. It is worthwhile to ask a critical colleague or peer to review the manuscript (I got the chapters of my recent book reviewed by my former students and trainees).

These days, manuscripts cannot only be written or keyed in on a computer but also dictated (smartphones have a voice recording option). While a good secretary is a valuable asset, devices and software that transcribe handwritten or dictated texts into a word document are a great help.

13.6 Format of the Text

By and large, the structure and format of each chapter should be uniform. In multi-author books, the editors should provide general guidance to authors on the content, outline and size of each chapter. The size of various chapters may vary, depending on the relative importance of each topic. This should be decided well in advance particularly with multi-author or contributory books. For example, a textbook of general surgery that contains a large number of chapters may be grouped in sections, e.g. upper and lower gastrointestinal, hepato-pancreato-biliary, head and neck, vascular and endocrine.

Each chapter has a title and starts with an introduction, which is followed by sections and subsections. For example, a chapter dealing with a disease may have subsections on its epidemiology, aetiology, pathogenesis, pathology, clinical features, differential diagnosis, management and prevention, in addition to the related investigations and the results. A chapter on an operative procedure may include subsections on the indications and contraindications of the procedure, preparation of the patient, gadgets and technique to be used, tips, complications and follow-up.

Every subsection should be divided into paragraphs, each dealing with one idea. One should preferably write short sentences (15–20 words each). As far as possible, one should use simple, everyday language that is easily understood (*see also* Chap. 14). Technical terms, even if obvious and apparently familiar, must be explained at first mention in each chapter. Tables, charts, algorithms, images (with labels) and line drawings provide information beyond the text and add to the book's appearance and appeal. Bulleted key points can be used to summarize important messages. For students who are likely to appear in examinations, a question–answer section or one or more illustrative cases may be of additional value.

The author (or editor, in the case of a multi-author book) must read through the final draft to minimize any major overlaps between chapters, repetition of material, omissions (topics not covered in any of the chapters) and, more importantly, contradictions.

13.7 Copyright

Copyright is the exclusive right to own and distribute an original creative work (intellectual property). Others who wish to use the work have to pay for or at least acknowledge its use. The copyright of a book usually remains with the author but may be assigned to the publisher. In the case of multi-author books, the publishers usually insist that the authors transfer the copyright of their individual chapters to them. Like any other copyrighted material, books also face the problem of pirated editions (cheaper prints, photocopies) (*see also* Chap. 10 on 'Copyright issues' and Chap. 24 on 'Scientific fraud and other types of misconduct').

13.8 Publishing

Getting a book published is much more difficult than writing it. If the purpose of writing a book is to have name and fame, or to satisfy one's ego, self-funded publishing is an option. However, if the purpose is to educate or to make money, the book needs to reach (be bought by) a large number of readers. This requires a good distribution network and marketing strategy, for which the author will have to take the help of a professional publisher (and distributor).

Sometimes publishers invite and commission an author to write a book on a mutually agreed topic. But mostly authors submit their manuscript to prospective publishers for consideration. The selected publisher should be suitable in terms of the book's subject matter and marketing capacity. It helps to opt for a reputed publishing house, which already has a few bestsellers on its list. However, a desirable course is to discuss the idea of the book with an editor of the prospective publishing house and develop it in terms of its marketing potential.

13.9 Book Proposal

The publisher usually asks the author to submit a proposal that includes a synopsis of the book, detailed table of contents, one or two sample chapters, approximate size (number of words or pages and figures and tables), target readership, time frame and author's professional details (including previously published books). The proposal will have a chance of quicker evaluation if the author can provide details of competing books and marketing channels (such as forthcoming conferences, student strength for the proposed book).

Once the proposal has been accepted, the publisher sends the author an agreement, which is signed by both parties. Most agreements have a standard format. However, the author may need to do some bargaining with respect to a few specifics, such as the royalty (ranges from 5 to 15%, usually 10%), number of free copies for the author, complimentary copies for the contributors in the case of multi-author works, subsidized copies and advance payment (if any).

13.10 Production

The production process is usually looked after by the publisher. However, the author's suggestions could be useful in terms of the size, format and binding of the book, quality of the paper, cover design, layout, page format, margins or space on each page, choice of text for the header and footer (book title, chapter title, name of author), etc. Print-on-demand publishing—i.e. printing a specified number of copies to fulfil an order—has enabled publishers to save on inventory. This technology is particularly suited to expensive books and those with a limited market.

13.11 Promotion

On publication, the book is brought to the notice of prospective readers (buyers). Publishers (distributors) promote a book by displaying it on their websites, in bookshops and at their stalls in book fairs and at conferences. They also advertise the book in journals and other (related) books and at places where a large number of potential buyers gather. The author/publisher also sends a copy of the book to journals for review. Complimentary copies are usually sent to peers, leaders, opinion-makers, teachers and examiners, who may directly or indirectly promote and recommend the book to students and the libraries of medical institutions/hospitals. Corporate houses (the pharmaceuticals and equipment industries) may be approached to sponsor copies for free distribution among students and medical practitioners.

13.12 Digital Publishing

A CD or DVD may accompany the print version of a book. Digital, online or web or electronic publishing (e-publishing) reduces the costs of printing, storage, shipping and distribution. For this reason, publishers of e-books are able to offer a higher (25–50%) royalty to authors. For instance, Amazon.com offers a royalty of 70% on e-books priced between US$2.99 and US$9.99 and of 55% on those priced outside this range. Some popular distributors of e-books are Amazon Kindle, iBooks (Apple) and BookBay.com. E-books can be read on various tablet devices, e.g. Amazon Kindle and Sony Reader, or downloaded as a PDF file on a computer.

13.13 Revision

The contents of a biomedical text may need to be revised every few years to incorporate new information and knowledge, correct mistakes and make good any deficiencies in the original writing. The frequency of revision would vary according to the type and subject of the book. Readers should be encouraged to provide the author with feedback on the book. Favourable excerpts from book reviews may be included in subsequent editions. Sometimes, all copies of the initial print are sold out sooner than expected, and the book is reprinted (without revisions).

13.14 Chapter in a Book

Multi-author books are common in biomedical sciences as one author is not expected to cover all aspects of a subject. In such cases, one or more editors are generally made responsible for anchoring the project. The editor(s) of such books are expected to give the author of each chapter clear instructions on the scope, structure and length of their contribution. To minimize the chance of any topic being left uncovered and of unnecessary duplication or contradiction, each author should be provided a detailed outline of the book.

13.15 Summary

Academicians and biomedical scientists, especially clinical practitioners, are often reluctant to write a book because they think it will take a lot of time, and the venture may not succeed. However, if they discuss the marketability of their proposal with potential publishers and then work to a plan, writing a book can be a satisfying experience.

Beyond Substance: Grammar, Syntax and Style

Usha Raman

> *'Writing is an art, but so far as scientific articles are concerned, that art should be restricted to telling the story accurately, simply, clearly and concisely. There is no place here for rhetoric, fancy, or inflated periods'.*

—Editorial, *The Canadian Medical Association Journal*, June 1937.

That description, written 80 years ago, sums up just what is expected of medical or scientific writing. The purpose of scientific writing is to promote understanding, to explain method and to provide a logically constructed pathway to a certain conclusion. Scientific writing is not only an art but also a craft—and one that needs much care. Its objective is to reduce the writing to its bare bones rather than clothe it with impressive language.

14.1 Substance Versus Style

The substance versus style debate is not new. In 1790 Lavoisier noted, 'It is impossible to dissociate language from science or science from language', adding that there is no other way to bring a concept or an idea into being than through language [1]. Scott Montgomery, writing at the beginning of this century, says that 'there are no boundaries, no walls, between the doing of science and the communication of it;

U. Raman
Department of Communication, University of Hyderabad, Hyderabad, India

© The National Medical Journal of India 2018
P. Sahni, R. Aggarwal (eds.), *Reporting and Publishing Research in the Biomedical Sciences*, https://doi.org/10.1007/978-981-10-7062-4_14

communicating is the doing of science' [2]. And we also have the opening quote to this chapter, written in 1937.

Some scientists might ask, 'Why talk about style and grammar when discussing scientific communication? Isn't it enough to just do good science? Doesn't content matter more than form?' Of course, the matter (or content) *does* matter—the idea, the act and the result are of primary importance. Earlier chapters in this book have emphasized the need for a framework in which to communicate scientific information, or, put another way, they discuss style as a structure and style as prescribed in a journal's instructions to authors. This chapter goes beyond these narrower definitions and discusses style at the micro level—the way in which words are chosen and arranged in a sentence to communicate effectively and make that communication a pleasure to read.

It is this seamless and essential relationship between the doing of science and its description that makes style and form so important. Those who truly wish others to understand the work they have done, and also grasp the meaning their work has for science and society, must pay attention to the way in which they communicate. Journal editors are also concerned about these issues (*see* page 125).

14.2   Why Worry About Style?

Scientific writing is often criticized for being dull and inelegant. It frequently places an undue burden on the reader, who must work hard to understand the content. Some scientists believed that the importance of a piece of work was inversely proportional to the number of people who could understand it! No one will agree with such an esoteric view today, because science is undeniably an international, interdisciplinary enterprise, with its members coming from a diversity of cultural, social and linguistic backgrounds. It is, therefore, imperative for scientific communication to leave no room for misunderstanding and misapprehension. Take a look at the following example:

> *Achromobacter xylosoxidans*, found in a wide variety of aquatic, soil and rhizosphere environments, is an aerobic, non-fermentative Gram-negative bacillus. *A. xylosoxidans* is frequently confused with other Gram-negative non-fermentative rods, especially *Pseudomonas* species, in clinical specimens and, therefore, we may underestimate its role as a significant pathogen.

Now take a look at this modified version:

> *Achromobacter xylosoxidans* is an aerobic, non-fermentative Gram-negative bacillus found in a wide variety of aquatic, soil and rhizosphere environments. (*The word order has been changed.*) In clinical specimens, *A. xylosoxidans* can be confused with other non-fermentative Gram-negative rods, especially *Pseudomonas* species, so its role as a significant pathogen may be underestimated. (*The relationship between the elements of the sentence is more clearly specified.*)

A few changes in the order of words in the first sentence, along with some substitutions ('frequently confused' with 'can be confused') and alterations in case (from passive to active in the last sentence) make the revision easier to understand on the first reading. Also, moving the phrase 'in clinical specimens' to the start of the second sentence makes it clear that the emphasis is shifting from the organism to a clinical situation.

Scientific writing differs little from most other forms of academic writing, except that greater detail is expressed in a shorter, more direct and blander style. It is perhaps constrained by the style conventions of individual journals through the instructions to authors that govern everything from units of measurement to punctuation.

An argument in support of our concerns about style is that the editors of medical journals are clearly troubled by it. A survey of journal editors [3] found that manuscripts were rejected for the following reasons, some of which are directly related to language and style:

- Irrelevant topic or topic of limited interest
- No new information
- *Lack of connection between introduction, objectives and conclusions*
- *Misleading argumentation*
- Weak methodology
- *Unfocused, incoherent text*
- Flawed design

The italicized items relate to the *manner* in which the material has been *presented* and not the material itself. Good scientific writing addresses these concerns. Good scientific style is nothing more than good science expressed in clear English that is grammatically and syntactically correct. Scientific literature is produced in several languages, but there is little disagreement that English is the major language of international science. However, in some parts of the world, scientists use English as a second or third language. They may have a good working knowledge of English but are often not comfortable enough with the language to become efficient or effective communicators. Manuscripts are often returned by journal editors with the comment: 'Please have the language corrected by a professional English editor'. The quality of science tends to be judged—or perhaps masked—by the quality of the writing.

The best scientific writing is characterized by brevity (conciseness), coherence and clarity. Quality is achieved by adhering to the rules of standard grammar and usage and by developing a knack for the rhythm (cadence) of language—a rhythm that is just as important in scientific prose as it is in poetry. Language with a desirable rhythm allows the meaning to emerge without difficulty. Writing that lacks an acceptable rhythm, or proceeds in a discordant fashion, resembles noise; this hinders the process of reading and can make it difficult to understand the meaning.

There are no shortcuts to becoming a good writer of scientific manuscripts. You should be as well versed in grammar as the English schoolteacher or the college grammarian and as sensitive to the meanings of words and their nuances as the creative writer. However, at the same time, it is important to note that the best scientific writing makes style invisible. It is transparent because the purpose of style is not to make the reader pause and wonder at the beauty of the expression; it is to clarify the meaning of the words without letting their arrangement interfere with the reader's comprehension.

Let us look at the attributes of style more closely. How can we ensure that they become part of the way we write? How can we cultivate a good style and consciously develop the elements that make our work readable and understandable?

14.3   Solving the Style Puzzle

As noted above, the purpose of style is to achieve clarity in explanation, describe processes and outcomes with precision and link arguments and evidence in a logical, systematic way that allows the reader to (i) replicate what you have done, (ii) apply your results in a different context or (iii) understand how your work relates to the larger body of knowledge. To do this, a writer must first follow the conventions described elsewhere in this book; these provide clear guidelines on where and how different types of information fit into a paper. Once this has been done, however, it is important to look at the manuscript at the micro level and see if it 'does the job' with regard to the four tenets of style—clarity, brevity, precision and cohesion.

14.3.1 Clarity

Clarity means clearness or the quality of being clear. Scientific communication must, above all, be clear. It must tell the reader exactly what is in the writer's mind— no more, no less. Complex ideas need not be expressed in complex language. In fact, a difficult idea should be expressed simply. Sometimes, we fall into the trap of using unnecessarily long or complicated words when much simpler ones would do just as well. For instance, some complex words/terms that can be replaced by simpler ones include elucidate (explain), proximal (close/near) and utilize (use).

Of course, there may be specific instances in which the more complex term is more suitable. For instance, when describing the allocation of subjects to two arms of a clinical trial, it is more appropriate to use the word 'randomized' than 'allocated'; the former describes a particular form of allocation where every subject has an equal chance of entering either arm, thus making the conclusions more robust.

Clarity comes from following a chronology that is logical or easy to understand, keeping subject (noun) and action (verb) close together and delineating all the necessary steps in an argument or description. We often make false assumptions about the reader's level of knowledge or understanding and skip a few steps in the processes we describe. The trick is to select points in your journey that provide a clear picture to the uninitiated reader—both in terms of what you did and how your argument emerged.

> Seven of 8 patients of keratitis were treated with a combination of ciprofloxacin and cefazolin and in 4 of these, the infection resolved, while one received a combination of ciprofloxacin and ceftazidime. (*Too many ideas in one sentence.*) The treatment was then modified to either amikacin or ceftazidime or a combination of both in the remaining patients. (*Remaining of 7 or 4?*)

In the above example, the first sentence could easily be split into two without taking away from the meaning or missing out on the information provided.

> Seven of 8 keratitis patients were treated with a combination of ciprofloxacin and cefazolin. In 4 of these 7, the infection resolved. The remaining patient received a combination of ciprofloxacin and ceftazidime. (*It was not clear what had happened to this one—it is useful to add this information.*) The 3 patients in whom the infection did not resolve were then treated with amikacin, ceftazidime or both (one each). (*More specific.*)

Here are some ways to enhance the clarity of your writing:

- Choose short words rather than long ones.
- Choose specific terms instead of vague or general ones.
- Express just one major idea in each sentence.
- Follow a chronological order.

14.3.2 Brevity

Brevity means expressing much in few words. Professional and academic literature is growing at an alarming rate and our busy lives make it difficult to keep up with the output. So the shorter a piece of writing is, the more likely it is to be read. If one can say something in fewer words and make just as much sense (and impact), then that is the way to say it. Most journals lay down strict word limits for submissions, so avoid the temptation to describe *everything* that you did in your laboratory, every nuance of the discovery or idea, and every connection that emerged.

One simple way to write briefly is to just cut down on unnecessary words and lengthy phrases. We often use bloated phrases ('based on the fact that' instead of 'because') or say things in roundabout ways ('one and the same' instead of 'alike'), simply because it seems to sound more impressive. But look at the following two paragraphs, and think about which one gets to the point quicker. Is any information lost in the shorter paragraph?

> It is well known that topical steroids are freely available as over-the-counter medications. Therefore, it is important that consumers be educated about the proper use and possible side-effects of steroid ointments, drops and salves. (37 words)

> Topical steroids are freely available over the counter. Therefore, it is important to educate consumers about their proper use and possible side-effects. (23 words)

14.3.3 Precision

Precision means exactness. In all areas of science, exactness—or precision—is required. We do not want to know vague details about an experiment or a case; we want to know exactly what happened and how and what sense it made. Vagueness may result from not using the right words or by not making the relationships between elements/phenomena clear. Sometimes, precision is compromised because the writer takes too much time to get to the point. The following sentences illustrate how brevity and the logical ordering of words can make for greater precision and clarity.

Long: The data were compiled and compared between the two groups undergoing different treatment modalities using the Fisher's exact test/independent sample test.

Shorter: Data from the two treatment groups were compared using Fisher's exact test/independent sample *t*-test.

14.3.4 Coherence

Coherence means the logical linking of words and ideas. When words are not arranged in a logical manner, or when ideas do not seem to flow in a meaningful sequence, the text lacks coherence. Simply changing the position of a phrase can make all the difference, as in the example below:

Although safe and effective technologies are available that could restore normal vision to a large majority of those affected, because of the backlog of cases to be operated upon, and the growing numbers of cataract cases due to the increase in life expectancy, the cataract burden is increasing annually.
...
Although safe and effective technologies are available that could restore normal vision to a large majority of those affected, the cataract burden continues to increase annually *because of the backlog of cases to be operated upon*, and an increase in life expectancy.

Coherent writing gives the reader a clear indication of what the sentence is setting out to do—make an argument, provide evidence, list a series of causes, etc. One should avoid constructing sentences in which the focus becomes clear only at the end:

Attitudes towards childhood ailments, perceptions of the causes of such ailments, and the socioeconomic status of the family are all factors which influence healthcare-seeking behaviour.

Instead, if one begins this way, the intention is clear right from the start:

Factors that influence healthcare-seeking behaviour include attitudes toward childhood ailments perceptions of the causes of such ailments, and the socioeconomic status of the family.

In the second sentence, the main idea (factors influencing healthcare-seeking behaviour) is placed first, and this is an important rule of good scientific writing. The reader needs to be 'led into' the sentence with the right kind of signposts. Note there is little change in the length of the sentence.

Other signposts that help readers along are transitional phrases—words that signal shifts in time, point of view, place, etc. When the action shifts from the laboratory to the field, for instance, it is important to signal this shift so that the reader can make that switch smoothly as he/she reads on. Transitional phrases include 'On the other hand…', 'In a different context…', 'Meanwhile…', 'Previously/Earlier…' and so on. The appropriate use of such transitional phrases lends coherence and continuity to the text.

14.4   Some General Points on Style

Concerns about style usually emerge in the later drafts of a manuscript. The writer is initially preoccupied with arranging the content, including all appropriate references and data, and making sure that clear evidence supports the main arguments.

As you revise a document, begin to look at it from the reader's point of view. To take a critical look at your writing as a piece of communication, you need to step back from the content and your own involvement in its creation. Spend some time rereading each sentence, and keep in mind the following rules.

14.4.1 Place the Main Idea First

As described above, sentences are easier to understand if they are 'framed' in the right way. The first few words of the sentence should convey what it is about and the information that will follow.

14.4.2 Use Specific Words: Avoid Nominalization (Changing Verbs and Adjectives to Nouns)

We often fall into the trap of using bloated and complex nouns when verbs will do just fine. For example, why say 'we held a discussion' (noun) when we can say 'we discussed' (verb)? Why say 'very large' when we can provide the exact dimensions? Why say 'measurement of the temperature was carried out twice a day'? Is it not better to say 'the temperature was measured twice a day'?

14.4.3 Use Active Voice

This is a rule that is often broken in scientific writing, much to the detriment of comprehension. Is there any doubt that the second sentence is easier to grasp than the first?

- The questionnaire was administered by a team of field workers.
- A team of field workers administered the questionnaire.

However, it is not always right to use the active voice, as the following cases show.

- *The following is a typical situation, requiring no agent.*
  - – Amniotic membrane is used as a substrate.
- *In this case, the active verb would require an unnecessary agent, leading to an awkward sentence.*
  - – Scientists use amniotic membrane as a substrate.
- *The active voice accuses.*
  - – You violated the ethics code by your actions.
- *The passive voice avoids accusing.*
  - – The ethics code was violated by this action.
- *You need to emphasize the object.*
  - – The test has been used widely by geneticists.

14.4.4 Keep Your Sentences Short

Sentences should generally be 12–25 words long. Only occasionally does one need to use longer sentences, e.g. to express complex ideas.

14.4.5 Maintain the Appropriate Tense

As described in earlier chapters of this book, different tenses are used in different parts of the paper. The introduction and review of the literature are usually written in the present tense, whereas the methods and results sections are in the past tense. The discussion is usually in the present tense or a combination of present, future and conditional, as this is the section in which arguments and propositions are made.

14.4.6 Use Standard or 'Global' English

English has changed over the years and in day-to-day communication. Many varieties of the language are accepted or, perhaps more correctly, tolerated. However, in formal writing, standard English is still the norm. Weed out phrases and usages that are peculiar to India and may be considered archaic ('as per', 'in lieu of', 'albeit'). Study the language of the target journal and write accordingly. If you are writing for a British/American journal, use the appropriate spellings.

14.4.7 Prefer Positive Statements

Readers find it easier to understand statements about what was done/found rather than what was not done or not found, even if your findings are negative. For example, it is more emphatic to say 'The culture showed no growth of fungal species' rather than 'The culture did not show any growth of fungal species'. A minor change in the sentence makes all the difference. Another example of a positive statement that conveys a negative finding is 'We found no evidence of malignancy'. This is more direct than 'We did not find any evidence of malignancy'.

14.4.8 Use Parallel Construction

Similar elements in a sentence or a series of sentences should be structured in the same way. In other words, use the same grammatical form for similar elements. For instance, in the two sentences below, the second uses parallel construction:

- The features that favour this treatment regimen are its low cost, it is highly specific, and there are no side-effects (*not parallel*).
- The features that favour this treatment are its low cost and high specificity, and the absence of side-effects (*parallel construction*).

Parallelism makes a sentence easier to grasp at first reading. It is a more elegant and precise way of writing.

14.5 Cleaning Up the Document

After the first rush of writing the draft paper, it is best to set it aside for a few hours, or even days, and then read through it again for content, clarity and coherence. Distancing yourself somewhat from your work will usually give you the perspective required to perform a 'grammar triage' on the text. It is best to go through your own work with a fine-tooth comb before an unfriendly editor decides to slash it with his/her pen.

Basic issues of grammar and syntax are beyond the scope of this chapter, and there are a number of grammar texts and guides on usage to help a writer tackle these areas more than adequately. What is more important is to develop a sensitivity to questions of grammar so that improper language does not detract from the substance of the text.

When checking the grammar, pay attention to the following.

Use of nouns and specific terms: Mark abstract nouns and make sure that a sentence does not contain a series of nouns, as this could create confusion regarding the main subject of the sentence. You should also make sure that you use the word which best conveys the intended meaning. Several dictionaries list commonly misused words, and it may be a good idea to invest in one.

Pronouns: Go through the text with a red pen and circle all the pronouns, and then check if the nouns they refer to are close enough to be obvious to the reader. When you say 'it' or 'these', is it absolutely clear which entity one is referring to? Also ensure that the number and gender of the pronoun agree with the noun.

Verbs: Mark all forms of the verb 'to be' (am, is, was, were, will be), particularly when combined with a past participle (is desired, was placed, were derived), and check if they have been used correctly. Are they always needed? Forms of 'to be' tend to weaken a sentence and can often be substituted with a more active verb, as in the following sentences:

There are several studies *pointing to* this relationship.
Several studies *point to* this phenomenon.
The hypothesis was *found to be* supported.
The hypothesis *was supported*.

Modifiers: These are words or phrases that further explain or qualify a subject. Mark all restricting (small, almost, quite), intensifying (very, substantially) and absolute (best, completely, totally, finally) modifiers. Do they say what you really want them to say? Do all the modifiers relate to the noun? Is the relationship clear? Are the modifiers misleading in any way? For instance, do not use 'continual' (ongoing with gaps) when you mean 'continuous' (ongoing without gaps) or 'majority' (usually, more than 50%) when you mean 'a considerable amount' (a lot, but not more than half). For some modifier words, the meaning in day-to-day usage and in science differs (e.g. 'normal' distribution, 'random' allocation)—one must be very careful and only use the scientific meaning of the word.

Prepositions: Make sure that all the prepositions (words that express the relationship between a subject and object or two nouns) used are the most logical ones possible. Are you saying 'in' when you mean 'on' or 'above' when you mean 'upon'? Limit the number of prepositional phrases in a sentence to two or three, e.g. 'The cultures were placed *in* a petri dish *at* a particular temperature *for* 3 days'.

Connectives: Check all the coordinating and correlative conjunctions to make sure that the joined elements are parallel in structure and form (*see* note on parallelism above). Are the elements in a sentence really connected or should you split them into two sentences? Do they relate in the same way to the main subject of the noun?

Sentence structure: Read through the text again to make sure there are no incomplete sentences. Take a look at the following sentences:

We tested the efficacy of two broad-spectrum antibiotics.
One of which recently entered the market.

The second part of the example is a fragment. It needs to be connected to the first part by substituting the period with a comma:

We tested the efficacy of two broad-spectrum antibiotics, one of which recently entered the market.

Run-on sentences, where two complete sentences are improperly combined, can also be a problem, as seen below:

Five slides were prepared with solution REB, six slides were prepared with solution TRP. (*Wrong*)

Five slides were prepared with solution REB, *while* six slides were prepared with solution TRP. (*Correct*)

Finally, read through the text once more, asking yourself the following questions:

- Have I said what I wanted to say?
- Have I said it as briefly as possible?
- Have I said it as clearly as possible?
- Have I said it as efficiently and forcefully as possible?

If you can answer 'Yes' to all these questions, your paper is probably ready to go.

Scientific style is ultimately about getting the message across to your intended audience in the best way possible. The reader should not have to pause over a sentence or puzzle over a phrase. To develop as a writer, it is most useful to develop the ability to read critically. One can also learn from the writing of professionals, those who do it well and with elegance. When you read a good article in a journal, think about what makes it good: is it the content alone or is it something more? That something more is the invisible polish known as style.

References

1. Aronson S. Style in scientific writing. Curr Contents. 1978;2:5–16.
2. Montgomery S. The Chicago guide to communicating science. Chicago: University of Chicago Press; 2003.
3. Noble KA. Publish or perish: what 23 journal editors have to say. Stud Higher Educ. 1989;14:97–102. https://doi.org/10.1080/03075078912331377642. Accessed online.

Suggested Reading

A variety of writing guides are available on the web: http://www.writing.engr.psu.edu/workbooks/intro.html; http://abacus.bates.edu/~ganderso/biology/resources/writing/HTWgeneral.html; http://www.excellent-proofreading-and-writing.com/scientific-style.html#axzz1xZKvDKME.

For a comprehensive discussion on style, word usage and other confusing issues related to academic writing, see http://www.ung.si/~sstanic/teaching/CIS/Stevens-Subtleties_of_Scientific_Style.pdf.

Strunk W Jr, White EB. The elements of style. 4th ed: Longman; 1999.

The Council of Science Editors (www.councilscienceeditors.org) links to a number of useful sites on grammar, style, scientific format and publication ethics.

Authorship and Acknowledgements

15

Rajeev Kumar

Biomedical writing serves two equally important purposes. The first is to inform peers about the outcomes of one's research; the second is to get recognition for that work. Several well-defined, self-explanatory rules, such as honesty, truthfulness and reproducibility, govern the conduct and publishing of research. However, the description of who qualifies as an author is more complex, which makes authorship one of the most vexed issues in the biomedical publication process.

Ideally, a biomedical publication aims to benefit science and humankind, yet authorship is often the primary reason why research is conducted and reported. The premiums linked with being an author are many. In academic medicine, authorship results in recognition among peers and career progression. Most academic institutions require a person to have a certain minimum number of publications for promotion to a higher position. Appointments and awards are often linked to the number and nature of publications an applicant has garnered. Grants for research also depend on previous scientific output, measured in terms of the number and quality of published papers.

Besides these well-known rewards, authorship can bring monetary benefits. Published research may hasten the acceptance of new drugs and devices, and the authors of such publications may stand to benefit from the consequent financial gains to the pharmaceutical industry. These potential benefits may drive the desire to be an author and result in conflicts of opinion about who deserves authorship in a manuscript. On the other hand, there is a growing concern about some persons who contribute to a manuscript, but specifically avoid being identified with it, the so-called 'hidden' or 'ghost' authors. This stems from their intention to hide their conflict of interest with the reported results—conflicts that would undermine the reader's faith in the findings.

R. Kumar
Indian Journal of Urology and Department of Urology, All India Institute of Medical Sciences, New Delhi, India

© The National Medical Journal of India 2018
P. Sahni, R. Aggarwal (eds.), *Reporting and Publishing Research in the Biomedical Sciences*, https://doi.org/10.1007/978-981-10-7062-4_15

15.1   Who Should Be an Author?

The primary principle behind authorship in biomedical journals is one of taking responsibility. The International Committee of Medical Journal Editors (ICMJE) recognizes that credit for authorship may be associated with academic and (potential) financial benefit. It places an important responsibility on all those listed as authors, by stating that 'contributors credited as authors (should) understand their role in taking responsibility and being accountable for what is published' [1]. Thus, while authorship has its rewards, it comes with the responsibility of vouching for the authenticity of the published work and the potential liability of any misconduct that may have occurred. This position of the ICMJE recalls an earlier statement by Richard Miner Hewitt who, as far back as 1954, wrote 'Thou shalt not allow thy name to appear as a co-author unless thou hast some authoritative knowledge of the subject concerned, hast participated in the underlying investigation, and hast laboured on the report to the extent of weighing every word and quantity therein' [2].

To make these principles objective and easier to apply, the ICMJE recommends that authors of biomedical manuscripts must fulfil four criteria [1]. All authors must have (1) made substantial contributions to conception and design, acquisition of data or analysis and interpretation of data, (2) participated in drafting the article or revising it critically for important intellectual content, (3) approved the final version to be published and (4) agree to be accountable for all aspects of the work. The fourth criterion was added to the ICMJE Recommendations in 2014. It places an additional responsibility on authors to ensure that any suspicion of misconduct is appropriately investigated and that they can identify who is responsible for each part of the published work (*see also* Chap. 24).

Several biomedical journals insist on authors providing a checklist wherein they confirm that they fulfil these criteria individually. These guidelines are in no way restrictive, as we shall see in a later example. They allow for a large degree of freedom as to who may be included as an author. However, anyone considered to be an author has a responsibility—they must publically defend their results. This makes published research more trustworthy.

Attention to the concept of responsibility and accountability for authors has grown in the past few decades. Most biomedical journals are now published on the Internet. For many journals, the archives have also been digitized. This allows for a much wider access to scientific papers than existed in the past and makes it easier to search for specific text strings. Inappropriate research, unexplainable results, plagiarism and duplicate publications are now far easier to detect. Such discovery results in journals seeking clarification from the authors, and those responsible for misconduct may face censure.

15.2   Who Should Not Be an Author?

The most common examples of individuals who do not fulfil the ICMJE criteria for authorship are senior colleagues, grant providers, data gatherers, laboratory supervisors and writing assistants—all of whom may have facilitated the conduct or publication of a piece of research but were not actually involved in it. For example, let us consider a very large study that reports questionnaire-based survey outcomes with three authors, all of whom are busy clinicians. An astute reader would question the ability of these authors to conduct the survey on their own. In this case, acknowledging the surveyors who collected the data would serve to strengthen the credibility of the manuscript. Collecting data would not fulfil the ICMJE criteria for authorship but acknowledging their work is suitable recognition for their services (*see also* page 138).

15.2.1 Order of Authors

In manuscripts with multiple authors, the order of the names can be contentious. The three names that are generally believed to carry more responsibility are the first, the last and that of the corresponding author. Several academic institutions give preferential credit to the first author and the corresponding author. This is because it is considered that the first author is the major contributor to the work, whereas the corresponding author is the senior author or team leader who conceived and supervised the research. This general perception is also common among authors. Zbar and Frank [3] surveyed 362 authors of published manuscripts on the perceived importance of the first and last authors. The first-named authors were considered seven times more likely to have conducted the research, written the manuscript and fulfilled the ICMJE criteria for authorship, whereas the last authors were perceived to be senior supervisors or heads with little contribution to the paper. Studies are often quoted using the first author's name, and this adds to the recognition received by the first author [4].

Though the key role of the first author is almost universally accepted, most journals do not confer any specific credit on the corresponding author. For journals, the corresponding author is simply the individual who deals with the editorial office on behalf of all the authors during the period of manuscript processing. Some journals will ask for one of the authors to be a guarantor for the integrity of the data in the paper (*see also* Chap. 17 on 'Manuscript preparation', Table 17.2, page 162).

In the references to a paper, most journals list only the first three or six authors; this too is a point that authors consider when deciding the order of names in a manuscript.

In large multi-author papers, authorship may be credited to the name of a group. The authorship line may list only the principal authors directly responsible for the manuscript, while others are included under the group name. Indexing services such as PubMed may list the entire group if their names are provided elsewhere in the manuscript.

15.3 Acknowledgements

As mentioned earlier, the Acknowledgements section of a manuscript lists persons who contributed to the study or manuscript preparation but do not qualify as authors. The most common inclusions here are writing assistants, statistical consultants, heads of departments who allow use of their resources and medical illustrators. Such individuals must be listed in the Acknowledgements section of the manuscript and their specific contribution mentioned. This is a transparent way of determining who did what. Written approval for the acknowledgement should be sought from each individual as listing a contribution can imply an endorsement of the content of the manuscript. Several journals now insist that individuals so named must also provide written approval for their listing.

Financial support may also be acknowledged here, though some journals may list these separately in the conflict of interest or funding statement.

15.4 Authorship Problems

15.4.1 Guests and Ghosts

Published research influences the practice of medicine and patient outcomes. It also determines the professional standing of scientific authors. More importantly, it can impact on the financial status of pharmaceutical companies and device manufacturers who may have invested heavily in a new molecule or device. A favourable report can often mean the difference between bankruptcy and financial windfall—motives that may be sufficiently strong to cloud ethical conduct. Peer-review is a process designed to substantiate the scientific content of a manuscript while avoiding conflicts of interest and ensuring transparency. However, the scientific community depends on the honesty of the authors since it is not possible to physically verify all data reported in a study. 'Guest' and 'ghost' authors are two entities that compromise this honesty.

Guest authors. These are individuals who are credited as authors despite their not fulfilling the criteria for authorship. The most common beneficiaries of this practice, also called 'gift authorship', are senior members of the academic department from where the manuscript originates. They may have permitted the study to be conducted or even helped acquire funds, but their role does not fulfil the criteria for authorship. In some cultures, 'gift authorship' is common practice and a way of thanking senior colleagues. In other situations, such authorship is the norm—and failure to follow this norm may adversely affect the junior author's career.

While such authorship may not impact on the scientific merit of the manuscript, it creates an expert where none exists. If a department publishes ten papers, all from different research teams but with a common senior author, the senior author may soon become recognized as an expert and have the potential to influence decision-making on a subject he knows little about. This is detrimental to science as it limits growth opportunities for the real researchers and helps create 'fake experts'.

Of greater concern is the fact that the fate of a manuscript can be affected by the names of the authors it carries. Manuscripts by senior, well-known researchers have a greater likelihood of acceptance for publication and of inducing change in clinical care. Thus, guest authorship by a senior researcher may represent an attempt to 'buy' influence for a paper that it would not otherwise have received. Such authors are often under obligation to present and publicize these manuscripts at various fora and are in a position to greatly shape policy and decision-making.

The Council of Science Editors (CSE) identifies these two categories separately, i.e. 'honorary or gift authorship' and 'guest authorship' [5].

Ghost authors. This refers to the non-listing of individuals who qualify to be authors. There are two situations where this can occur. The first (a relatively benign one) is where a professional writer drafts and revises the manuscript in return for a monetary payment but is not listed or acknowledged. This usually happens when the actual researchers have to write in a non-native language. It also happens when researchers have limited time available and need help in drafting the manuscript. Such ghost authors may not fulfil the criteria for authorship but their contribution must be acknowledged. This is important because such writers may have influenced the interpretation of the results or have a conflict of interest. For instance, a professional writer working for a pharmaceutical company may present the interpretation or discussion of a drug trial in a more favourable light than the results would warrant.

The second, and more serious, concern with ghost authorship is intentional omission of names of authors who are known to have strong conflicts of interest with the contents of a manuscript. Evident conflicts of interest between authors and content always dilute the impact of a manuscript, no matter how robust the methodology or results. This is most relevant in industry-funded research where the impact of positive findings may be less if it were known that one of the authors has a major financial stake in the outcome. Omitting the names of such authors from the manuscript byline may increase its acceptability by reviewers and readers.

15.4.2 Inclusion and Exclusion

It is not surprising that authorship problems are common. In a forerunner of this book, the late Dr. S.R. Naik discussed the historical issues surrounding authorship [6]. He noted that, in the past, authorship of medical articles was often limited to one person. This would generally be the senior researcher who would have written the manuscript herself. However, research has now moved to a phase where it is not possible for a single researcher to do the entire work and write the manuscript for publication. Single author publications are now limited to editorials or opinion pieces. Multiple-author publications raise issues of who should and who should not be included as an author and the sequence in which their names should appear.

Research is conceived and designed by senior academics, but the work is mostly done by their junior colleagues. The work often involves several people and departments and requires approval and supervision by multiple authoritative heads. It may last for a number of years during which individual contributors may change. The authorship of such manuscripts has an inherent potential for conflict. Should individuals who contributed in the past but are no longer working be included as authors on the manuscript? Should all laboratories who contributed to data in the manuscript be included? When the main researcher leaves midway and the work is completed by another person, who should be the first author? If a guarantor joined in the latter half of a project, can he vouch for the authenticity of the entire work? No guidelines exist for resolving such concerns, and decisions are subject to individual interpretation. Some of these questions are addressed in the following examples.

15.4.3 Prevention and Cure

The most effective method of limiting controversies about authorship is primary prevention. Whenever research involving multiple people is done, questions of authorship should be decided at the outset. At this stage, the agreement may be relatively broad-based. For instance, if a group of clinicians and laboratory scientists agree to work on a problem together, they may decide that the clinical researcher would write the clinically oriented manuscripts and the basic researcher would handle the technology articles. Authorship may also be decided before beginning work on each individual manuscript. At times, institutions have predefined guidelines for researchers to follow. Not only does this limit the possibility of conflict, it also helps define each individual's role in the research and the preparation of the manuscript. The concept of 'contributorship' is becoming increasingly common with some biomedical journals; it requires all authors to clearly define their contribution before the journal begins to evaluate a manuscript.

Considering the potential risk associated with being listed as an author, i.e. liability for any misconduct identified at a later stage, it is important that all authors consent to both their placement and relative position on the authorship byline before the manuscript is submitted to a journal. After submission, most journals do not allow changes to the authorship list (such as addition, deletion or alteration in the order of names) without good reason and approval from all the authors.

Despite efforts at avoiding authorship disputes, these do occur. Such disputes can be resolved through discussions among all concerned. Several organizations have developed suggestions and flow charts to address these issues. These include the ICMJE guidelines on universal requirements for manuscripts submitted to biomedical journals [1], the Committee on Publication Ethics (COPE) report on handling authorship issues [4, 7], the World Association of Medical Editors (WAME) statement on authorship disputes [8] and the COPE position statement on responsible research publication [9]. All these guidelines recommend equating authorship with responsibility and deciding who the authors will be before the research work is started or written up.

15.4.4 Example 1

Clinician **A** joins an academic clinical department as a trainee under clinician **B**. Sometime later, **B** asks **A** to study the levels of a cytokine in a particular disease. **A** prepares the first draft of the protocol. **B** discusses this proposal with **D** who heads the laboratory that works on cytokine research, and the latter suggests some useful changes in the protocol. **C**, who is a trainee with **D**, conducts the laboratory analysis and interpretation. At the end of the study, **A** writes up the manuscript and gives it to **B** for comments. Who should be listed as an author?

As per the ICMJE guidelines, **A** would fulfil all four criteria if he approves the final manuscript and should qualify as an author. **B** has contributed to the concept and is critically reviewing the manuscript; if he approves the final version and takes responsibility, he would also be an author. **C** has contributed to data acquisition and interpretation and thus fulfils the first criterion; but if he does not contribute to the manuscript preparation and approval or accept responsibility, he will only be acknowledged and not listed as an author. However, if he does contribute to these three tasks, the flexibility of the ICMJE criteria would allow him to become an author. **D** has contributed to the concept and design by suggesting improvements in the study design and thus fulfils the first criterion; as with **C**, being listed as an author is dependent upon his contributing to the manuscript, approving its content and accepting responsibility.

15.4.5 Example 2

A surgical department began using a new technique 10 years ago. Over the years, three surgeons have performed 100 such procedures. Two of the surgeons have moved to a different institution. The third surgeon, who remains at the parent institution, decides to write a paper based on the experience of these 100 cases. Should the previous two surgeons be included as authors?

Legally, the data on patients is owned by the institution where the work was conducted. The surgeons who previously operated cannot lay claim to this data. As departments grow, the data gathered will increase, so previous contributors cannot *expect* to be considered for authorship. However, their inclusion as authors would depend on the judgement of the current surgeon and the institutional review board that permits collection and publication of the data. If the two surgeons had helped develop a novel procedure, it would be unethical not to include them. Similarly, if their contribution to the data (the patients that they cared for) constitutes the bulk of the experience, they should be included. Authorship in these cases must follow the ICMJE guidelines in that the previous surgeons must contribute to the manuscript and approve the final version. Not only does this give credit where it is due, it is also scientifically important. The surgeons who developed the procedure, or performed surgery on the largest number of patients, are likely to be in a better position to analyse the data and interpret the findings. The manuscript must communicate their experience so that the readers may learn from them.

The recent modification of the ICMJE authorship criteria specifically warns against excluding individuals who may qualify for authorship by stating that 'all individuals who meet the first criterion should have the opportunity to participate in the review, drafting, and final approval of the manuscript' [1].

15.5   Summary

Authorship enables individuals to get credit for their research. However, this credit is associated with responsibility because only the authors know the facts of the research. Readers depend on the authors' integrity since the reported data are not always easy to verify. The ICMJE criteria lay down a useful framework for defining authorship. At the same time, they also allow sufficient flexibility so that all contributors get due credit.

References

1. International Committee of Medical Journal Editors (ICMJE). Recommendations for the conduct, reporting, editing, and publication of scholarly work in medical journals. 2014. http://icmje.org/recommendations. Accessed 1 May 2015.
2. Hewitt RM. Exposition as applied to medicine: a glance at the ethics of it. JAMA. 1954;156:477–9.
3. Zbar A, Frank E. Significance of authorship position: an open-ended international assessment. Am J Med Sci. 2011;341:106–9.
4. Albert T, Wager E. How to handle authorship disputes: a guide for new researchers. The COPE Report 2003; pp. 32–34. http://www.publicationethics.org/files/2003pdf12.pdf. Accessed 1 May 2015.
5. Council of Science Editors (CSE). White paper on publication ethics. http://www.council-scienceeditors.org/resource-library/editorial-policies/white-paper-on-publication-ethics. Accessed 1 May 2015.
6. Naik SR. Authorship and acknowledgements. In: Naik SR, Aggarwal R, editors. Communication for biomedical scientists. New Delhi: Indian Council of Medical Research; 2003. p. 45–7.
7. Committee on Publication Ethics (COPE). Flowcharts. http://www.publicationethics.org/resources/flowcharts. Accessed 1 May 2015.
8. World Association of Medical Editors (WAME). Policy statements. http://www.wame.org/about/policy-statements#Authorship. Accessed 1 May 2015.
9. Wager E, Kleinert S. Responsible research publication: International standards for authors. http://www.publicationethics.org/files/International%20standards_authors_for%20website_11_Nov_2011.pdf. Accessed 1 May 2015.

How to Choose the Right Journal

16

Shobna J. Bhatia

Authors of a scientific manuscript wish their paper to be published in a journal and then read, used and cited by their peers. However, there can be many stumbling blocks in this process. One such impediment is submitting the manuscript to an inappropriate journal. At one extreme, it may result in a journal editor summarily rejecting the manuscript without even commissioning an external peer review; this results in the need to resubmit the manuscript to another journal and a consequent delay in publication. At the other extreme, the paper may be published in a journal that is rarely accessed or read by those interested in the work. Either way, the authors' efforts to disseminate their knowledge have been frustrated.

Selecting a journal that publishes papers in one's field of study is a priority—a good choice increases the likelihood of your manuscript being published and read by the right people. The selection process needs some experience and entails both hard work and seeking guidance from your peers. This chapter discusses some of the main points that authors should consider when choosing a journal for submitting their work.

16.1 When to Choose a Journal

A tentative decision about the choice of a journal should be made as soon as one starts writing the paper. Different journals follow somewhat different styles for the writing and formatting of manuscripts. Hence, knowing the style and format of the journal you wish to publish your work in can save time and effort spent later in adapting your generic manuscript to its style.

S. J. Bhatia
Department of Gastroenterology, Seth GS Medical College and KEM Hospital,
Mumbai, India
e-mail: sjb@kem.edu

© The National Medical Journal of India 2018
P. Sahni, R. Aggarwal (eds.), *Reporting and Publishing Research in the Biomedical Sciences*, https://doi.org/10.1007/978-981-10-7062-4_16

Some scientists start thinking about a target journal for their proposed study even when writing the research protocol. If the protocol and plan of research work are prepared according to the requirements of a particular journal, one is already a step ahead when it comes to the final writing of the paper. However, one must remember that such meticulous planning does not ensure that an article will be accepted for publication in the preferred journal; it is important to have a shortlist of three or four journals when you start writing.

16.2   Factors Influencing the Choice of a Journal

Several factors influence the choice of a journal for a particular manuscript (Box 16.1). Each of these is individually discussed below, though some are interrelated.

> **Box 16.1 Factors Affecting Choice of Journal for Publication of a Biomedical Manuscript**
> - Novelty of the research topic or findings
> - Scope of the journal: general medical versus narrow and specialized
> - Geographical focus of the journal: international versus regional
> - Quality and prestige of the journal:
>   - Inclusion in literature databases
>   MEDLINE/PubMed
>   Other databases, e.g. Embase, Science Citation Index (Web of Science), etc.
>   - Impact factor and related measures
>   - Perception of researchers in the field
>   - Duration of publication
>   - Editor and editorial team
>   - Peer review process
> - Authors' objectives for manuscript publication
> - Journal's readership and availability
> - Journal's policies:
>   - Journals subject coverage and types of papers published
>   - Manuscript length, number of tables, figures and authors, etc.
>   - Journal's turnaround time
>   - Publication charges (including page or colour charges)

16.2.1 Novelty of the Research Topic or Finding

A key determinant in the choice of a journal is the authors' own assessment of the importance of their work. Most research falls into two categories: (1) incremental research (i.e. research that builds on existing knowledge) or (2) replication of work that has been done previously. Manuscripts dealing with incremental research are considered more important, since these advance science, i.e. they improve our understanding of a disease or its treatment. Hence, a manuscript that adds to existing knowledge is more likely to be considered favourably by a high-impact journal.

Replication of findings is an important concept in biomedical sciences. But journal editors are not always interested in manuscripts based on work carried out in previous studies. A replication study on a topic of recent or current global interest might be accepted in a top- or medium-level journal as their readers are interested in looking for articles that deal with similar problems from all over the world. However, once many articles on a particular topic have been published, new ones are considered less favourably, unless they have a new message. These may evince greater interest if a very different population group is reported on, and particularly if your results differ from those recorded in, previous papers. Hence, you need to choose a journal, based on how much similar work has already been published, by descending an informal pecking order of journals in the field if there are already many replicative publications.

It is rare for a piece of research to be truly innovative and represent a conceptual advance. Such work can impact both future research and the clinical management of a disease. However, there is always the possibility that the findings or reasoning followed in such original work will turn out to be unfounded and fail to influence science in the long run. Innovative work often challenges existing knowledge and dogmas and may face resistance from peers. An element of chance operates for such papers. If the work is perceived as novel and is appreciated by the peer reviewers and the editorial team, it may be published in a high-impact journal, such as *Science* or *Nature*. For instance, the article describing the discovery of hepatitis C virus was published in *Science* [1]. On the other hand, the paper describing the discovery of *Helicobacter pylori* (then called *Campylobacter pyloridis*) was rejected as an original article. The report was published as a letter in *The Lancet* [2] in 1983; in 2005 the authors received the Nobel Prize for their work!

16.2.2 Scope of the Journal: General Medical Versus Narrow and Specialized

Another important point to be considered early is whether to submit a manuscript to a journal that covers a broad subject area of biomedical research, i.e. publishes articles related to one or more broad specialties (e.g. *New England Journal of Medicine, Lancet, BMJ*) or science (*Science, Nature, Proceedings of the National Academy of Sciences of USA*) or to one that focuses on a narrow field (e.g. *Esophagus, Fetal and Pediatric Pathology*).

Journals with a wider scope usually have a large readership. They have a higher frequency of publication and faster turnaround times, both from submission to acceptance and from acceptance to publication. However, the wider the scope of a journal, the more submissions it receives, and the harder it is to get published in it. It is worth remembering that though general medical journals have a wide readership, they may not be read by many specialists; hence their editors often do not encourage the publication of highly specialized papers. If your manuscript addresses a specialist topic, a specialist journal is more likely to publish it. Also, these journals are read by specialists; hence, if your paper addresses their interest, they are more likely to read it.

If your research is multidisciplinary, there may be a wider range of journals that you could consider for publication. In such cases, one needs to carefully consider the target reader groups. For instance, a paper that addresses the pathophysiology of a particular disease could be sent to a more clinically oriented journal in an attempt to emphasize the clinical relevance of the work. On the other hand, if the work is unlikely to be understood by clinicians, it may be better to submit it to a basic science journal.

While writing your paper, you would have read papers that report work similar to your own. The journals in which these studies were published might be the most appropriate for your manuscript too. Hence, scanning the list of references in your paper could help you identify journals that would consider publishing your work.

16.2.3 Geographical Focus of the Journal: International Versus Regional

Another important issue is whether your work is relevant internationally or only to a limited geographical area. In the latter instance (e.g. for studies on tropical diseases), publishing in a regional journal may well be the best way for your message to reach the population, scientists and physicians located in that area. In addition, a top international journal might well reject your manuscript, but a lower-ranking regional journal is more likely to accept it.

The reverse is also true. Submitting a manuscript of wide interest to a local or national journal will restrict your message and deprive others of the benefit that they could have from reading your paper.

16.2.4 Quality and Prestige of a Journal

Prestige of an author often depends on the quality and prestige of the journal in which their papers are published. So how does one judge the quality or prestige of a journal? Though difficult to quantify, each field of science has its own, 'unwritten' pecking order of journals based on their perceived prestige. Several factors appear to influence this subjective measure of prestige.

Inclusion in literature databases. A crucial factor is whether a journal is indexed and available in a public database. The foremost example for biomedical literature is MEDLINE, run by the National Library of Medicine, USA. There are similar databases for specific subareas of biomedicine (e.g. *Embase* for pharmacology, drug research and toxicology, *CINAHL* for nursing and allied health sciences). The *Science Citation Index* is important because it is the basis for determining a journal's impact factor (*discussed below*).

MEDLINE currently includes around 5600 journals—a small fraction of all the biomedical journals published worldwide. Its managers use stringent criteria for selecting journals for inclusion in the database. These include the scope and coverage of a subject, the quality of content, editorial quality in terms of peer review and selection of articles, production quality, types of journal content, international contribution, etc. Several of these criteria relate to journal quality. Hence, journals included in this database are believed to be more prestigious than those that are not. This database also has a wide reach; its search engine, PubMed (www.ncbi.nlm.nih.gov/Pubmed), is the de facto starting point for all biomedical researchers to search the published literature. It also includes abstracts of articles and links to the various journal sites hosting the complete article. Inclusion in MEDLINE increases the visibility and accessibility of a journal and the articles it publishes. These are reasons enough to encourage a prospective author to publish in a journal that is included in the MEDLINE database.

Science Citation Index is a database that indexes citations between journals. It records the number of times a published journal article has been cited by papers in other journals. In recent years, developments in technology have allowed the database to expand (Science Citation Index Expanded). It is accessed via the Web of Science Core Collection and includes nearly 6500 journals across 150 disciplines of science, medicine and technology, from the year 1900 to the present. In general, this database is more restrictive in its coverage than MEDLINE, and a journal's inclusion is generally associated with greater prestige.

Impact factor. The impact factor of a journal is a numerical measure based on citation data included in the *Science Citation Index*. Published annually, it is widely perceived as a measure of journal 'quality'. It is calculated using two elements: 'the numerator, which is the number of citations in the current year to any items published in a journal in the previous 2 years, and the denominator, which is the number of substantive articles (source items) published in the same 2 years' [3].

For instance, the impact factor of a journal for the year 2014 is the average number of citations received by papers published in 2012 and 2013 during the year 2014 divided by the number of 'citable' papers published in the journal in the years 2012 and 2013 (Box 16.2). The numerator includes all citations to any articles published in the 2-year period, whereas the denominator includes only the articles published in the 2-year period that are considered 'citable' as defined by the publisher. Citable articles include research articles, reviews and other longer articles, whereas editorials, commentaries and letters to the editor are excluded. Other types of articles may be less easily categorized.

Box 16.2 Calculation of the Impact Factor of a Journal
Let us assume that:

Number of citable papers published in a journal during the year 2012 = A1
Number of citable papers published in a journal during the year 2013 = A2
Number of citations to the above papers in journals in the Science Citation
    Index during the year 2014 = B

Then: impact factor of the journal for 2014 = B/(A1 + A2).
(Impact factor is expressed up to three digits after the decimal point)

The impact factor was originally developed to help librarians decide which journals to buy for their libraries [4]. However, over the years, it has been used not only to compare journals, but also to assess research outputs of individuals and institutions. These latter uses are clearly inappropriate; however, even as a measure of journal quality, the impact factor has a number of limitations. First, the impact factors vary widely between scientific disciplines and fields, so direct comparisons are not truly valid; for instance, journals in fast-moving areas such as immunology have much higher impact factors than those in traditional fields such as physiology. Second, review articles often receive a disproportionately large number of citations compared to original research; thus, journals with a large number of review articles tend to have higher impact factors. Furthermore, the number of citations varies greatly for different papers published in a particular journal, with a large proportion of articles receiving no citation; the use of arithmetic mean for such data is fraught with problems. Finally, the impact factors are subject to manipulation [5, 6].

Similar journal indices have been developed which try to correct for some of the limitations of the impact factor, such as the Eigenfactor score, Article Influence Score and SCImago Journal Ranking. However, all indices must be used very carefully when trying to assess a journal's quality or prestige.

An author selecting a journal for a paper must remember that journals with a higher impact factor or another measure of quality have higher rejection rates, and hence the selection of a target journal depends on a match between the quality of one's work and the perceived quality of the journal.

Perception of researchers in the field. Scientists who regularly publish papers 'know' which journals advance knowledge in their particular area. They consider these journals to be prestigious, even though they might not have a high-impact factor. Thus, a journal's prestige is often determined more by subjective assessment of its quality than on the more objective measures derived from calculations!

Duration of publication. Several new journals are launched every year; a few of these survive, while others drop out with time. To begin with, most journals are not indexed, and it may take a few years before even a successful publication is listed in electronic databases. This implies that new journals are viewed with caution, and their prestige tends to be lower than that of journals with a long track record of publication.

Editor and editorial team. The respect that the editor and members of the editorial advisory board have in a particular field is an important criterion by which to judge a journal. An editorial board whose members are international, experienced and reputed enhances a journal's prestige.

Peer-review process. Peer review refers to a process whereby the findings of scientific research are reviewed for their quality by other researchers in the same or related fields. These peer reviewers are often external reviewers who advise journal editors on whether a manuscript should be published or not (*see* Chap. 21 on 'Editorial process and peer-review'). The peer-review process is the mechanism that ensures the quality of the published record. Despite its several limitations, it helps weed out manuscripts that report poor science and improves the quality of reporting in those articles that are finally published.

Peer-reviewed journals are generally considered to be of a higher quality. This distinction has become even more marked with the advent of several online-only journals, which publish manuscripts without a peer review or just a perfunctory review. Some journals exist primarily for the purpose of making money from author fees without providing author services; such 'predatory journals and publishers' should be avoided. It is important to find out if a journal to which you are planning to submit your paper has a credible peer-review process—something which can be verified by asking one's colleagues whether they or someone they know has ever been invited to review a paper for the journal [7, 8].

16.2.5 Authors' Objectives for Manuscript Publication

Another factor is your publishing objective and whether a particular journal would help you achieve this goal. Your primary aim should be to reach the readership your research is most likely to benefit or interest.

If you are an academic or basic science researcher, you will be interested in not only having your article read but also in having it cited. You will hope that your paper will be published in a journal that is likely to be cited by others (e.g. *Gastroenterology* or *Gut* for work related to gastroenterology); this would help in advancing your academic career. The reviewers of your next grant application, who possibly read these journals, will then be more likely to be familiar with your previous work.

On the other hand, if your work is primarily related to patient care, e.g. guidelines or algorithm for the management of a disease, then the aim is to get practitioners to read it, and citation is far less important. Your target journal should be one read by a larger number of practitioners in your field and not a top academic publication, from which your paper is likely to be returned with a barrage of discouraging comments.

If your main goal is to reach as many readers as possible, an open access journal may prove to be the best option. Open access allows anyone to read your article, online and free of charge, and this increases the likelihood of your paper being cited. However, you may have to pay for publication (*see below*).

An article with immediate application—say, for reasons related to public health—would be suitable for a journal with an early online option or fast-track publication. In recent years, most of the papers about disease outbreaks, (e.g. SARS, H1N1 influenza and Ebola) were published in such journals.

If your institution prefers articles to be published (and promoted) in an 'indexed' journal (usually taken as meaning 'indexed in MEDLINE'), you can consider only those journals that are so indexed. Similarly, if the agency that funded your research insists that the research must be publicly available, you are obliged to submit your paper to an open access journal. Such funding agencies would often pay the journal's publication charges.

16.2.6 Readership of a Journal

The number and nature of potential readers of a journal are important considerations as you want your work to reach as many people as possible.

Journals vary widely in their circulation. A journal with a larger circulation may be expected to reach more people and have a larger readership. Similarly a journal that many libraries subscribe to will also carry the message to a larger audience. In today's electronic era, when most readers access journal articles online, the idea of circulation has been replaced by that of online accessibility—particularly the ability to be read without the need to pay at the time of access. Thus, a journal offered to libraries as part of a publisher package may be preferable to a journal with a limited online presence.

The nature of a journal's readership is even more important than the number of readers as authors are often interested in reaching one or more niche group(s). Journals published by national or international organizations of such experts are a good avenue for such papers as members normally receive a hard copy of the journal as well as online access. Even individuals without access can often find a colleague who does have access. In developing countries such as India, several associations publish journals from their own resources and make them free online to everyone.

16.2.7 Policies of a Journal

Once you have identified a few potential journals for your paper, the next stage is to find out more about their policies, as these may directly affect the suitability of your paper for a particular journal. Policies about manuscript handling are published at least in the first issue of each volume and on the journal's website.

The information one should look for includes (1) the editorial aims of a journal: the subject coverage, research focus and whether the readership of the journal is mainly academicians, researchers and/or practitioners, (2) types of papers published, (3) limits on length of manuscripts and the number of figures and/or tables, (4) turnaround time, (5) any charges payable by authors, etc. Occasionally, there may be other issues—for instance, a journal may require their authors to have registered a clinical trial before starting their study or have made their protocol publicly available—if you did not do this, you cannot submit your manuscript to that particular journal.

Journals subject coverage and types of papers published. All journals provide guidance about their subject coverage and focus. They also provide detailed information on the types of manuscript they publish; for instance, some journals do not publish review articles, while others will only publish them if they have been solicited. Potential authors should write to the editorial office of such a journal and confirm whether or not the journal is interested in the subject matter of their review (and the particular authors writing on it!). A journal may not publish certain types of articles—for example, case reports, non-human studies, etc. Make sure in advance that the journal you have identified publishes the type of manuscript you have written.

Manuscript length, number of tables, figures and authors. Many journals have a restriction on the overall length of the manuscripts they will consider. If your paper is based on a large study and it exceeds the word limit, this is not the journal for your work.

Similarly, a journal may limit the number of figures and tables for certain types of paper (e.g. case reports). If your paper requires several figures, e.g. a description of novel pathological changes in a disease that needs a series of photomicrographs, it would be best to send the paper to a journal that will accept the number of figures you wish to publish. The same reasoning applies if you are preparing a case report of a multisystem disease; several specialties may have played an important role, but the journal limits the number of contributors it is willing to list as authors.

Journal's turnaround time. This can be difficult to predict but can vary from a few days to a few months. The publication time can be gauged from the dates of receipt, acceptance and final publication, which are printed on the first or last page of every article. Many journals also publish a performance report every few years, and this indicates the number and types of articles a journal receives, the acceptance rate and turnaround time.

If you wish your manuscript to be published quickly, you should send it to a journal with a quick turnaround—the advantage being that if the article is rejected, the response arrives within a couple of weeks, and you can then submit the article to another journal. Journals with the highest publication frequency (weekly or biweekly) usually have shorter waiting periods than quarterly journals. Many journals today have an online component; check whether the journal will post articles online as soon as they are approved for publication, even if the printed version is not available for a while. This helps to disseminate the message in your article much earlier than the final printed version. The advantages of rapid publication in a lower-ranked journal outweigh the potential credit of being published by a higher-ranked journal.

Publication charges. Biomedical journals do not pay the authors of research articles and often require authors to pay for publication. Some journals charge the authors only if their manuscript includes colour pictures or exceeds a certain length (e.g. if the number of pages in the printed paper exceeds a certain predefined number). However, the advent of 'open access journals' has seen many journals charge for all the original papers they publish (*see* Chap. 19 on 'Open access journals'). The authors have to pay these charges after the manuscript has been accepted for publication. In exchange, the articles are freely available to readers. Some journals allow authors to retain a degree of copyright to their work (*see* Chap. 10 on 'Copyright issues'). There are journals that even charge authors in advance for reviewing the manuscript irrespective of whether the paper is finally accepted for publication.

The submission or publication fees for a paper can vary widely and may exceed US$ 2000 per article. Journals assume that these charges will be paid out of institutional funds or research grants. However, if the agency that funded your research does not cover such charges or if the work was not funded, you need to think very hard about following the 'author pays model' (and pay from your personal funds!). However, negotiation is an option that might result in a complete or partial waiver of publication charges, particularly if the work was done in a limited-resource setting or if the funding agency does not cover such charges. Hence, it is useful to look up the websites of potential journals for various possibilities before making a choice.

It is important to remember that journals levying a charge for publishing a manuscript are not necessarily of a high quality.

16.3 Summary

When searching for a suitable journal for your manuscript, begin by considering a large number of possibilities, and try to arrive at a short list of three to four journals. No one journal will have all the features you are looking for but do not compromise on quality and inclusion in reputed international databases—with the latter being a surrogate marker of the former. Selecting the most appropriate journal may take some time, experience and effort—of visiting the library, discussing with peers and going through the instructions to authors. However, the effort is worthwhile, especially if your paper gets accepted by the first journal you send it to and then reaches your intended readers.

Alternatively, you could discuss with a colleague who is 'knowledgeable'—having published several papers. You could use websites that help authors choose a journal for publication by providing keywords and abstract. One such website is JANE (Journal/Author Name Estimator: http://www.biosemantics.org/jane); at a nominal cost, it provides not only a journal selection feature but also helps to search for similar articles which may help you to build up the References section.

Finally, it is a good idea to identify your second- and third-choice journals in case your paper is rejected from your first-choice journal. Many authors try to initially target their paper to a journal somewhat higher in the pecking order than the one they expect it to be published in. If the 'higher' journal accepts the manuscript, they have scored a bonus; if it doesn't, they can then revise the paper using the comments they receive and send it to their second-choice journal ... until it is finally accepted. Aiming too high though can be a problem—repeated rejection may break your resolve to publish and waste time.

References

1. Choo QL, Kuo G, Weiner AJ, Overby LR, Bradley DW, Houghton M. Isolation of a cDNA clone derived from a blood-borne non-A, non-B viral hepatitis genome. Science. 1989;244:359–62.
2. Marshall BJ, Warren JR. Unidentified curved bacilli on gastric epithelium in active chronic gastritis. Lancet. 1983;321:1273–5.
3. Garfield E. Journal impact factor: a brief review. CMAJ. 1999;161:979–80.
4. Garfield E. The history and meaning of the journal impact factor. JAMA. 2006;295:90–3.

5. Amin M, Mabe M. Impact factors: Use and abuse. Elsevier Perspectives in Publishing October 2000; revised 2007. http://www.elsevier.com/framework_editors/pdfs/Perspectives1.pdf. Accessed 25 April 2015.
6. Wilhite AW, Fong EA. Coercive citation in academic publishing. Science. 2012;335:542–3.
7. Clark J. How to avoid predatory journals—a five-point plan. BMJ Blogs. http://blogs.bmj.com/bmj/2015/01/19/jocalyn-clark-how-to-avoid-predatory-journals-a-five-point-plan/. Accessed 9 Sept 2015.
8. Principles of transparency and best practice in scholarly publishing. http://www.wame.org/about/principles-of-transparency-and-best-practice. Accessed 9 Sept 2015.

Suggested Reading

Guthrie J, Parker L, Gray R. From thesis to publication. In: Burton S, Steane P, editors. Surviving your thesis. London: Routledge; 2004. p. 232–47.
Smyth J, Verweij J, D'Incalci M, Balakrishnan L. The art of successful publication. ECCO 13 workshop report. Eur J Cancer. 2006;42:434–6.
Tomaska L. Teaching how to prepare a manuscript by means of rewriting published scientific papers. Genetics. 2007;175:17–20.

Manuscript Preparation: The ICMJE Recommendations

17

Ana Marušić

By the time you have reached this chapter, you would have learnt how to write a good report of your research and address most of the publication requirements and standards. And then, when you have a draft of your manuscript and have picked the right journal, it is time to check whether the manuscript format is suitable for the target journal. This may be the time when you will learn about or are advised to consult something that has been usually (and quite mysteriously) called URMs— Uniform Requirements for Manuscripts. It may be too late, especially if you have done a clinical trial and written an article to then realize that the requirement for the submission of such a report to the journal of your choice is the registration of your trial before the enrolment of the first patient. So, the URMs are something to be aware of and informed about before starting research.

17.1 What Are the URMs?

URMs was the term used until 2014 for Uniform Requirements for Manuscripts— Guidance for Manuscript Preparation and Responsible Editing and Publishing, produced by the International Committee of Medical Journal Editors (ICMJE) [1]. These guidelines had become known as 'The Uniform Requirements' or 'URMs'. The title was changed in 2014 to the Recommendations for the Conduct, Reporting, Editing, and Publication of Scholarly Work in Medical Journals, to reflect the fact that ICMJE provides recommendations for best practices and does not impose strict rules. The ICMJE Recommendations address not only manuscript preparation but

A. Marušić
Journal of Global Health and Department of Research in Biomedicine and Health, University of Split School of Medicine, Split, Croatia

University of Edinburgh, Edinburgh, Scotland, UK

© The National Medical Journal of India 2018
P. Sahni, R. Aggarwal (eds.), *Reporting and Publishing Research in the Biomedical Sciences*, https://doi.org/10.1007/978-981-10-7062-4_17

155

also several other aspects of editing and publishing health research. In this chapter we will use the term URMs because it is still used commonly among authors and editors. The ICMJE Recommendations are widely accepted by biomedical journals: the list of journals that have officially contacted the ICMJE to request listing as a journal following the guidelines (available at *http://icmje.org/journals-following-the-icmje-recommendations/*) currently has over 2000 journals. Although the journals themselves do not always keep up with the latest updates of the URMs, as shown in several studies [2, 3], the URMs are a standard and authoritative guide for manuscript preparation in medicine.

If you are a prospective author of a manuscript, this chapter will not help you make a perfect submission to a journal—you will need to read the URMs very closely and go back to your manuscript to check whether you have addressed all the issues that journals and their editors consider to be important. This chapter aims to convey the importance of careful manuscript preparation and submission to a journal: when your manuscript is well written, references are in order, correctly written, and in a uniform style; tables and figures are clear and uniformly formatted; and the reviewers and editors will not be distracted by technical imperfections and stylistic flaws and will be able to concentrate on judging the excellence of your work. Also, by following the best publication practices outlined in the URMs, such as those on authorship, conflict of interest, and trial registration, you will make sure that your research report is endowed with due integrity and accountability.

17.2   History of the URMs

To understand the current publishing standards outlined in the URMs, it is good to know how they came about and how they developed. The best, most comprehensive (and only!) history of the URMs was written by one of the founding members of the ICMJE, Edward J. Huth, former editor of the *Annals of Internal Medicine*, and Kathleen Case, long-term secretary of the ICMJE, also from the *Annals of Internal Medicine* [4]. Their article about the establishment of the ICMJE, and creation and development of the URMs, written in 2004 on the occasion of the 25th anniversary of URMs, is a fascinating story about the reasons why the ICMJE and its URMs were conceived in 1978 and came into being in 1979. Most young researchers reading this book would not even imagine that the roots of these well-known guidelines were related to typing machine technology in the 1960s. At that time, the authors typed their manuscripts in triplicate on a typing machine and sent these to a journal by surface mail. Each journal had a specific and often widely varying style, particularly in writing the references [5]. The story goes that the URMs were created as a response to the demands of a secretary to a researcher in Seattle, USA, who complained about the need to retype a manuscript each time it was rejected by one journal and had to be submitted to a new one (remember, this happened in 1968, at the time of typing machines, albeit already electrical). The researcher in question was advised by the librarian to write to the editors of major US journals and ask them whether they could use the same format for references, which would then save time for authors and for journal staff. And that was the start of the ICMJE, at first called the International Steering Committee. The group met for the first time in Vancouver in 1978 (hence the common term for ICMJE: 'the Vancouver group'). Table 17.1 presents a detailed history of the changes to the URMs and policy statements from the ICMJE up to 2004 [4].

The first action of the editors was to address the reference style and provide basic guidelines for manuscript formatting (paper size, components of the title page, manuscript sections and abbreviations for units, statistical terms, chemicals, and journal titles). The first URMs were published in 1979. The purpose of such a guideline was that member journals agreed that they would accept all submitted manuscripts for

Table 17.1 Versions of the Uniform Requirements for Manuscripts submitted to Biomedical Journals (URMs) and the separate statements up to 2003[a]

Year	Change in URMs
1979	**URMs first edition** Covered physical properties for manuscripts, including paper size; such components as title page, abstract, page numbers, tables, and illustrations; the content appropriate to sections (Introduction, Methods, and Results); acceptable abbreviations (units, statistical terms, substances, and journal titles); and the submission process Formats for references were similar to those for Index Medicus, but the year of publication followed the journal title, and the closing pagination was shortened
1982	**URMs second edition** Included a statement on prior and duplicate publication; other changes were minor
1987	**Retraction of research findings** 'Expressions of Concern' text was added in 1997
1988	**Editorial freedom and integrity**
1988	**URMs third edition** Further defined authorship criteria. Section on acknowledgements defined types of credit and permissions needed. Use of International System of Units (SI) was recommended. Abbreviations list was eliminated. Section on statistics was added and use of confidence intervals emphasized
1989	**Confidentiality** **The role of the correspondence column**
1991	**Competing manuscripts based on the same study** **Order of authorship** **Guidelines for the protection of patients' rights to anonymity**
1991	**URMs fourth edition; revised in 1993, 1994** Presentation of a paper at a meeting does not constitute prior publication, nor do press reports of the meeting. Order of authorship is a joint decision of the co-authors. Word limits for structured abstracts added. Number of authors cited in a reference reduced from seven to six (plus 'et al.'). Reference examples greatly expanded, from 14 to 34. List of participating journals deleted The 1993 revision noted that electronic publication was considered publication. Corporate authorship was subject to the same criteria as individual authorship. A section on manuscripts on diskette was added. The 1994 revision introduced the term redundant publication and described remedies. Secondary publication was described as acceptable under some conditions
1992	**Definition of a peer-reviewed journal**

(continued)

Table 17.1 (continued)

Year	Change in URMs
1993	Medical journals and the popular media Conflicts of interest (editorial comment, 2001)
1994	**Advertising** **Supplements**
1997	**URMs fifth edition; revised in 1999, 2000, 2001** Revisions included putting some of the separate statements in the URMs. Issues to consider before submitting a manuscript included duplicate publication, secondary publication, and privacy. Some editors may choose to publish notes on what each author contributed; authors may wish to explain how the order of authors was determined; some journals limit the number of authors. Care should be taken when describing race or ethnicity, because the terms are ambiguous. Methods used in clinical trials and for review articles should be described. Claims of economic benefit should not be included without data. Written permission is needed for use of personal communications and in-press articles. Reference examples were expanded to include more legal material and electronic formats In 2000, revisions included stronger statements on preliminary release of information to the press and reporting guidelines for specific study designs, with a reference to the CONSORT guidelines. Authorship criteria were revised to include responsibility for 'appropriate portions' of the text, not all of it; one or more authors, not necessarily all, should take responsibility for the work as a whole; acquisition of data is considered an authorship-worthy contribution; editors were urged to publish information about the contributions of each author. How and why experimental subjects were selected should be described, and stronger warnings about use of ethnic descriptors were added
2000	**Project-specific industry support for research**
2001	**Policies for reporting biomedical journal information on the Internet**
2003	**Current version** A heavily reorganized and edited version with emphasis on ethical and procedural issues. All separate statements have been incorporated into the document. Authorship criteria more strict. The statements on conflicts of interest were greatly expanded, especially those on industry funding. The section on formats for references is replaced with a hypertext link to *www.nlm.nih.gov/bsd/uniform_requirements.html*

[a]Reproduced with permission, Council of Science Editors (CSE), from the article by Huth and Case in *Science Editor* [4]

editorial and/or peer-review processing if they were written (and typed) in the URMs format, regardless of the style used by the individual journal.

From today's point of view, when a click in a reference management software can format references to your desired journal style, it may appear surprising that the first years of the ICMJE were dedicated to passionate discussions on whether to use the 'Harvard system' of citing references in the text (author-year system) or a numerical system—the so-called Vancouver style; the latter finally won as the preferred reference format in biomedical journals [4].

In the 1980s, when the ICMJE had resolved the controversies of reference styling, the group's focus shifted to ethical issues in editing and publishing—duplicate publications, retractions, authorship, confidentiality, protection of patient's anonymity, conflicts of interest, and industry support for research and advertising [4, 6]. Today, the URM's full title is Recommendations for the Conduct, Reporting, Editing, and Publication of Scholarly Work in Medical Journals [1].

17.3   Current Policies in the URMs

The latest update to the URMs is from 2014 [1]. After 2004, two major changes to the URMs had an important impact on clinical trials worldwide.

17.3.1 Registration of Clinical Trials

In 2004, the ICMJE put forth its statement on mandatory registration of clinical trials as a prerequisite for manuscript submission [7]. This statement provided a major push for already existing calls for greater transparency of clinical trials and helped shape current medical publishing as well as legal standards of clinical trials in many countries [8, 9]. The current update of the URMs also acknowledges the rapid development of trial registration practices, including mandatory posting of trial results at specific websites in some countries [8].

For the authors, regardless of the country they come from and national legal requirements for clinical trials, the ICMJE registration policy means that they have to register their trial before the enrolment of the first patient. There are many trial registries, from the largest one in the USA, *ClinicalTrials.gov*, to many smaller national registries, but it is important to choose a registry that is fully open to the public [1, 10]: 'The registry must be accessible to the public at no charge'. It must be open to all prospective registrants and managed by a not-for-profit organization. There must be a mechanism to ensure the validity of the registration data, and the registry should be electronically searchable. Another requirement is indicating the registration number for the trial at the end of the abstract in the manuscript.

It is also important to keep in mind the definition of a clinical trial and related terms [1]: 'The ICMJE defines a clinical trial as any research project that prospectively assigns people or a group of people to an intervention, with or without concurrent comparison or control groups, to study the cause-and-effect relationship between a health-related intervention and a health outcome. Health-related interventions are those used to modify a biomedical or health-related outcome; examples include drugs, surgical procedures, devices, behavioural treatments, educational programmes, dietary interventions, quality improvement interventions, and process-of-care changes. Health outcomes are any biomedical or health-related measures obtained in patients or participants, including pharmacokinetic measures and adverse events. The ICMJE does not define the timing of first patient enrolment, but best practice dictates registration by the time of first patient consent.'

The ICMJE also recognizes the current legal requirement in some countries for mandatory registration of trial results [10]. The new URMs make it clear what is acceptable to post as results in a trial registry and what might be considered prior publication [1]. Thus: 'The ICMJE will not consider as prior publication the posting of trial results in any registry that meets the above criteria if results are limited to a brief (500 word) structured abstract or tables (to include patients enrolled, key outcomes, and adverse events).'

17.3.2 Uniform Conflict of Interest Declaration Form

The second major change in the URMs is the uniform declaration form for competing interests, which has been adopted by all ICMJE journals [11]. This means that each author has to declare both financial and nonfinancial conflicts of interest related to the submitted work and the author's research in general (*see* Chap. 23 on 'Conflicts of interest').

17.4 Future of URMs

In the future, we may expect to see further developments in trial registration policy, particularly in relation to posting results in public registries.

Another important task for the ICMJE will be the work on authorship definition. The history of the ICMJE authorship definition is also an interesting read (Table 17.2), and it is clear that there are still unresolved problems of authorship versus contributorship, ghost writing, and declarations of authorship contributions [12–14].

Table 17.2 History of the definition of authorship in the Uniform Requirements for Manuscripts submitted to Biomedical Journals (URMs) by the International Committee of Medical Journal Editors (ICMJE)[a]

URMs	Definition
1988, 1991	All persons designated as authors should qualify for authorship. Each author should have participated sufficiently in the work to take public responsibility for the content
	Authorship credit should be based only on substantial contributions to (a) conception and design or analysis and interpretation of data and to (b) drafting the article or revising it critically for important intellectual content and on (c) final approval of the version to be published. Conditions (a), (b), and (c) must all be met. Participation solely in the acquisition of funding or the collection of data does not justify authorship. General supervision of the research group is also not sufficient for authorship. Any part of an article critical to its main conclusions must be the responsibility of at least one author
	A paper with corporate (collective) authorship must specify the key persons responsible for the article; others contributing to the work should be recognized separately (*see* Acknowledgements)
	Editors may require authors to justify the assignment of authorship
1994	*The following statement was added*:
	The order of authorship should be a joint decision of the co-authors. All authors should meet the previously mentioned basic criteria. Because the order of authorship is assigned in different ways, its meaning cannot be inferred accurately unless it is stated by the authors. Authors may wish to add an explanation of the order of authorship in a footnote. In deciding on order, authors should be aware that many journals limit the number of authors listed in the table of contents and that the National Library of Medicine (NLM) lists only the first ten authors in MEDLINE

Table 17.2 (continued)

URMs	Definition
1995	All persons designated as authors should qualify for authorship. The order of authorship should be a joint decision of the co-authors. Each author should have participated sufficiently in the work to take public responsibility for the content.
	Authorship credit should be based only on substantial contributions to (a) either conception and design or else analysis and interpretation of data and to (b) drafting the article or revising it critically for important intellectual content, and on (c) final approval of the version to be published. All three conditions must be met. Participation solely in the acquisition of funding or the collection of data does not justify authorship. General supervision of the research group is also not sufficient for authorship. Any part of an article critical to its main conclusions must be the responsibility of at least one author
	Editors may require authors to justify the assignment of authorship.
	Increasingly, multicentre trials are attributed to a corporate author. All members of the group who are named as authors, either in the authorship position below the title or in a footnote, should fully meet the criteria for authorship as defined in the 'Uniform requirements'. Group members who do not meet these criteria should be listed, with their permission, under Acknowledgements or in an appendix (*see* Acknowledgements)
1997	All persons designated as authors should qualify for authorship. Each author should have participated sufficiently in the work to take public responsibility for the content.
	Authorship credit should be based only on substantial contributions to (a) conception and design or analysis and interpretation of data and to (b) drafting the article or revising it critically for important intellectual content and on (c) final approval of the version to be published. Conditions (a), (b), and (c) must all be met. Participation solely in the acquisition of funding or the collection of data does not justify authorship. General supervision of the research group is not sufficient for authorship. Any part of an article critical to its main conclusions must be the responsibility of at least one author.
	Editors may ask authors to describe what each contributed; this information may be published
	Increasingly, multicentre trials are attributed to a corporate author. All members of the group who are named as authors, either in the authorship position below the title or in a footnote, should fully meet the above criteria for authorship. Group members who do not meet these criteria should be listed, with their permission, in the Acknowledgements or in an appendix (*see* Acknowledgements)
	The order of authorship should be a joint decision of the co-authors. Because the order is assigned in different ways, its meaning cannot be inferred accurately unless it is stated by the authors. Authors may wish to explain the order of authorship in a footnote. In deciding on the order, authors should be aware that many journals limit the number of authors listed in the table of contents and that the NLM lists in MEDLINE only the first 24 plus the last author when there are more than 25 authors

(continued)

Table 17.2 (continued)

URMs	Definition
2004–2006	Authorship credit should be based on (1) substantial contributions to conception and design or acquisition of data or analysis and interpretation of data, (2) drafting the article or revising it critically for important intellectual content, and (3) final approval of the version to be published. Authors should meet conditions 1, 2, and 3.
	When a large, multicentre group has conducted the work, the group should identify the individuals who accept direct responsibility for the manuscript. These individuals should fully meet the criteria for authorship defined above, and editors will ask these individuals to complete journal-specific author and conflict-of-interest disclosure forms. When submitting a group author manuscript, the corresponding author should clearly indicate the preferred citation and should clearly identify all individual authors as well as the group name. Journals will generally list other members of the group in the acknowledgements. The NLM indexes the group name and the names of individuals the group has identified as being directly responsible for the manuscript. Acquisition of funding, collection of data, or general supervision of the research group, alone, does not justify authorship.
	All persons designated as authors should qualify for authorship, and all those who qualify should be listed.
	Each author should have participated sufficiently in the work to take public responsibility for appropriate portions of the content.
	Some journals now also request that one or more authors, referred to as 'guarantors', should own responsibility for the integrity of the work as a whole, from inception to published article, and for that information to be published.
	Increasingly, authorship of multicentre trials is attributed to a group. All members of the group who are named as authors should fully meet the above criteria for authorship.
	The order of authorship on the byline should be a joint decision of the co-authors. Authors should be prepared to explain the order in which authors are listed.
2007	*The section on the order of authorship changes to*:
	The group should jointly make decisions about contributors/authors before submitting the manuscript for publication. The corresponding author/guarantor should be prepared to explain the presence and order of these individuals. It is not the role of the editors to make authorship/contributorship decisions or to arbitrate conflicts related to authorship.
2008–2009	*The section on large, multicentre groups changes to*:
	When a large, multicentre group has conducted the work, the group should identify the individuals who accept direct responsibility for the manuscript. These individuals should fully meet the criteria for authorship/contributorship defined above, and editors will ask these individuals to complete journal-specific author and conflict-of-interest disclosure forms. When submitting a manuscript authored by a group, the corresponding author should clearly indicate the preferred citation and identify all individual authors as well as the group name. Journals generally list other members of the group in the Acknowledgements. The NLM indexes the group name and the names of individuals the group has identified as being directly responsible for the manuscript; it also lists the names of collaborators if they are listed in the Acknowledgements.
2014	*The definition of authorship changes to*:
	The ICMJE recommends that authorship be based on the following four criteria:
	• Substantial contributions to the conception or design of the work; or the acquisition, analysis, or interpretation of data for the work; AND
	• Drafting the work or revising it critically for important intellectual content; AND
	• Final approval of the version to be published; AND
	• Agreement to be accountable for all aspects of the work in ensuring that questions related to the accuracy or integrity of any part of the work are appropriately investigated and resolved.
	In addition to being accountable for the parts of the work he or she has done, an author should be able to identify which co-authors are responsible for specific other parts of the work. In addition, authors should have confidence in the integrity of the contributions of their co-authors.

[a]Reproduced with permission, *Medical writing* (formerly *The write stuff*), from the article by Marušić and Marušić [6]. Adapted to include the recent change in the definition [1]

The future of the URMs or the ICMJE Recommendations, as these are now known, will be as interesting as its past.

References

1. International Committee of Medical Journal Editors (ICMJE). Recommendations for the conduct, reporting, editing, and publication of scholarly work in medical journals. Updated December 2014. http://icmje.org/recommendations/browse/. Accessed 3 May 2015.
2. Wager E. Do medical journals provide clear and consistent guidelines on authorship? Med Gen Med. 2007;9:16.
3. Hopewell S, Altman DG, Moher D, Schulz KF. Endorsement of the CONSORT statement by high impact factor medical journals: a survey of journal editors and journal 'instructions to authors'. Trials. 2008;9:20.
4. Huth EJ, Case K. The URM: twenty-five years old. Sci Editor. 2004;27:17–21.
5. Porcher FH. Reference practices of biomedical journals: uniform requirements style or not. CBE Views. 1986;9:30–9.
6. Marušić A, Marušić M. A contribution to the authorship debate: can we trust definitions and declarations? The Write Stuff. 2010;19:14–7.
7. De Angelis C, Drazen JM, Frizelle FA, Haug C, Hoey J, Horton R, et al.; International Committee of Medical Journal Editors (ICMJE). Clinical trial registration: a statement from the International Committee of Medical Journal Editors. Lancet. 2004;364:911–12.
8. Califf RM, Zarin DA, Kramer JM, Sherman RE, Aberle LH, Tasneem A. Characteristics of clinical trials registered in ClinicalTrials.gov, 2007–2010. JAMA. 2012;307:1838–47.
9. Viergever RF, Ghersi D. The quality of registration of clinical trials. PLoS One. 2011;6:e14701.
10. Laine C, Horton R, DeAngelis CD, Drazen JM, Frizelle FA, Godlee F, et al. Clinical trial registration: looking back and moving ahead. Lancet. 2007;369:1909–11.
11. Drazen JM, Van Der Weyden MB, Sahni P, Rosenberg J, Marusic A, Laine C, et al. Uniform format for disclosure of competing interests in ICMJE journals. Lancet. 2009;374:1395–6.
12. Marušić A, Bošnjak L, Jerončić A. A systematic review of research on the meaning, ethics and practices of authorship across scholarly disciplines. PLoS One. 2011;6:e23477.
13. Bošnjak L, Marušić A. Prescribed practices of authorship: review of codes of ethics from professional bodies and journal guidelines across disciplines. Scientometrics. 2012;93:751–63.
14. Marušić A, Hren D, Mansi B, Lineberry N, Bhattacharya A, Garrity M, et al. Five-step authorship framework to improve transparency in disclosing contributors to industry-sponsored clinical trial publications. BMC Med. 2014;12:197. http://www.biomedcentral.com/1741-7015/12/197. Accessed 3 May 2015.

Reporting Guidelines: A Framework for Clarity and Transparency

Larissa Shamseer and David Moher

'Researchers excel at being creative and scientifically credible, but they aren't necessarily good communicators and writers.'

—Paul Hébert, Former Editor-in-Chief, *Canadian Medical Association Journal*

18.1 Introduction

Complete and transparent reporting is imperative when assessing the validity of reported treatment effects and other findings of health research. A study's methods should be described in enough detail so that they can be replicated, the analyses should follow the protocol, and the results should be provided in sufficient detail to be incorporated into future research, meta-analyses and practice guidelines. Complete and transparent reporting enables clinicians and others to make better, more informed healthcare decisions; it also reduces waste in healthcare research. Transparent reporting is an integral part of the research process and helps the reader judge whether good science has been used. For instance, without a description of the methods used to control internal validity (e.g. randomization, blinding) and external validity (e.g. definition of the population under study), the reader is left to ponder whether the reported effect of treatment is accurate and applicable to his/her own patients.

In an ideal world, healthcare decisions are based on the highest quality evidence, and such evidence is based on information gathered from all available studies. Data

L. Shamseer (✉) • D. Moher
Clinical Epidemiology Program, Ottawa Hospital Research Institute, Ottawa, ON, Canada

School of Epidemiology, Public Health and Preventative Medicine, University of Ottawa, Ottawa, ON, Canada
e-mail: lshamseer@ohri.ca; dmoher@ohri.ca

© The National Medical Journal of India 2018
P. Sahni, R. Aggarwal (eds.), *Reporting and Publishing Research in the Biomedical Sciences*, https://doi.org/10.1007/978-981-10-7062-4_18

from research studies are effectively translated into maximum health benefits when they are presented in an accurate, complete and useable format. Such clarity enables readers to understand exactly how the research was conducted, what was found, how reliable the findings are and how they fit into the wider context of existing knowledge.

18.2   The Healthcare Knowledge Process

Generating, aggregating, reporting and implementing health research is a complex process. For pharmaceuticals, the framework followed is something like this. Basic scientific innovation leads to several drugs being tested in a variety of animal models. Successful drugs are then tested in the 'first in human' studies, and those that seem effective in and well tolerated by the target population without substantial harm are evaluated using a gold-standard design—the randomized controlled trial (RCT). Several trials of the same compound may lead to a systematic review of its likely therapeutic benefit, as well as economic evaluation as part of a health technology assessment. Clinicians then use these results as a prescription guide in everyday practice. The results are also used by policymakers to calculate prescription costs in official drug benefit programmes. The description above assumes, naively, that all research findings are available to interested readers and that what is published, after peer-review, is of high enough quality that the descriptions of the methods and findings are clear, accurate and transparent, enabling readers to use the information. Unfortunately, much research is wasted as it cannot be reused.

18.3   Preventable Waste in Research

It is estimated that US$ 200 billion is spent globally on biomedical research every year [1], and about one million research publications are produced annually. One goal of this huge expenditure is to improve the health of patients suffering from various diseases and/or conditions. However, it is estimated that over 85% of this large investment is lost in the form of preventable waste which accrues over several stages of the research process (Table 18.1) [2–6]. Chalmers and Glasziou assert that, 'while some waste is inevitable and bearable, current levels of waste are intolerable' [1].

Waste first occurs in the research process when research agendas and questions fail to address the needs and priorities of patients [7]. For instance, nondrug systematic reviews produced by the Cochrane Collaboration are more frequently accessed than reviews of drug interventions. Yet, despite this, less funding is available to support nondrug research, and researchers are left with little choice about what to study [1].

Second, unnecessary and poorly designed research is frequently undertaken. Research is often unnecessarily duplicated because systematic reviews of existing

Table 18.1   Types of waste generated in the research and reporting process

1. Related to relevance of research questions to clinicians and patients [2]
    (a) Failure to address high-priority questions
    (b) Failure to assess important outcomes
    (c) Failure to involve clinicians and patients in setting research agendas
2. Related to appropriateness of study design and methods [3]
    (a) Designing studies without prior systematic reviews of existing evidence (applies to >50% of studies)
    (b) Failure to take adequate steps to reduce bias (e.g. allocation concealment) (applies to >50% of studies)
3. Related to research regulation and management [4]
    (a) Disproportionate regulatory approval compared to the conceivable risks to research participants
    (b) Inefficient management of the procedural conduct of research
4. Related to access to full data and publication [5]
    (a) Failure to publish in full (nearly 50% of studies)
    (b) Biased underreporting of studies with negative results
5. Related to unbiased nature and usability of study reports [6]
    (a) Failure to describe trial interventions sufficiently (over 30%)
    (b) Failure to report planned study outcomes (over 50%)
    (c) Failure to interpret new research findings in the context of systematic assessment of other relevant information

Adapted from Macleod MR, Michie S, Roberts I, Dirnagl U, Chalmers I, Ioannidis JPA, et al Biomedical research: Increasing value, reducing waste. Lancet 2014;383:101–4

evidence are overlooked. Initiatives such as the prospective registration of clinical trials (www.clinicaltrials.gov) and systematic reviews before starting research (www.crd.york.ac.uk/prospero/) should help reduce redundancy and increase the transparency of research. In addition, some researchers do not pay adequate attention to methods that control for bias; reports of RCTs have shown inadequate or unclear documentation of randomized sequence generation, allocation concealment, and blinding—all factors that may lead to biased estimates of intervention effects (Fig. 18.1) [8, 9].

More waste accumulates when research findings and publications are not made available or accessible to those who need them for future research. Research with disappointing results takes longer to publish [10] and is generally less likely to be published—particularly if a study uncovers a harmful effect of a treatment [11]. This is a direct form of unscientific and unethical misconduct for which researchers should be held accountable; a recent consensus statement in the UK shows the seriousness of the situation [12].

Of particular importance to the reporting of research is the final pillar of waste, which results from the production of research reports that are biased and unusable. As described in detail below, research reports are filled with poor or selective reporting. Poorly reported studies not only fail to clearly and transparently inform readers about the methods and findings of research but also obscure true representation of

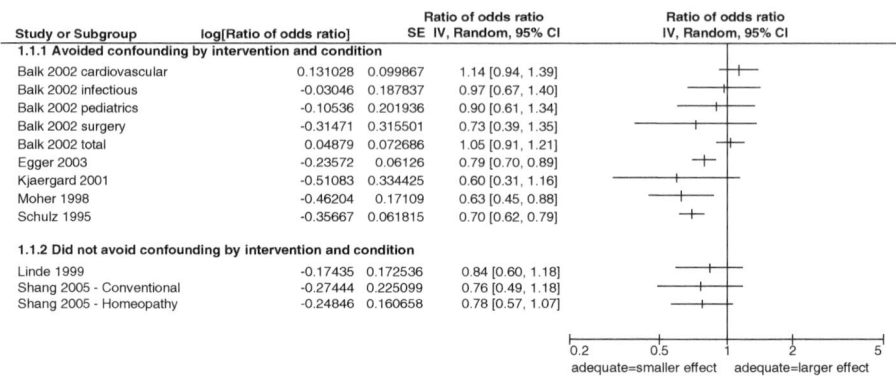

Fig. 18.1 Studies of controlled trials with adequate concealment of allocation compared with inadequate/unclear concealment of allocation across different interventions and conditions—ratio of odds ratios (Odgaard-Jensen J, Vist GE, Timmer A, Kunz R, Akl EA, Schünemann H, *et al.* Randomisation to protect against selection bias in healthcare trials. *Cochrane Database Syst Rev* 2011 Apr 13;(**4**):MR000012. doi: 10.1002/14651858.MR000012.pub3)

the methodological quality of a study, which too may be poor. Ambiguous reporting can make a poorly described study barely distinguishable from a poorly designed and/or poorly conducted study; so the results of even well-conducted studies can be lost to their users.

18.4   Moral Obligation of Good Reporting

Inadequate reporting is unacceptable and unethical at many levels. It is particularly unfair to patients who participate in research assuming that all studies are published and well reported so that the findings can be used in healthcare decision-making [13, 14]. Furthermore, the public expects research (particularly that which is publicly funded) to be conducted to the highest possible standards. Unfortunately, there are substantial failures in how research is reported. This is an objectionable and inefficient manner of running a multibillion dollar enterprise.

18.5   The Extent of Poor Reporting

Many publications lack clarity, transparency and completeness in how the authors actually carried out their research; this problem is endemic and affects all areas of health research. Up to a third of the most-cited clinical research seems to encounter problems when being replicated [15]. This is indicative of a serious, systemic issue in how research is reported.

In a follow-up to a study that evaluated the reporting quality of trials published in Indian medical journals, the reporting of 13 CONSORT checklist items, including key elements related to bias (e.g. sequence generation, allocation concealment, blinding), showed no improvement over the 3-year period between 2004–2005 ($n = 151$) and 2007–2008 ($n = 145$) [16]. In both years, there were no trials that completely reported all the 13 selected items, and only four were completely reported in more than 50% of trials. For some items, the proportion of adequately described trials significantly declined over time (i.e. blinding: −17%, 95% CI −6% to −28%). Allocation concealment—a fundamental aspect of RCTs—was the least often reported item, with only 16% of trials reporting it during 2004–2005 and 21% doing so in 2007–2008.

In another study, Mignini and Khan reviewed 30 systematic reviews of animal studies and 45 laboratory bench studies and found that many failed to report key details such as review hypothesis (77%), details of the search strategy (41%) and assessment of study heterogeneity (85%) [17].

Glasziou and colleagues assessed descriptions of administered treatments for both clinical trials and systematic reviews ($n = 80$) for which summaries were published over 1 year (October 2005 to October 2006) in *Evidence-Based Medicine*—a journal targeted at physicians working in primary care and general medicine [18]. Treatment descriptions were inadequate in half ($n = 41$) of the original published articles, making their replication and use in clinical practice difficult, if not impossible. Perhaps a more interesting finding of this study is that, when authors were asked to provide more details about reported treatments, 52 of 59 authors responded, and descriptions improved from being 46% complete to 76% complete [18].

While the reporting of research has shown some improvement over time, gains have been small and relative and do not represent a fundamental change in alleviating an unsustainable situation. For instance, though the proportion of RCTs that adequately described sequence generation showed a 62% relative increase between 2000 and 2006, still only 34% of RCTs in 2006 reported this item adequately [19]. A similar situation exists with descriptions of sample size calculation and allocation concealment; both of these showed improvements over time but were still being reported fewer than 50% of the time as of 2006. Primary outcome description fared slightly better with 52% of trials providing adequate descriptions in 2006 compared to 45% in 2000. The description of blinding in RCTs did not appear to improve with time.

Over 50% of RCTs have major deficiencies in reporting these essential elements; their interpretation and use by readers are consequently limited. These are just a few examples of a large and serious problem with the literature [20, 21], indicating the general failure in the quality of reporting of health research.

18.6 Consequences of Inadequate Reporting

For several reasons inadequate reporting is an obstacle to evidence-based clinical practice. Studies that lack details about their conduct and findings stand little chance of being meaningfully included in syntheses of evidence, such as systematic reviews; thus, they will not inform clinical practice and healthcare policies. However, if such studies are included, inappropriate and inefficient clinical decision-making might occur. It is not uncommon to find comments in the discussion sections of systematic reviews such as 'A further 11 (studies) that met the inclusion criteria had to be excluded because of poor data reporting' [22]. In addition, the quality of reporting of included studies is often so poor that the results have to be interpreted cautiously, such as 'Care should be taken in interpreting the above studies as failure to show benefit in a series of small, poorly reported studies does not mean that the anti-staphylococcal interventions could not be helpful in eczema' [23]. Such negative conclusions lead to wastage of a lot of time spent in reviewing the available literature and affects the content and quality of clinical practice guidelines and adversely impacts the care patients receive.

In a seminal meta-epidemiological study, Schulz and colleagues examined the methodological quality of 250 controlled trials from 33 meta-analyses in the Cochrane Pregnancy and Childbirth Database for associations between aspects of methodology and estimated treatment effects [24]. They found that trials in which concealment was either inadequate or was unclear (not reported at all or incompletely reported) yielded significantly larger estimates of treatment effects ($p < 0.001$) than those trials that reported adequately concealed treatment allocation. Odds ratios were exaggerated by 41% for inadequately concealed trials and by 30% for unclearly concealed trials. These results showed that adequately concealed treatment allocation is an essential bias-limiting element of RCTs and provided the first compelling link between inadequate methods, as reported, and biased estimates of treatment effectiveness. This result has been confirmed by other studies [8], and, more recently, other serious reporting biases have been recognized.

18.7   Efforts to Improve the Reporting of Research

Over the past decade or more, there have been several efforts to improve the quality of reporting of research studies. Guidelines and checklists have been developed as a simple, low-technology solution to help authors produce complete, accurate and clear reports of their research. These sets of rules or principles guide authors towards the best practices in a particular area. More than 200 reporting guidelines address different study types or aspects of studies (e.g. reporting harms). They usually specify a minimum set of information needed for a complete and transparent account of what was done and what was found during a research study and particularly concentrate on those aspects that might have introduced bias into the research. Ninety-seven per cent of existing reporting guidelines contain a checklist of reporting criteria [25]. (*See* Box 18.1 for more on checklists).

> **Box 18.1 The Importance of Checklists**
> A checklist is a common cognitive device that can help complete a task [26]. When adhered to, checklists have transformed entire industries [27]. In clinical medicine, checklists can save many lives. One example is the World Health Organization's Surgical Safety Checklist. When used by surgical teams in both developing and developed countries, there were clinically and statistically important decreases in morbidity and mortality [28]. Similarly, a checklist to improve intensive care saved 1500 lives and US$ 100 million in healthcare costs over an 18-month period [29]. Checklists can reduce waste in healthcare spending, resulting in more efficient patient care. Checklists for reporting are yet to see widespread success; perhaps they are perceived as a tool that stifles author expertise and autonomy.

The term 'reporting guideline' has not been formally defined, but a working definition has been created, based on the collective experience of the EQUATOR (Enhancing the QUAlity and Transparency Of health Research) Network executive for use in their research initiatives. It states that a reporting guideline typically consists of a checklist of minimum items to be reported, sometimes accompanied by a flow diagram and/or explicit text to guide authors in reporting a specific type of research, developed using explicit methodology, involving a consensus process [25, 30]. Some guidelines also provide readers with the evidence and rationale behind each item along with examples of adequate reporting of items from existing literature [31–33].

18.8   The CONSORT Statement

RCTs have been the focus of scrutiny because of their direct impact on healthcare. To rectify inadequacies in reporting, the Consolidated Standards of Reporting Trials (CONSORT) statement (www.consort-statement.org) was developed after two groups of researchers (including clinical trialists, statisticians, epidemiologists and biomedical editors) campaigned for better reporting standards [34, 35]. The original CONSORT statement provided authors of RCTs with a standard way to report their findings. It emerged in 1996 [36] and since then has been updated twice [37, 38]. CONSORT 2010—the latest iteration—comprises a 25-item checklist (Table 18.2) and a flow diagram (Fig. 18.2) to help authors document the flow of participants through a trial. It is also accompanied by an explanatory document that contains examples of good reporting and an explanation of each checklist item [31].

CONSORT has shown a durability and uptake seen by few other scientific products. It was recently named one of the major milestones in health research methods over the past century by the Patient-Centered Outcomes Research Institute (PCORI) [39]. Furthermore, it has been informally established as the model after which

Table 18.2 CONSORT 2010 checklist (Schulz 2010)[a] [38]

Section/topic	Item no.	Checklist item	Reported on page no.
Title and abstract			
	1a	Identification as a randomised trial in the title	
	1b	Structured summary of trial design, methods, results and conclusions (for specific guidance, *see* CONSORT for abstracts)	
Introduction			
Background and objectives	2a	Scientific background and explanation of rationale	
	2b	Specific objectives or hypotheses	
Methods			
Trial design	3a	Description of trial design (such as parallel, factorial) including allocation ratio	
	3b	Important changes to methods after trial commencement (such as eligibility criteria), with reasons	
Participants	4a	Eligibility criteria for participants	
	4b	Settings and locations where the data were collected	
Interventions	5	The interventions for each group with sufficient details to allow replication, including how and when they were actually administered	
Outcomes	6a	Completely defined prespecified primary and secondary outcome measures, including how and when they were assessed	
	6b	Any changes to trial outcomes after the trial commenced, with reasons	
Sample size	7a	How sample size was determined	
	7b	When applicable, explanation of any interim analyses and stopping guidelines	
Randomization: sequence generation	8a	Method used to generate the random allocation sequence	
	8b	Type of randomization; details of any restriction (such as blocking and block size)	
Allocation concealment mechanism	9	Mechanism used to implement the random allocation sequence (such as sequentially numbered containers), describing any steps taken to conceal the sequence until interventions were assigned	
Implementation	10	Who generated the random allocation sequence, who enrolled participants, and who assigned participants to interventions	
Blinding	11a	If done, who was blinded after assignment to interventions (e.g. participants, care providers, those assessing outcomes) and how	
	11b	If relevant, description of the similarity of interventions	

Table 18.2 (continued)

Section/topic	Item no.	Checklist item	Reported on page no.
Statistical methods	12a	Statistical methods used to compare groups for primary and secondary outcomes	
	12b	Methods for additional analyses, such as subgroup analyses and adjusted analyses	
Results			
Participant flow (a diagram is strongly recommended)	13a	For each group, the numbers of participants who were randomly assigned, received intended treatment and were analysed for the primary outcome	
	13b	For each group, losses and exclusions after randomization, together with reasons	
Recruitment	14a	Dates defining the periods of recruitment and follow-up	
	14b	Why the trial ended or was stopped	
Baseline data	15	A table showing baseline demographic and clinical characteristics for each group	
Numbers analysed	16	For each group, number of participants (denominator) included in each analysis and whether the analysis was by original assigned groups	
Outcomes and estimation	17a	For each primary and secondary outcome, results for each group and the estimated effect size and its precision (such as 95% confidence interval)	
	17b	For binary outcomes, presentation of both absolute and relative effect sizes is recommended	
Ancillary analyses	18	Results of any other analyses performed, including subgroup analyses and adjusted analyses, distinguishing prespecified from exploratory	
Harms	19	All important harms or unintended effects in each group (for specific guidance *see* CONSORT for harms)	
Discussion			
Limitations	20	Trial limitations, addressing sources of potential bias, imprecision and, if relevant, multiplicity of analyses	
Generalizability	21	Generalizability (external validity, applicability) of the trial findings	
Interpretation	22	Interpretation consistent with results, balancing benefits and harms and considering other relevant evidence	

(continued)

Table 18.2 (continued)

Section/topic	Item no.	Checklist item	Reported on page no.
Other information			
Registration	23	Registration number and name of trial registry	
Protocol	24	Where the full trial protocol can be accessed, if available	
Funding	25	Sources of funding and other support (such as supply of drugs), role of funders	

Source: Schulz KF, Altman DG, Moher D; CONSORT Group. CONSORT 2010 statement: Updated guidelines for reporting parallel group randomized trials. *Ann Intern Med* 2010;**152:**726–32

Templates of the CONSORT 2010 checklist in MS Word and Adobe PDF format are available to download at http://www.consort-statement.org/consort-2010

[a]We strongly recommend reading this statement in conjunction with the CONSORT 2010 Explanation and Elaboration for important clarifications on all the items. If relevant, we also recommend reading CONSORT extensions for cluster randomized trials, non-inferiority and equivalence trials, non-pharmacological treatments, herbal interventions, and pragmatic trials. Additional extensions are forthcoming: for those and for up to date references relevant to this checklist, see www.consort-statement.org

subsequent guidelines have been developed (e.g. STARD [Standards for Reporting of Diagnostic Accuracy], STROBE [Strengthening the Reporting of Observational Studies in Epidemiology] for reporting cohort, case–control and cross-sectional studies, PRISMA [Preferred Reporting Items for Systematic Reviews and Meta-Analyses]). Several 'extensions' of the main CONSORT statement have been developed to address the reporting of other trial designs (i.e. cluster trials), special interventions (e.g. non-pharmacological) and different types of data (e.g. harms). While it is not a specific intent of CONSORT, some suggest that CONSORT may even impact the way trials are designed [40].

18.9 EQUATOR Network

In 2006, a small group of methodologists who had been responsible for pioneering and propelling the area of research reporting (including leading members of the CONSORT initiative) came together to launch the EQUATOR Network (www.equator-network.org). EQUATOR is an overarching, international initiative that promotes reporting guidelines to improve the accuracy, transparency and reliability of published health research [41].

The EQUATOR Network hosts a Library for Health Research Reporting, which includes the rapidly accumulating numbers of reporting guidelines; these are identified through extensive, quarterly MEDLINE searches. Over half of the existing guidelines have emerged in the past 5 years. The EQUATOR Network Library classifies guidelines according to the study designs they address, making it an easily searchable resource for authors preparing studies with different designs. The

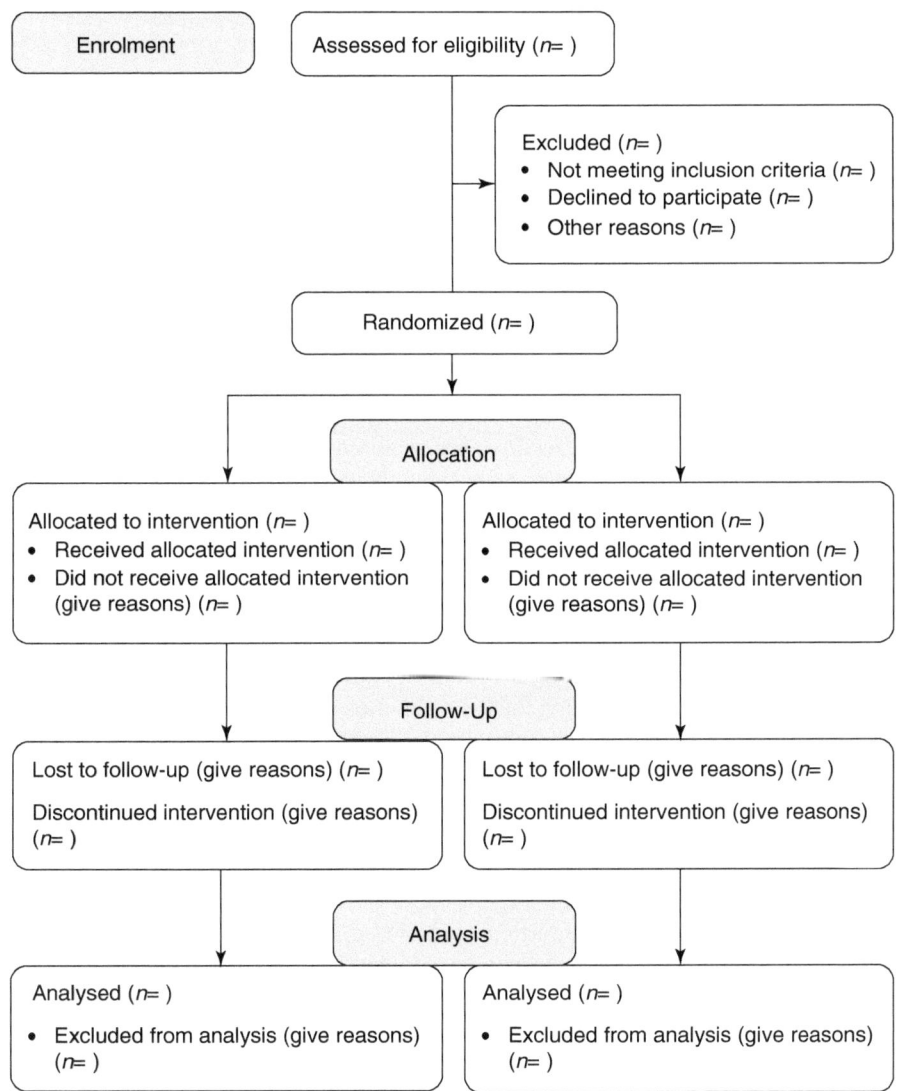

Fig. 18.2 CONSORT 2010 Flow Diagram (Schulz KF, Altman DG, Moher D; CONSORT Group. CONSORT 2010 statement: Updated guidelines for reporting parallel group randomized trials. *Ann Intern Med* 2010;**152:**726–32)

EQUATOR Network also carries out other reporting guideline-related activities: it (1) assists in the development, dissemination and implementation of robust reporting guidelines; (2) actively promotes the use of reporting guidelines and good research reporting practices through an education and training programme; (3) conducts regular assessments of how journals implement reporting guidelines; and (4) regularly audits the quality of reporting across the health research literature [42].

18.10 Reporting Guideline Development

In 2011, members of the EQUATOR group analysed the development process of 81 reporting guidelines [25]. This systematic review revealed inconsistencies in the way many guidelines had been developed. For instance, while all guidelines stated that they were 'consensus-based', 28% did not provide details about how a consensus was achieved. Those that did used a formal questionnaire (i.e. Delphi), an informal method or a combination of both. Half of the guidelines did not report on how their development was funded, and only 56% indicated that they searched for existing guidance before starting the development process. A description of guideline development is crucial to understanding and gauging the credibility of a guideline and a potential factor in its successful uptake, as can be seen from the example of CONSORT and its 'descendants'.

The EQUATOR Network executive has acquired much experience in developing numerous, successful guidelines, and they have proposed an 18-step process (Table 18.3) for developers to follow when developing a reporting guideline [43]. This process generally includes (1) identifying the need and means to develop the guideline; (2) conducting a Delphi survey to gain input from a large number of stakeholders, some of whom will be invited to participate in a smaller consensus-focused meeting; (3) holding a meeting of experts to gain consensus on guideline items and content; (4) developing the reporting guideline and related documents for publication; and (5) encouraging the dissemination of a guideline and evaluating its impact. Since its emergence in February 2010, this informal 'guidance' has been accessed nearly 10,000 times—a remarkable indication of its usefulness.

18.11 The Role of Journals in Adherence to Guidelines

The mere publication of a reporting guideline does not guarantee its success in improving the transparency and accuracy of what is published; to that end, journal editors have a crucial role to play as gatekeepers of the published literature. In 1979, the International Committee of Medical Journal Editors (ICMJE, www.icmje.org) began providing guidance on reporting for authors—the Uniform Requirements for Manuscripts submitted to Biomedical Journals [44]. The guidance (since updated) has seen many successes in improving the publishing of medical research and has facilitated the standard registration of clinical trials. In 1996, ICMJE endorsed the CONSORT statement and recommended that authors should use it when submitting papers of clinical trials to member journals. Other organizations such as the World Association of Medical Editors (WAME) and Committee on Publication Ethics (COPE) have also made formal endorsements of CONSORT.

Some journal editors now use reporting guidelines to complement their existing advice on writing. Such 'endorsement' takes the form of a supportive statement in a journal's 'Instructions to authors' and encourages or requires authors to submit a completed checklist to ensure that all guideline items have been addressed in their manuscript. Few guideline groups have the resources to track the use of their

Table 18.3 Recommended steps for developing a health research reporting guideline

Step	Item number	Detail
Initial steps	1	Identify the need for a guideline
	1.1	Develop new guidance
	1.2	Extend existing guidance
	1.3	Implement existing guidance
	2	Review the literature
	2.1	Identify previous relevant guidance
	2.2	Seek relevant evidence on the quality of reporting in published research articles
	2.3	Identify key information related to the potential sources of bias in such studies
	3	Obtain funding for the guideline initiative
Pre-meeting activities	4	Identify participants
	5	Conduct a Delphi exercise
	6	Generate a list of items for consideration at the face-to-face meeting
	7	Prepare for the face-to-face meeting
	7.1	Decide size and duration of the face-to-face meeting
	7.2	Develop meeting logistics
	7.3	Develop meeting agenda
	7.3.1	Consider presentations on relevant background topics, including summary of evidence
	7.3.2	Plan to share results of Delphi exercise, if done
	7.3.3	Invite session chairs
	7.4	Prepare materials to be sent to participants prior to meeting
	7.5	Arrange to record the meeting
The face-to-face consensus meeting itself	8	Present and discuss results of pre-meeting activities and relevant evidence
	8.1	Discuss the rationale for including items in the checklist
	8.2	Discuss the development of a flow diagram
	8.3	Discuss strategy for producing documents; identify who will be involved in which activities; discuss authorship
	8.4	Discuss knowledge translation strategy
Post-meeting activities	9	Develop the guidance statement
	9.1	Pilot test the checklist
	10	Develop an explanatory document (E&E)
	11	Develop a publication strategy
	11.1	Consider multiple and simultaneous publications
Post-publication activities	12	Seek and deal with feedback and criticism
	13	Encourage guideline endorsement
	14	Support adherence to the guideline
	15	Evaluate the impact of the reporting guidance
	16	Develop Website
	17	Translate guideline
	18	Update guideline

Source: Moher D, Schulz KF, Simera I, Altman DG. Guidance for developers of health research reporting guidelines. *PLoS Med* 2010 Feb 16;**7(2):**e1000217. doi: 10.1371/journal.pmed.1000217

guideline, but it is known that over 600 journals have formally endorsed CONSORT—probably the most endorsed guideline to date.

Peer-reviewers also have a role to play in upholding and implementing reporting standards. The academic community has depended heavily on peer-review as a trustworthy mechanism of determining the most meritorious and methodologically sound research. However, poor reporting can obscure the true quality of research design and conduct, and this leaves the reviewer with an extraordinarily difficult task. At present, there is little evidence to support the usefulness of peer-review [45, 46], although some recent studies show that using reporting guidelines in the peer-review process does improve the quality of the published manuscript [47–49].

Some reporting guideline checklists include a right-most column in which authors are expected to report the page number of their manuscript on which a specific checklist item is described. This is intended to help authors ensure each checklist item is addressed and to aid peer-reviewers in locating reported text for each item within a document. However, this is not the best system for peer-reviewers to identify reporting inadequacies as they still have to search through much printed matter to locate the exact text that describes a checklist item. When multiple items are listed separately but reported together or vice versa, this problem is compounded, since it may be unclear exactly what content pertains to each item.

18.12 Impact of Reporting Guidelines

There have been many reports evaluating the impact of reporting guidelines. Two systematic reviews assessing both CONSORT and all other guidelines as a group are described below.

The completeness of reported trials has been assessed in at least 50 evaluative studies [50]. The review by Turner et al. assessed whether the completeness of reporting differed across trials published in journals that endorsed and did not endorse CONSORT or between periods before and after the endorsement of CONSORT within a journal or cohort of journals. Trials that adhered to the CONSORT (2001) checklist were significantly better reported, and this finding has remained robust over time [50, 51]. Although this might seem encouraging, reports of RCTs are still much less useful than they should be. Many key elements of trial design and results are still being reported at exceedingly low levels, even when published in journals that endorse CONSORT. For instance, the reporting of allocation concealment is adequate in only 45% of trials published in endorsing journals (22% in non-endorsers)—a suboptimal level for a methodologically crucial aspect of an RCT. Many other key methodological items are well reported in fewer than 50% of trials in endorsing journals.

Randomized trials are only a small proportion of the literature on the evaluation of medical interventions [52, 53]. However, these are a much more familiar study design to both researchers and readers. Also, the CONSORT guidelines were the first to be developed. Hence, the poor reporting of randomized trials does not bode well for guidelines for other study designs that are less prominent than

CONSORT. Those guidelines have ostensibly been less well received, implemented and adhered to. A review characterizing the impact of reporting guidelines other than CONSORT found that only 9 of 101 included guidelines had been evaluated by 26 evaluations meeting inclusion criteria: the *BMJ* checklist, CONSORT for harms outcome, CONSORT for herbal interventions, STARD, STRICTA, STROBE, QUOROM and PRISMA [54]. Only 13 evaluations had enough data for meta-analysis. No significant differences in the completeness of reporting between endorsers and non-endorsers, or before and after endorsement for any items (or sum of items) were observed for any guidelines except PRISMA; it appears to be associated with better overall reporting of systematic reviews based on three evaluations. In contrast to the volume of studies evaluating CONSORT ($n = 50$) and RCTs assessed for completeness of reporting ($n = 16,604$), there is little evidence from which to draw conclusions about the effectiveness of reporting guidelines other than CONSORT. One major limitation of the review was that authors of evaluations considered guideline publication to be the 'intervention' of interest rather than guideline endorsement and, therefore, did not evaluate the primary outcome (completeness of reporting) using the lens of endorsement. This illustrates the general problem that endorsement is variable even among CONSORT-endorsing journals [55, 56].

The impact of reporting guidelines, however, should not be understated and can be seen in other ways as well. For instance, the CONSORT statement and elaboration papers are among the most widely cited scientific contributions of all time (over 5300 citations, excluding self-citation). CONSORT 2010 is among the top 1% of article-level content contained in the Public Library of Science (www.plos.org). In addition to CONSORT 2010, three other reporting guidelines are among the top-cited papers in the 100 most-referenced journals (across all fields) since 2007. These are STROBE for reporting cohort, case–control and cross-sectional studies [33, 57], PRISMA [32, 58] and STARD [59, 60]. Their importance has been reiterated by journal editors but the extent of their endorsement is yet to be described.

18.13   Common Reporting Guidelines

Several editors indicate particular interest in a few specific reporting guidelines. These are described in Table 18.4.

18.14   Importance of Reporting Research Protocols

A well-described protocol helps detect the recently identified problem of reporting bias [61–64]. Selective reporting of outcomes, for instance, can only be identified when readers are able to compare planned versus reported outcomes. Chan and colleagues first described selective reporting in trials through a comparison of 48 protocols of RCTs that were funded by the Canadian Institutes of Health Research (CIHR) and their 68 associated publications [65]. More than one in every three primary outcomes (40%) differed between the protocol and full publication, and statistically

Table 18.4 Common reporting guidelines for health research

Reporting guideline	Type of study	When and how to use
CONSORT	Parallel-group randomized trial	For reporting trials comparing efficacy between treatments and/or control
CONSORT extension for harms	Randomized trial with harms as an outcome	For reporting randomized trials measuring harms-related outcomes
CONSORT extension for non-pharmacological interventions	Randomized trial of non-pharmacological intervention	For reporting trials evaluating at least one non-pharmacological intervention as a treatment arm
CONSORT extension for cluster randomized trials	Cluster randomized trial	For reporting randomized trials in which groups of patients are randomized rather than individuals
CONSORT extension for non-inferiority and equivalence trials	Non-inferiority and equivalence trials	For reporting randomized trials intended to determine whether one intervention is no worse than another or whether at least two interventions are therapeutically similar
PRISMA	Systematic review and meta-analysis	For reporting systematic reviews that may or may not contain meta-analyses or meta-analyses not contained within reviews
STROBE	Observational study	For reporting cohort, case–control and cross-sectional studies
STARD	Diagnostic accuracy study	For reporting studies reporting diagnostic tests

positive efficacy outcomes were nearly three times more likely to be reported than non-significant efficacy outcomes. This finding has been confirmed in subsequent studies that compared planned to completed methods, and there is now compelling evidence that selective reporting overestimates the benefits of treatments [61].

The preparation and availability of a protocol also offer research teams an opportunity to ensure that a study is carefully planned and that what is planned is explicitly documented before the study starts, thus promoting accountability, research integrity and transparency of the eventual report. A protocol preparation process may also reduce arbitrariness in decision-making by allowing researchers to anticipate potential problems before they transpire. To this end, two reporting guidelines initiatives have emerged to facilitate the complete documentation of research protocols for randomized trials (the 'SPIRIT' initiative [66, 67]) and for systematic reviews and meta-analyses (the 'PRISMA-P' initiative) [68, 69].

18.15 Summary

Poor reporting is not always an indication of poorly designed research, although the two can be inextricably linked [70]. In some cases, poor reporting may indicate a lack of understanding of the need to document methodological aspects of studies related to an increased risk of bias. It is therefore important that elements considered essential in the reporting of trials should be incorporated in the design of trials. Prospective study registration in one of the clinical trial registries and the newly launched international registry for systematic reviews (PROSPERO) is one such step. These initiatives are closely linked to both the earlier CONSORT and PRISMA reporting guidelines and to the subsequent SPIRIT and PRISMA-P guidelines for protocols.

Thus, paying attention to reporting guidelines not only helps authors report their research completely, transparently, and accurately but may also help improve the study design during the planning of research. These effects should result in a reduced risk of bias in research.

References

1. Macleod MR, Michie S, Roberts I, Dirnagl U, Chalmers I, Ioannidis JPA, et al. Biomedical research: increasing value, reducing waste. Lancet. 2014;383:101–4.
2. Chalmers I, Bracken MBM, Djulbegovic B, Garattini S, Grant J, Gülmezoglu AM, et al. How to increase value and reduce waste when research priorities are set. Lancet. 2014;383:156–65.
3. Ioannidis JPA, Greenland S, Hlatky MA, Khoury MJ, Macleod MR, Moher D, et al. Increasing value and reducing waste in research design, conduct, and analysis. Lancet. 2014;383:166–75.
4. Al-Shahi Salman R, Beller E, Kagan J, Hemminki E, Phillips RS, Savulescu J, et al. Increasing value and reducing waste in biomedical research regulation and management. Lancet. 2014;383:176–85.
5. Chan A-WA, Song F, Vickers A, Jefferson T, Dickersin K, Gøtzsche PC, et al. Increasing value and reducing waste: addressing inaccessible research. Lancet. 2014;383:257–66.
6. Glasziou P, Altman DG, Bossuyt P, Boutron I, Clarke M, Julious S, et al. Reducing waste from incomplete or unusable reports of biomedical research. Lancet. 2014;383:267–76.
7. Tallon D, Chard J, Dieppe P. Relation between agendas of the research community and the research consumer. Lancet. 2000;355:2037–40.
8. Pildal J, Hróbjartsson A, Jørgensen KJ, Hilden J, Altman DG, Gøtzsche PC. Impact of allocation concealment on conclusions drawn from meta-analyses of randomized trials. Int J Epidemiol. 2007;36:847–57. Erratum in: Int J Epidemiol 2008;37:422.
9. Odgaard-Jensen J, Vist GE, Timmer A, Kunz R, Akl EA, Schünemann H, et al. Randomisation to protect against selection bias in healthcare trials. Cochrane Database Syst Rev. 2011;(4):MR000012. https://doi.org/10.1002/14651858.MR000012.pub3.
10. Hopewell S, Clarke M, Stewart L, Tierney J. Time to publication for results of clinical trials. Cochrane Database Syst Rev. 2007;(2):MR000011.
11. Hopewell S, Loudon K, Clarke MJ, Oxman AD, Dickersin K. Publication bias in clinical trials due to statistical significance or direction of trial results. Cochrane Database Syst Rev. 2009;(1):MR000006. https://doi.org/10.1002/14651858.MR000006.pub3.
12. A consensus statement on research misconduct in the UK. BMJ. 2012;344:e1111. https://doi.org/10.1136/bmj.e1111.
13. Moher D. Reporting research results: a moral obligation for all researchers. Can J Anaesth. 2007;54:331–5.
14. Groves T. Enhancing the quality and transparency of health research. BMJ. 2008;337:a718. https://doi.org/10.1136/bmj.a718.
15. Ioannidis JP. Contradicted and initially stronger effects in highly cited clinical research. JAMA. 2005;294:218–28.
16. Tharyan P, George AT, Kirubakaran R, Barnabas JP. Reporting of methods was better in the Clinical Trials Registry–India than in Indian journal publications. J Clin Epidemiol. 2013;66:10–22. https://doi.org/10.1016/j.jclinepi.2011.11.011.

17. Mignini LE, Khan KS. Methodological quality of systematic reviews of animal studies: a survey of reviews of basic research. BMC Med Res Methodol. 2006;6:10.
18. Glasziou P, Meats E, Heneghan C, Shepperd S. What is missing from descriptions of treatment in trials and reviews? BMJ. 2008;336:1472–4. https://doi.org/10.1136/bmj.39590.732037.47.
19. Hopewell S, Dutton S, Yu LM, Chan AW, Altman DG. The quality of reports of randomised trials in 2000 and 2006: comparative study of articles indexed in PubMed. BMJ. 2010;340:c723. https://doi.org/10.1136/bmj.c723.
20. Duff JM, Leather H, Walden EO, LaPlant KD, George TJ Jr. Adequacy of published oncology randomized controlled trials to provide therapeutic details needed for clinical application. J Natl Cancer Inst. 2010;102:702–5. https://doi.org/10.1093/jnci/djq117.
21. de Vries TW, van Roon EN. Low quality of reporting adverse drug reactions in paediatric randomised controlled trials. Arch Dis Child. 2010;95:1023–6. https://doi.org/10.1136/adc.2009.175562.
22. Nolte S, Wong D, Lachford G. Amphetamines for schizophrenia. Cochrane Database Syst Rev. 2004;(4):CD004964.
23. Birnie AJ, Bath-Hextall FJ, Ravenscroft JC, Williams HC. Interventions to reduce Staphylococcus aureus in the management of atopic eczema. Cochrane Database Syst Rev. 2008;(3):CD003871. https://doi.org/10.1002/14651858.CD003871.pub2.
24. Schulz KF, Chalmers I, Hayes RJ, Altman DG. Empirical evidence of bias. Dimensions of methodological quality associated with estimates of treatment effects in controlled trials. JAMA. 1995;273:408–12.
25. Moher D, Weeks L, Ocampo M, Seely D, Sampson M, Altman DG, et al. Describing reporting guidelines for health research: a systematic review. J Clin Epidemiol. 2011;64:718–42. https://doi.org/10.1016/j.jclinepi.2010.09.013.
26. Winters BD, Gurses AP, Lehmann H, Sexton JB, Rampersad CJ, Pronovost PJ. Clinical review: checklists—translating evidence into practice. Crit Care. 2009;13:210. https://doi.org/10.1186/cc7792.
27. Gawande A. The checklist manifesto: how to get things right. New York: Metropolitan Books; 2010.
28. Haynes AB, Weiser TG, Berry WR, Lipsitz SR, Breizat AH, Dellinger EP, et al. A surgical safety checklist to reduce morbidity and mortality in a global population. N Engl J Med. 2009;360:491–9. https://doi.org/10.1056/NEJMsa0810119.
29. Pronovost P, Needham D, Berenholtz S, Sinopoli D, Chu H, Cosgrove S, et al. An intervention to decrease catheter-related bloodstream infections in the ICU. N Engl J Med. 2006;355:2725–32. Erratum in: N Engl J Med 2007;356:2660.
30. Shamseer L, Stevens A, Skidmore B, Turner L, Altman DG, Hirst A, et al. Does journal endorsement of reporting guidelines influence the completeness of reporting of health research? A systematic review protocol. Syst Rev. 2012;1:24. https://doi.org/10.1186/2046-4053-1-24.
31. Moher D, Hopewell S, Schulz KF, Montori V, Gøtzsche PC, Devereaux PJ, et al. CONSORT 2010 explanation and elaboration: updated guidelines for reporting parallel group randomised trials. BMJ. 2010;340:c869. https://doi.org/10.1136/bmj.c869.
32. Liberati A, Altman DG, Tetzlaff J, Mulrow C, Gøtzsche PC, Ioannidis JP, et al. The PRISMA statement for reporting systematic reviews and meta-analyses of studies that evaluate health care interventions: explanation and elaboration. PLoS Med. 2009;6:e1000100. https://doi.org/10.1371/journal.pmed.1000100.
33. Vandenbroucke JP, von Elm E, Altman DG, Gøtzsche PC, Mulrow CD, Pocock SJ, et al. Strengthening the Reporting of Observational Studies in Epidemiology (STROBE): explanation and elaboration. PLoS Med. 2007;4:e297.
34. Call for comments on a proposal to improve reporting of clinical trials in the biomedical literature. Working Group on Recommendations for Reporting of Clinical Trials in the Biomedical Literature. Ann Intern Med. 1994;121:894–5.
35. A proposal for structured reporting of randomized controlled trials. The Standards of Reporting Trials Group. JAMA. 1994;272:1926–31. Erratum in: JAMA 1995;273:776.

36. Begg C, Cho M, Eastwood S, Horton R, Moher D, Olkin I, et al. Improving the quality of reporting of randomized controlled trials. The CONSORT statement. JAMA. 1996;276:637–9.
37. Moher D, Schulz KF, Altman DG, CONSORT. The CONSORT statement: revised recommendations for improving the quality of reports of parallel group randomized trials. BMC Med Res Methodol. 2001;1:2.
38. Schulz KF, Altman DG, Moher D, CONSORT Group. CONSORT 2010 statement: updated guidelines for reporting parallel group randomized trials. Ann Intern Med. 2010;152:726–32. https://doi.org/10.7326/0003-4819-152-11-201006010-00232.
39. Gabriel SE, Normand SL. Getting the methods right—the foundation of patient-centered outcomes research. N Engl J Med. 2012;367:787–90. https://doi.org/10.1056/NEJMp1207437.
40. Williams HC. Cars, CONSORT 2010, and clinical practice. Trials. 2010;11:33. https://doi.org/10.1186/1745-6215-11-33.
41. Simera I, Moher D, Hirst A, Hoey J, Schulz KF, Altman DG. Transparent and accurate reporting increases reliability, utility, and impact of your research: reporting guidelines and the EQUATOR Network. BMC Med. 2010;8:24. https://doi.org/10.1186/1741-7015-8-24.
42. Simera I, Altman DG. Writing a research article that is 'fit for purpose': EQUATOR Network and reporting guidelines. Evid Based Med. 2009;14:132–4. https://doi.org/10.1136/ebm.14.5.132.
43. Moher D, Schulz KF, Simera I, Altman DG. Guidance for developers of health research reporting guidelines. PLoS Med. 2010;7(2):e1000217. https://doi.org/10.1371/journal.pmed.1000217.
44. International Steering Committee of Medical Editors. Uniform requirements for manuscripts submitted to biomedical journals. Br Med J. 1979;1:532–5.
45. Jefferson T, Rudin M, Brodney Folse S, Davidoff F. Editorial peer review for improving the quality of reports of biomedical studies. Cochrane Database Syst Rev. 2007;(2):MR000016.
46. Demicheli V, Di Pietrantonj C. Peer review for improving the quality of grant applications. Cochrane Database Syst Rev. 2007;(2):MR000003.
47. Cobo E, Cortés J, Ribera JM, Cardellach F, Selva-O'Callaghan A, Kostov B, et al. Effect of using reporting guidelines during peer review on quality of final manuscripts submitted to a biomedical journal: masked randomised trial. BMJ. 2011;343:d6783. https://doi.org/10.1136/bmj.d6783.
48. Cobo E, Selva-O'Callagham A, Ribera JM, Cardellach F, Dominguez R, Vilardell M. Statistical reviewers improve reporting in biomedical articles: a randomized trial. PLoS One. 2007;2:e332.
49. Hirst A, Altman DG. Are peer reviewers encouraged to use reporting guidelines? A survey of 116 health research journals. PLoS One. 2012;7:e35621. https://doi.org/10.1371/journal.pone.0035621.
50. Turner L, Shamseer L, Altman DG, Weeks L, Peters J, Kober T, et al. Consolidated standards of reporting trials (CONSORT) and the completeness of reporting of randomised controlled trials (RCTs) published in medical journals. Cochrane Database Syst Rev. 2012;(11):MR000030. https://doi.org/10.1002/14651858.MR000030.pub2.
51. Plint AC, Moher D, Morrison A, Schulz K, Altman DG, Hill C, et al. Does the CONSORT checklist improve the quality of reports of randomised controlled trials? A systematic review. Med J Aust. 2006;185:263–7.
52. Funai EF, Rosenbush EJ, Lee MJ, Del Priore G. Distribution of study designs in four major US journals of obstetrics and gynecology. Gynecol Obstet Invest. 2001;51:8–11.
53. Scales CD Jr, Norris RD, Peterson BL, Preminger GM, Dahm P. Clinical research and statistical methods in the urology literature. J Urol. 2005;174(4 Pt 1):1374–9.
54. Stevens A, Shamseer L, Weinstein E, Yazdi F, Turner L, Thielman J, et al. Relation of completeness of reporting of health research to journals' endorsement of reporting guidelines: systematic review. BMJ. 2014;348:g3804.
55. Altman DG. Endorsement of the CONSORT statement by high impact medical journals: survey of instructions for authors. BMJ. 2005;330:1056–7.

56. Hopewell S, Altman DG, Moher D, Schulz KF. Endorsement of the CONSORT Statement by high impact factor medical journals: a survey of journal editors and journal 'Instructions to Authors'. Trials. 2008;9:20. https://doi.org/10.1186/1745-6215-9-20.

57. von Elm E, Altman DG, Egger M, Pocock SJ, Gøtzsche PC, Vandenbroucke JP, STROBE Initiative. Strengthening the Reporting of Observational Studies in Epidemiology (STROBE) statement: guidelines for reporting observational studies. BMJ. 2007;335:806–8.

58. Moher D, Liberati A, Tetzlaff J, Altman DG, PRISMA Group. Preferred reporting items for systematic reviews and meta-analyses: the PRISMA statement. BMJ. 2009;339:b2535. https://doi.org/10.1136/bmj.b2535.

59. Bossuyt PM, Reitsma JB, Bruns DE, Gatsonis CA, Glasziou PP, Irwig LM, et al. Towards complete and accurate reporting of studies of diagnostic accuracy: the STARD initiative. Standards for Reporting of Diagnostic Accuracy. Clin Chem. 2003;49:1–6.

60. Bossuyt PM, Reitsma JB, Bruns DE, Gatsonis CA, Glasziou PP, Irwig LM, et al. The STARD statement for reporting studies of diagnostic accuracy: explanation and elaboration. Clin Chem. 2003;49:7–18.

61. Dwan K, Altman DG, Cresswell L, Blundell M, Gamble CL, Williamson PR. Comparison of protocols and registry entries to published reports for randomized controlled trials. Cochrane Database Syst Rev. 2011;(1):MR000031. https://doi.org/10.1002/14651858.MR000031.pub2.

62. Kirkham JJ, Dwan KM, Altman DG, Gamble C, Dodd S, Smyth R, et al. The impact of outcome reporting bias in randomised controlled trials on a cohort of systematic reviews. BMJ. 2010;340:c365. https://doi.org/10.1136/bmj.c365.

63. Kirkham JJ, Altman DG, Williamson PR. Bias due to changes in specified outcomes during the systematic review process. PLoS One. 2010;5:e9810. https://doi.org/10.1371/journal.pone.0009810.

64. Dwan K, Altman DG, Arnaiz JA, Bloom J, Chan AW, Cronin E, et al. Systematic review of the empirical evidence of study publication bias and outcome reporting bias. PLoS One. 2008;3:e3081. https://doi.org/10.1371/journal.pone.0003081.

65. Chan AW, Krleza-Jerić K, Schmid I, Altman DG. Outcome reporting bias in randomized trials funded by the Canadian Institutes of Health Research. CMAJ. 2004;171:735–40.

66. Chan AW, Tetzlaff JM, Altman DG, Laupacis A, Gøtzsche PC, Krleža-Jerić K, et al. SPIRIT 2013 statement: defining standard protocol items for clinical trials. Ann Intern Med. 2013;158:200–7. https://doi.org/10.7326/0003-4819-158-3-201302050-00583.

67. Chan AW, Tetzlaff JM, Gøtzsche PC, Altman DG, Mann H, Berlin JA, et al. SPIRIT 2013 explanation and elaboration: guidance for protocols of clinical trials. BMJ. 2013;346:e7586.

68. Moher D, Shamseer L, Clarke M, Ghersi D, Liberati A, Petticrew M, et al. Preferred reporting items for systematic review and meta-analysis protocols (PRISMA-P) 2015 statement. Syst Rev. 2015;4:1. https://doi.org/10.1186/2046-4053-4-1.

69. Shamseer L, Moher D, Clarke M, Ghersi D, Liberati A, Petticrew M, et al. Preferred reporting items for systematic review and meta-analysis protocols (PRISMA-P) 2015: elaboration and explanation. BMJ. 2015;349:g7647.

70. Soares HP, Daniels S, Kumar A, Clarke M, Scott C, Swann S, Djulbegovic B, Radiation Therapy Oncology Group. Bad reporting does not mean bad methods for randomised trials: observational study of randomised controlled trials performed by the Radiation Therapy Oncology Group. BMJ. 2004;328:22–4.

Open Access Journals

19

Trish Groves

19.1 Introduction

The American sociologist Robert K. Merton has argued that science is underpinned by four moral elements: communalism (where scientists give up intellectual property rights in exchange for recognition and esteem), universalism (where truth is evaluated in terms of universal criteria), disinterestedness (where scientists are rewarded for acting in ways that appear to be selfless) and organized scepticism (where all ideas must be tested and are subject to rigorous, structured, community scrutiny) [1]. To put it more simply, scientific advances involve sharing and peer review of research questions that have been objectively tested.

For the largely public and charitable funders of research and other scholarly work, open access publishing maximizes the influence and reach of the research findings of their grantees. Moreover, it ensures that publicly funded work is widely available.

For authors, open access greatly facilitates the communal sharing of their scientific work, increases their audience and potentially widens the influence of their work. To many authors, however, the open access model may seem to be just another hurdle to publication of their research and other scholarly work. Not only do they have to do good work, write it up nicely, follow increasingly complex instructions to authors and survive peer review; now they also have to pay a fee to get their accepted articles published.

For readers, open access to scientific information can help to greatly increase their knowledge. Yet, for many readers of medical journals, the concept of 'open access' is irrelevant. As long as they can freely read online the articles that they want to read, they do not care how access was provided or who paid for it. After all, most information on the internet is free anyway.

T. Groves
BMJ and BMJ Open, London, UK
e-mail: tgroves@bmj.com

© The National Medical Journal of India 2018
P. Sahni, R. Aggarwal (eds.), *Reporting and Publishing Research in the Biomedical Sciences*, https://doi.org/10.1007/978-981-10-7062-4_19

19.2   Philosophy and History of Open Access to Academic Literature

Open access in its purest sense—making scholarly information available to every-one—has been around for at least as long as public libraries, the earliest of which in Europe opened at London's Guildhall in 1425. It is hardly a new idea in India either: Mahatma Gandhi's publication *Hind Swaraj* (1909) was translated into English a year later as *Indian Home Rule* and published with 'No rights reserved' [2].

But, these days, 'open access' implies unrestricted online access, a concept that has been in existence for about 20 years. The world's first website was launched in August 1992 at info.cern.ch. With rapid growth of the World Wide Web over the following decade came the idea that articles reporting publicly funded research, particularly in health sciences, ought to be accessible to anyone, irrespective of the ability to pay.

This idea became a movement in December 2001 at an international meeting in Budapest, Hungary, convened by the Open Society Institute (the institute was established in 1993 by investor and philanthropist George Soros, whose foundation aims to develop and support democracies and to foster open societies; http://www.soros.org). Two months later, 16 participants from that meeting signed a statement launching the Budapest Open Access Initiative (http://www.soros.org/openaccess/read) and asserting that:

> 'An old tradition and a new technology have converged to make possible an unprecedented public good. The old tradition is the willingness of scientists and scholars to publish the fruits of their research in scholarly journals without payment, for the sake of inquiry and knowledge. The new technology is the internet. The public good they make possible is the worldwide electronic distribution of the peer-reviewed journal literature, and completely free and unrestricted access to it by all scientists, scholars, teachers, students, and other curious minds. Removing access barriers to this literature will accelerate research, enrich education, share the learning of the rich with the poor and the poor with the rich, make this literature as useful as it can be, and lay the foundation for uniting humanity in a common intellectual conversation and quest for knowledge.'

The initiative called on institutions and individuals to help open up access to peer-reviewed journal articles and preprints and to remove price barriers (online paywalls). Two complementary strategies would achieve such open access: 'self-archiving' of articles in open electronic repositories and publication in open access journals.

Since 2001, the statement has been signed by more than 6000 supporters world-wide and has been reinforced by numerous other statements and initiatives, including the Bethesda Statement on Open Access Publishing (http://www.earlham.edu/~peters) and the Berlin Declaration on Open Access to Knowledge in the Sciences and Humanities, both launched in 2003 (http://www.zim.mpg.de/openaccess-berlin). The Indian National Science Academy immediately signed the Berlin Declaration, and the Indian Medlars Centre [the ICMR-NIC Centre for Biomedical Information, established by the National Informatics Centre (NIC) and the Indian Council of Medical Research (ICMR)] started hosting open access versions of many Indian medical journals [3].

That same year, two biomedical publishers—the Public Library of Science (PLoS, using charitable funding) and BioMed Central (using venture capital)—launched and developed the 'author-pays' model of open access publishing where the publisher levies fees to publish accepted peer-reviewed articles. Soon after that, two large funders of research—the Howard Hughes Medical Institute in the United States and the Wellcome Trust in the United Kingdom—pledged to cover their grantees' open access fees. The *BMJ* (*British Medical Journal*), already a partly open access journal for several years, said on the occasion: 'open access publishing had taken off' [4].

In 2006 at a workshop on electronic publishing and open access at the Indian Institute of Science, Bangalore—and supported by the Open Society Institute—policymakers and research scientists from India, China, Brazil and South Africa adopted a model national open access policy for developing countries (Box 19.1).

Box 19.1 National Open Access Policy for Developing Countries: India's Policy
The Government of India expects the authors of papers reporting publicly funded research to maximize the accessibility, usage and applications of their findings. To this end:
As a condition for research funding, the government:

1. Requires electronic copies of any research papers that have been accepted for publication in a peer-reviewed journal and are supported in whole or in part by government funding, to be deposited in an institutional digital repository [IR] immediately upon acceptance for publication
2. Encourages government grant holders to provide open access to their deposited papers immediately upon deposit
3. Encourages government grant holders to publish in a suitable open access journal where one exists

Source: http://www.ncsi.iisc.ernet.in/OAworkshop2006/

19.3 What Exactly Is Open Access?

'Free access' and 'open access' are not the same thing. Peter Suber, professor of philosophy at Earlham University and director of Harvard University's Open Access Project, has for many years been the world's leading advocate and blogger about open access to scholarly content. In his excellent, authoritative introduction to the concept and logistics of open access (http://www.earlham.edu/~peters/fos/overview.htm), he explains that 'free access' lifts price barriers, whereas 'open access' lifts at least some barriers to reusing published content without having to obtain explicit permission from the copyright holder(s). The ability to share and reuse scholarly articles, or at least some of the text and illustrations they contain, is vital for teaching, learning and research. It has advantages for authors as well as readers.

Open access makes reuse easier to do quickly and affordably, with proper and full attribution of the original source.

Open access does not apply only to published information. Indeed, there is much valuable scholarly content that is never formally published in journals, monographs or books, and the open access movement has enabled scholars to share it and readers to find it.

19.4 Free Access

19.4.1 Free Access to Journals: Provided by Journal Owners and Publishers

Many journals are published online with free access to the full text of all contents. These journals tend to be set up and run by not-for-profit institutions and are edited by doctors and other academics who are not paid for their efforts. These may be hosted online by free publishing platforms such as Bioline International (which currently hosts 14 Indian medical journals published by Medknow Publications; http://www.bioline.org.br/journals) and the Journals Online project (which hosts journals in Bangladesh and Nepal; http://www.banglajol.info, http://www.nepjol.info). These not-for-profit platforms aim to reduce the knowledge gap between the world's south and north, help improve global understanding of health and build research capacity in less-developed countries.

Such journals do not intend to make money and cost (relatively) little to produce. They are often funded by public money because institutions recognize that high-quality free journals can be of great value to readers who want to keep up-to-date with local or regional developments in medicine and for whom the research evidence and education published in high-impact international medical journals are largely irrelevant. They may also be valuable to readers in other parts of the world facing similar challenges to public health and clinical practice. Free online access gives these journals a global reach and, importantly, also brings authors a much wider audience for their writing and research.

Some for-profit platforms also provide a range of free access. HighWire Press, which hosts many medical journals including the *BMJ* (bmj.com), claims to be the largest archive of free full-text science on earth (http://highwire.stanford.edu/lists/freeart.dtl). As of On the 25th of March, 2015, HighWire Press was 'assisting in the online publication of 2,434,604 free full-text articles and 7,659,003 total articles', with 31 websites with free trial periods, 124 completely free sites and 287 sites with free back issues (accessed on on the 25th of April, 2015).

19.4.2 Free Access to Journals: Provided by Publishers in Collaboration with Not-For-Profit Bodies

What about the journals—including those with global influence and high impact factors—that levy subscriptions to individuals and libraries? Students, academics and doctors in India and richer countries are often able to access such journals freely online within their universities or hospitals because the institutions' libraries have online subscriptions. But, when working in community or rural settings or at home or when accessing the internet via a mobile phone, tablet computer, or internet café, these professionals hit a journal paywall and cannot access articles without paying. Moreover, libraries and public institutions in many countries lack the funds to pay for journal subscriptions.

To plug these gaps, international publishers and other organizations are collaborating in a variety of ways to highlight and increase the visibility of freely available information and research on health. For example, every *BMJ* article published since the journal's first issue in October 1840 is available online at www.bmj.com. This archive was produced by digitally scanning 824,183 pages of the print journal. The process cost about $1 (£0.68; Euros 0.76) a page and was funded by the US National Library of Medicine (NLM) and the United Kingdom's Wellcome Trust and Joint Information Systems Committee. In addition to all *BMJ* research articles being openly accessible to all on the journal's website, all articles, both research and non-research, published in the journal between 1840 and July 2008 are also available free on PubMed Central (www.ncbi.nlm.nih.gov/pmc), without any registration.

Much wider collaborations between publishers include the International Network for the Availability of Scientific Publications (INASP, http://www.inasp.info/) and its Programme for the Enhancement of Research Information (PERii, http://www.inasp.info/file/98804148d71a72e2c691a2dda813aa45/perii-open-access.html). Perhaps the best known of these initiatives is, however, HINARI.

HINARI. In 2002, the World Health Organization (WHO) and several large publishers of health-related information and biomedical journals launched the HINARI programme (Health InterNetwork to Research Initiative, http://www.who.int/hinari/en/). HINARI is now part of Research4Life along with three other similar programmes—AGORA (focusing on agriculture), OARE (focusing on environment) and ARDI (focusing on applied science and technology).

HINARI gives health institutions in low-income countries free online access to content that elsewhere requires subscriptions. HINARI currently makes around 14,000 journals and 46,000 e-books in 30 different languages available to institutions in more than 100 countries (http://extranet.who.int/hinari/en/journals.php) (Fig. 19.1).

Local, not-for-profit health institutions in two groups of countries may register for access to publications through HINARI, with eligibility based on four factors: total gross national income (GNI) (World Bank figures); GNI per capita (World Bank figures); United Nations least developed country (LDCs) list; and human development index (HDI). Institutions in countries with at least one of the following criteria may be eligible for free access: inclusion in the LDCs; an HDI of less than 0.63; or GNI per capita at or below US$1600. Those countries that do not match at least one of the above criteria and with either a GNI per capita less than $5000 or HDI at or below 0.67 may be eligible to pay a fee of US$ 1000 per year (*see* lists of countries at http://www.who.int/hinari/eligibility/en/). But India, despite its poverty levels (http://data.worldbank.org/country/india), is not covered by HINARI because the participating publishers see it and other BRICS (Brazil, Russia, India, China and South Africa) countries as valuable emerging markets.

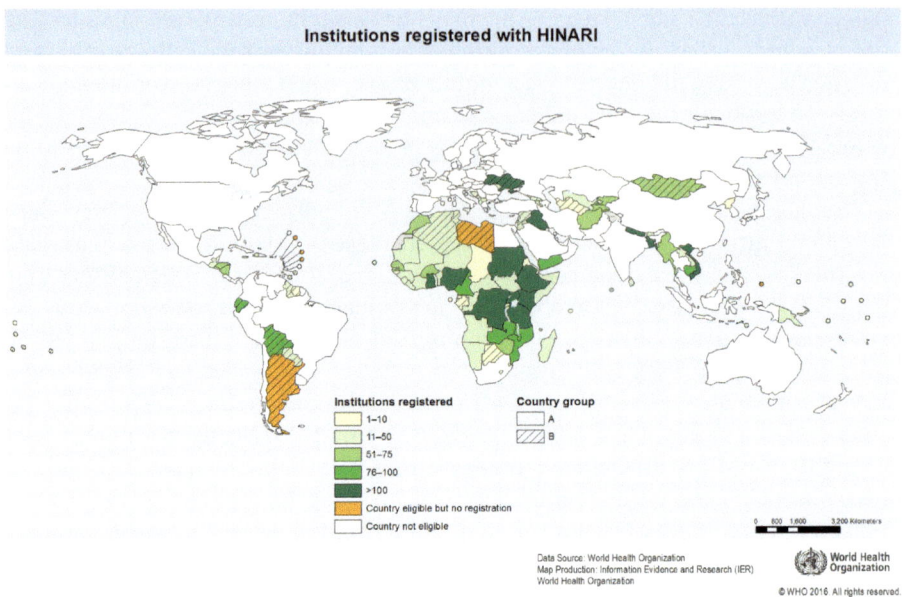

Fig. 19.1 Map of countries with HINARI access in 2016. Reprinted with the permission of WHO from http://www.who.int/hinari/Global_HINARI_registered_2016.png (accessed on 4 June 2016). The boundaries and names shown and the designations used on this map do not imply the expression of any opinion whatsoever on the part of the World Health Organization concerning the legal status of any country, territory, city or area or of its authorities, or concerning the delimitation of its frontiers or boundaries. Dotted and dashed lines on maps represent approximate border lines for which there may not yet be full agreement

19.4.3 Free Access to Journals: Provided by Governments

Many governments have invested in free portals to give academics in their countries free access to scholarly articles. The biggest repository of freely accessible biomedical journals and articles is PubMed Central® (PMC), launched in 2000 by the US government's National Center for Biotechnology Information (NCBI). When accessed in June 2016, PMC contained 3.9 million articles and the full text of more than 1800 journals (Fig. 19.2).

PMC is a free permanent digital archive of biomedical and life sciences journal literature at the US National Institutes of Health's National Library of Medicine (NIH/NLM), and it is free to everyone everywhere (http://www.ncbi.nlm.nih.gov/pmc/about/intro/). Journal literature is deposited in PMC by participating publishers, sometimes after a delay to allow the publishers to first make money from the 'paywall' (subscription barrier). And free access via PMC does not get around the journals' copyright protections for publishers and individual authors, and users still have to abide by the terms defined by copyright holders.

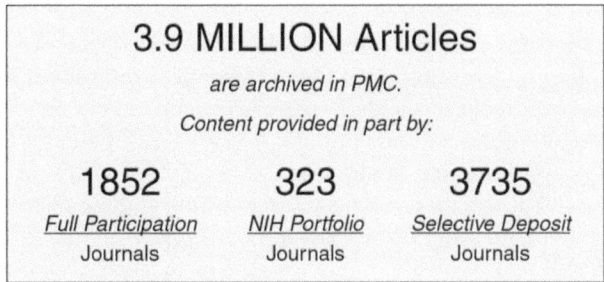

3.9 MILLION Articles

are archived in PMC.

Content provided in part by:

1852	323	3735
Full Participation Journals	*NIH Portfolio* Journals	*Selective Deposit* Journals

Fig. 19.2 Home page of PubMed Central showing the number of articles and journals indexed as on 4 June 2016

Given the importance of free access to both readers and authors in India, the National Informatics Centre (NIC) and Indian Council of Medical Research (ICMR) jointly established the ICMR-NIC Centre for Biomedical Information (the Indian Medlars Centre). From 1986 to 2009, the centre provided information support services to the medical research community and produced a bibliographic database (IndMED) that indexed more than 75 Indian medical journals (http://medind.nic.in/medindcf/medinda.shtml) and a portal (medIND) that provided free full-text access to 40 Indian medical journals. In 2010, the responsibility for maintaining, updating and improving these national resources was taken over by a new ICMR funded project: National Databases of Indian Medical Journals.

19.5 How Does Open Access Work?

Professor Peter Suber's 'very brief introduction to open access' is itself an open access document with a licence that allows free sharing with proper attribution (http://www.earlham.edu/~peters/fos/brief.htm), and it is well worth reproducing verbatim:

'Open-access (OA) literature is digital, online, free of charge, and free of most copyright and licensing restrictions. What makes it possible is the internet and the consent of the author or copyright-holder.

In most fields, scholarly journals do not pay authors, who can therefore consent to OA without losing revenue. In this respect, scholars and scientists are very differently situated from most musicians and movie-makers, and controversies about OA to music and movies do not carry over to research literature.

OA is entirely compatible with peer-review, and all the major OA initiatives for scientific and scholarly literature insist on its importance. Just as authors of journal articles donate their labour, so do most journal editors and referees participating in peer-review.

OA literature is not free to produce, even if it is less expensive to produce than conventionally published literature. The question is not whether scholarly literature can be made costless, but whether there are better ways to pay the bills than by charging readers and creating access barriers. Business models for paying the bills depend on how OA is delivered.

There are two primary vehicles for delivering OA to research articles: OA journals and OA archives or repositories (Box 19.2).

Box 19.2 A Brief Introduction to Open Access: Delivering Open Access

- OA archives or repositories do not perform peer review but simply make their contents freely available to the world. They may contain unrefereed preprints, refereed postprints or both. Archives may belong to institutions, such as universities and laboratories, or disciplines, such as physics and economics. Authors may archive their preprints without anyone else's permission, and a majority of journals already permit authors to archive their postprints. When archives comply with the metadata harvesting protocol of the Open Archives Initiative (OAI), then they are interoperable, and users can find their contents without knowing which archives exist, where they are located or what they contain. There is now open-source software for building and maintaining OAI-compliant archives and worldwide momentum for using it.

- OA journals perform peer review and then make the approved contents freely available to the world. Their expenses consist of peer review, manuscript preparation and server space. OA journals pay their bills very much the way broadcast television and radio stations do: those with an interest in disseminating the content pay the production costs upfront so that access can be free of charge for everyone with the right equipment. Sometimes this means that journals have a subsidy from the hosting university or professional society. Sometimes it means that journals charge a processing fee on accepted articles, to be paid by the author or the author's sponsor (employer, funding agency). OA journals that charge processing fees often waive them in cases of economic hardship. OA journals with institutional subsidies tend to charge no processing fees. OA journals can get by on lower subsidies or fees if they have income from other publications, advertising, priced add-ons or auxiliary services. Some institutions and consortia arrange fee discounts. Some OA publishers waive the fee for all researchers affiliated with institutions that have purchased an annual membership. There's a lot of room for creativity in finding ways to pay the costs of a peer-reviewed OA journal, and we're far from having exhausted our cleverness and imagination.'

The two main models are often called 'green' (where authors place their manuscripts, preprints or published articles in open access repositories) or 'gold', where publishers provide open access to journals' published articles (Fig. 19.3).

Many biomedical journals take yet another road, facilitating deposition of published articles in PMC after an initial period behind a paywall. Others are hybrid journals where some research is unlocked for a fee, for example, in the *BMJ* Group's specialist journals.

Suber also explains that the legal basis of open access is the expiration of copyright for old content or, for newer literature, consent of the copyright holder to allow free sharing and reuse. That consent is most easily conveyed by using a publication

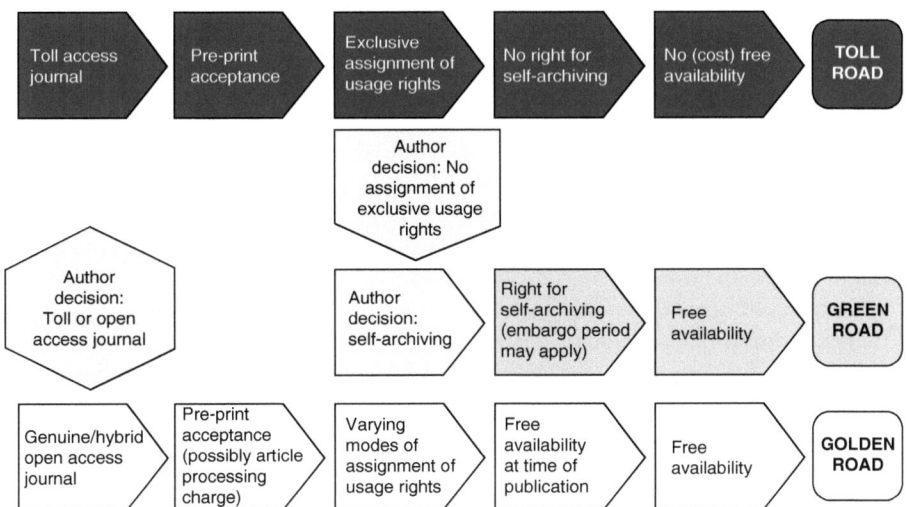

Fig. 19.3 Schematic diagram to show the different types of publication models [The Berlin Declaration http://oa.mpg.de/lang/en-uk/informationen-fur-autoren/open-access-publizieren/]

licence, and the most widespread (but not the only) types of licence are provided by Creative Commons, a US-based charitable organization (http://creativecommons. org/). Suber states that licences usually give consent to 'the unrestricted reading, downloading, copying, sharing, storing, printing, searching, linking, and crawling of the full-text of the work. Most authors choose to retain the right to block the distribution of mangled or misattributed copies. Some choose to block commercial re-use of the work. Essentially, these conditions block plagiarism, misrepresentation, and sometimes commercial re-use, and authorize all the uses required by legitimate scholarship, including those required by the technologies that facilitate online scholarly research.'

19.6   Open Access Fees

As gold open access journals do not charge the end users of their articles (the readers and subscribers), they usually instead seek article processing fees from the generators of articles (the authors and, if the reported work was funded, the funders).

The amount payable varies widely, with journals based in higher-income countries and those covering better-funded disciplines charging the most (http://www. rossmounce.co.uk/2012/09/04/the-gold-oa-plot-v0-2/) [5].

Critics of this 'author-pays' model of publishing worry that such payment introduces a conflict of interest for editors and threatens the objectivity of decision-making: the more research editors accept, the more money the journal will make. Some open access journals, including BioMed Central's *BMC Medicine Series*, *BMJ Open* and *The BMJ*, counter this by opening up the black box of peer review and posting reviewers' reports next to published papers. And many open access journals will consider requests to reduce or completely waive article processing fees if authors cannot pay: these include the PLoS journals, *The BMJ*, *BMJ Open* and *BioMed Central Journals*. Such journals ensure that all correspondence regarding payment of fees is handled only by administrative staff and that editors are oblivious to the authors' ability to pay. Even if the funding statement for a research paper mentions that the study was funded by, for example, the Wellcome Trust, the editor will not be able to tell if a fee will be payable: grants often have to cover several publications, and it is common for the authors to run out of money too soon.

Some gold open access journals, such as *PLoS One* and *BMJ Open*, rely entirely on peer-reviewers' judgements of the scientific quality and transparency of submitted articles. Editors do not judge articles' importance or contribution to knowledge but instead use bibliometrics and measures of online usage, share, and comment to tell whether published articles have proved useful to readers. The rapid growth of these journals suggests that authors and funders generally like this model, not least because these open access journals have lower thresholds for acceptance than traditional journals and yet have, increasingly, acceptable impact factors. Critics, however, worry that the lack of editorial filtering in such journals will lower the overall quality of the evidence base and lead to 'vanity publishing'.

Indeed, this model of publishing has allowed unscrupulous businesses to set up so-called 'predatory journals' which purport to offer peer review but have been shown to publish any submission, sometimes of very low quality or even unintelligible, for a fee. In response, the Committee on Publication Ethics (COPE), the Directory of Open Access Journals (DOAJ), the Open Access Scholarly Publishing Association (OASPA) and the World Association of Medical Editors (WAME) have compiled minimum criteria to assess journals seeking membership of their organizations (http://publicationethics.org/files/Principles_of_Transparency_and_Best_Practice_in_Scholarly_Publishingv2.pdf).

These principles of transparency and best practice in scholarly publishing may be used by any author, peer reviewer or other person who wishes to assess the trustworthiness and professionalism of a journal.

Another fear is that moving to this model would threaten the incomes of the professional societies that co-own and profit from traditional journals, thus reducing their ability to support activities for their members, such as continuing professional development. There is, perhaps, less widespread concern for the profits of the large international traditional publishers, whose income from institutional subscriptions and reprint sales would fall if they shifted to open access; however, it would not serve science well if their journals faltered.

A few journals levy submission fees instead of article processing fees: everyone has to pay on submission but at a much lower rate. The argument in favour of submission fees is that all authors contribute equally to the costs of peer review and publication, and there is no danger of a perverse incentive towards high acceptance rates. These journals offer no waivers, however, and it is not clear how funders and authors of rejected manuscripts feel about this model [6].

19.7 Open Access Mandates

If gold open access depended on authors opening their wallets, it would almost certainly fail. But many large funders now insist on open access—through either the green or gold route—to the outputs of work that they have funded and are willing to pay journals' article processing fees to ensure this. For an up-to-date list of funders' mandates, open access publishers and open access repositories visit the SHERPA (Securing a Hybrid Environment for Research Preservation and Access) website, initially established just for the United Kingdom but now a comprehensive, international resource (http://www.sherpa.ac.uk/index.html).

Governments, too, are increasingly supporting open access publishing. In July 2012, the UK government, the major public funder Research Councils UK and the Higher Education Funding Council for England (HEFCE) all announced policies that will greatly accelerate the shift to gold open access, while the European Commission recommended open access policies for the European Union member states and the Federal Research Public Access Act (FRPAA) headed to the US Congress [7]. In July 2015, the Fair Access to Science and Technology Research Act (FASTR), building on the failed FRPAA, was awaiting a full vote in the US Senate.

19.8 Gold and Hybrid Open Access Journals

Physics was the discipline that embraced open access most quickly and widely. Medicine was a lot slower. Having said that, within two and a half years of the birth of the web, the *BMJ* (*British Medical Journal*) had launched 'eBMJ' at www.bmj.com, and in 1998 the *BMJ* became one of the first journals to provide full free access to all of its contents. From 2005, bmj.com gradually introduced a paywall for non-research articles, so that income from subscriptions could support continuing free access to research articles. In 2010 the *BMJ* introduced article processing fees for research articles, which apply only when authors can claim the money back, in full, from whoever funded the research.

In their paper in *PLoS One*, the world's largest open access journal, Laakso and colleagues report on the development of open access journals from the early 1990s until 2009 [8]. By analysing a stratified sample of titles from almost 5000 journals listed in the Directory of Open Access Journals (http://www.doaj.org/) and a separate sample of pioneer open access journals, the authors showed that open access publishing had grown rapidly during the period 1993–2009 (Fig. 19.4).

During 2000–2009, the average annual growth rate was 18% for the number of open access journals and 30% for the number of articles therein, whereas the background annual growth in journal publishing in general over this period was reported as only 3.5%. The authors also noted that some journals made the transition during this period from subscription-only to hybrid or to full gold open access publishing models.

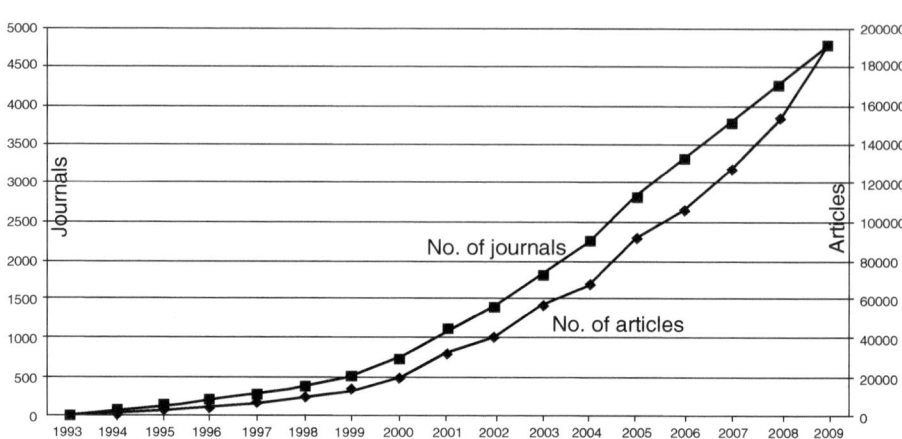

Fig. 19.4 The development of open access publishing 1993–2009 (available at doi: 10.1371/journal.pone.0020961; accessed on 28 April 2015)

Two information specialists looked at the status of Indian open access journals of all disciplines as listed in the Directory of Open Access Journals (DOAJ) and used citation rates from Google Scholar [9]. In March 2011, India was the fifth most prolific producer of open access journals (307 journals, with the majority—120—covering medical science), preceded by the United States (1200), Brazil (571), the United Kingdom (492) and Spain (381). Within Asia, India ranked much higher than Japan (105) and China (29). The growth rate of Indian open access journals increased greatly between 2006 and 2011. Of the top ten Indian journals by citation rate, six had adopted open access from 2010 onwards and before that they were available only in print and on subscription, with much lower citations rates.

Muthu Madhan and Subbiah Arunachalam reported further in 2011 that there were 360 Indian open access journals. Most of the papers published in these journals were written by Indian researchers, whereas India's contribution to the 'authors-pay' journals published by BioMed Central and PLoS was 'modest at best' [3]. The authors suggested that self-archiving in open repositories may still be an important option for India.

19.9 Open Access Repositories

Peter Suber, yet again, is a good source of information about open repositories for self-archiving, arguing that:

> 'green open access is less expensive than gold open access and can easily accommodate the full research output of a university, funding agency, or nation. Just as importantly, green open access can be mandated today and gold cannot. Because only about 30% of the world's peer-reviewed journals are open access, a policy requiring authors to publish in open access journals would limit their freedom to submit work to the journals of their choice. That could change if enough journals convert to open access, or enough adopt open access options, to become eligible for reimbursements for article processing charges from funders such as the RCUK. But gold open access isn't there yet.' [7]

Meanwhile, says Suber, every research-funding agency, public or private, and every university should require green open access for new peer-reviewed research articles by their grantees and faculty.

The Directory of Open Access Repositories (DOAR, http://www.opendoar.org) currently lists four Indian open repositories for articles and theses from medicine: the Digital Knowledge Repository of Central Drug Research Institute (http://dkr.cdri.res.in:8080/dspace/index.jsp), the Indian Academy of Sciences: Publications of Fellows (http://repository.ias.ac.in/), the Knowledge Repository Open Network (KNoor, http://dspaces.uok.edu.in:8080/jspui/) and OpenMED@NIC (http://openmed.nic.in/)—the last of these is an international archive of work in medical and allied sciences for anyone to archive their scientific and technical articles for free.

19.10 Data Sharing

The next frontier for open access is the sharing of data, not only of articles. There are compelling arguments that access to the full results of publicly funded research—and any research that will influence or change clinical practice or policy and thus, indirectly, individual or public health—is a moral good. Most research in medicine is publicly funded (even industry-funded clinical studies are usually conducted with publicly funded settings, patients and staff), and its output affects the general public as participants. Yet, it is becoming clear that published medical articles represent only one, rather skewed, view of the real evidence base. This is particularly troubling when this evidence gap applies to the results of randomized controlled trials of treatments and other health interventions [10].

In early 2011, major international funders of medical research jointly stated their support for the sharing of research data to improve public health (http://www.wellcome.ac.uk/About-us/Policy/Spotlight-issues/Data-sharing/Public-health-and-epidemiology/WTDV030690.htm; Box 19.3).

Box 19.3 Joint Statement of Major International Funding Agencies on Sharing of research data

The main principles in the statement are that data sharing should be:

- *Equitable:* Any approach to sharing of data should recognize and balance the needs of researchers who generate and use data, other analysts who might want to reuse those data and communities and funders who expect health benefits to arise from research.
- *Ethical:* All data sharing should protect the privacy of individuals and the dignity of communities while simultaneously respecting the imperative to improve public health through the most productive use of data.
- *Efficient:* Any approach to data sharing should improve the quality and value of research and increase its contribution to improving public health. Approaches should be proportionate and build on existing practice and reduce unnecessary duplication and competition.

In June 2012, the UK's Royal Society recommended that 'Scientists should communicate the data they collect and the models they create, to allow free and open access, and in ways that are intelligible, assessable and usable for other specialists … Where data justify it, scientists should make them available in an appropriate data repository' [11]. The report calls for, in time, mandatory publishing of data in a reusable form to support findings, more expertise in managing and supporting the use of digital data and new software tools to analyse data. It is time, says the report, to shift from a culture where 'many scientists still pursue their research through the measured and predictable steps in which they communicate their thinking within relatively closed groups of colleagues; publish their findings, usually in peer-reviewed journals; file their data and then move on.'

Many journals such as *Nature* and the PLoS journals already have policies that mandate sharing of raw data, but these are mostly in the fields of basic science and genetics. Sharing the data from medical research is a relatively new concept, and it is potentially hampered by the important need to protect patient's confidentiality and to first seek their permission [12]. However, it is possible to share anonymized datasets. To this end, since 2007, the *Annals of Internal Medicine* has asked authors to provide 'reproducible research' statements for every paper, declaring whether or not the authors will share raw and supplementary data and statistical code [13]. The *BMJ* followed suit and extended this approach. The *BMJ* and *BMJ Open* now ask authors to provide data sharing statements for every research paper, stating their intention to share data (or not) and, if so, to state how and where they will do this while protecting the participants' identities. Furthermore, authors of *BMJ* and *BMJ Open* research papers can share raw and supplementary datasets and statistical code through Dryad (http://datadryad.org/). *BMJ Open* is the first medical journal to partner with Dryad, an online repository which provides a permanent, citable and open access online home for datasets related to peer-reviewed, published articles in biosciences. Data deposition is integrated with the journal's manuscript submission system.

In January 2015, the US Institute of Medicine published an influential report *Sharing clinical trial data: Maximizing benefits, minimizing risk* that may encourage many more journals to embrace the idea of data sharing from clinical trials [14]. The report—produced by an expert international committee and informed by two large workshops and a public consultation—affirmed that data sharing from trials is in the public interest and recommended cultural and practical changes to make this happen.

Then, in January 2016, the International Committee of Medical Journal Editors (ICMJE) proposed that authors submitting a clinical trial to any ICMJE member journal must share with others the de-identified individual patient data (IPD) underlying the results (along with relevant metadata) no later than 6 months after publication. Data sharing should comply with a plan registered prospectively by the authors as a component of clinical trial registration. ICMJE said it would revise the draft policy in the light of invited comments and then implement the revised policy 1 year later (i.e. in 2017) [15].

19.11 Summary

Over the past 20 years, the Internet has allowed rapid development of thousands of new journals, shorter publication times and lengthened word limits and has greatly increased the reach of scholarly work. In turn, open access has increased the visibility and usability of those outputs and democratized their dissemination. This movement, ideally coupled with access to studies' raw datasets, creates huge possibilities for collaboration, advancement and understanding in science and medicine.

The last word should go to the participants at the Bangalore workshop in 2006 which led to the adoption of India's national policy on open access (http://www.ncsi.iisc.ernet.in/OAworkshop2006/). Their report said: 'The importance of access to the world's research information for the development of a strong economy and a vibrant research capability is widely acknowledged, yet financial barriers limit access by developing countries to the research information they need. Equally, the unique research carried out in countries representing 80% of the world's population is largely 'invisible' to international science because of economic or other constraints. The resolution of many of the world's problems, such as emerging infectious diseases, environmental disasters, HIV/AIDS or climate change, cannot be achieved without incorporation of the research from developing countries into the global knowledge pool.'

References

1. Merton RK. The normative structure of science. In: Merton RK, editor. The sociology of science: theoretical and empirical investigations. Chicago: University of Chicago Press; 1942. ISBN 0-226-52092-7.
2. Would Gandhi have been a Wikipedian? The Indian Express. 17 January 2012. http://www.indianexpress.com/news/would-gandhi-have-been-a-wikipedian/900506/0. Accessed 25 Apr 2015.
3. Muthu M, Subbiah A. Use made of open access journals by Indian researchers to publish their findings. Curr Sci. 2011;100:1297–306. http://cis-india.org/openness/blog/use-of-open-access-journals-for-publishing-findings. Accessed 25 Apr 2015.
4. Delamothe T, Smith R. Open access publishing takes off. BMJ. 2004;328:1–3. https://doi.org/10.1136/bmj.328.7430.1. http://www.ncbi.nlm.nih.gov/pmc/articles/PMC313879/. Accessed 25 Apr 2015.
5. Solomon DJ, Björk BC. Publication fees in open access publishing: sources of funding and factors influencing choice of journal. J Am Soc Information Sci Technol. Preprint. http://www.openaccesspublishing.org/apc/preprint.pdf. Accessed 25 Apr 2015.
6. Mark Ware Consulting. Submission fees—a tool in the transition to open access? Summary of report to knowledge exchange. 2010. http://www.knowledge-exchange.info/default.aspx?id=413. Accessed on 25 Apr 2015.
7. Suber P. Ensuring open access for publicly funded research. BMJ. 2012;345:e5184. https://doi.org/10.1136/bmj.e5184. Accessed 25 Apr 2015.
8. Laakso M, Welling P, Bukvova H, Nyman L, Björk BC, Hedlund T. The development of open access journal publishing from 1993 to 2009. PLoS One. 2011;6:e20961. https://doi.org/10.1371/journal.pone.0020961. http://www.ncbi.nlm.nih.gov/pmc/articles/PMC3113847/. Accessed 25 Apr 2015.

9. Mukherjee B, Mal BK. India's efforts in open access publishing. Library philosophy and practice. 2012. http://www.webpages.uidaho.edu/~mbolin/mukherjee-mal.htm. Accessed 25 Apr 2015.
10. Lehman R, Loder E. Missing clinical trial data. BMJ. 2012;344:d8158. https://doi.org/10.1136/bmj.d8158. Accessed 25 Apr 2015.
11. The Royal Society. Science as an open enterprise: open data for open science. 2012. http://royalsociety.org/uploadedFiles/Royal_Society_Content/policy/projects/sape/2012-06-20-SAOE.pdf. Accessed 25 Apr 2015.
12. Hrynaszkiewicz I, Norton ML, Vickers AJ, Altman DG. Preparing raw clinical data for publication: guidance for journal editors, authors, and peer reviewers. BMJ. 2010;340:c181. https://doi.org/10.1136/bmj.c181. Accessed on 25 Apr 2015.
13. Laine C, Goodman SN, Griswold ME, Sox HC. Reproducible research: moving toward research the public can really trust. Ann Intern Med. 2007;146:450–3.
14. Institute of Medicine. Sharing clinical trial data: maximizing benefits, minimizing risks. http://www.iom.nationalacademies.org/Reports/2015/Sharing-Clinical-Trial-Data.aspx.
15. Taichman DB, Backus J, Baethge C, Bauchner H, Leeuw PW, Drazen JM, et al. Sharing clinical trial data. BMJ. 2016;352:i255.

Electronic Publishing

20

Margaret Winker

The Internet has so fundamentally changed research and publishing—searching, collaborating, communicating, analysing, authoring, publishing, distributing, sharing and publishing business models—that it is difficult to recall how either process occurred without it. While the scope of change reaches far beyond what this chapter will cover, authors should be aware of some central issues related to electronic publishing. Most of this chapter pertains primarily to journal publishing, but the information on drafting content applies to any form of authoring.

20.1 Digital Publishing Business Models

Publishing research content is an important public good, but the process of editorial review, revision, editing and publishing and distribution incurs expenses that must be paid for in some way. When publishing was entirely print based, publishing models included member benefits from professional organizations, paid subscriptions, advertising and sponsorship and reprint purchases. Digital publishing added to this mix the cost of programming, conversion and hosting but also reduced costs related to postage, printing and distribution. Many aspects of publishing online business models, such as subscription sales, advertising and reprints, have grown out of similar print-based models. However, no single model may be sufficient to accommodate the rapid evolution of the marketplace, and publishing companies often diversify their revenue streams to accommodate the business shifts as they occur.

M. Winker
World Association of Medical Editors, Winnetka, IL, USA

Journals that rely on subscriptions, membership or pay-per-view for revenue are discussed below; open-access journals are discussed in detail in Chap. 19. Some journals provide a hybrid approach, permitting authors to pay to have their article freely available instead of the access-controlled default option. Authors choosing a journal should consider many qualities of a journal before submitting (*see also* Chap. 16), including whether open access is important for their research exposure and whether author fees (which may be part of publishing in an open-access journal or a hybrid journal and may appear as page or colour charges in a subscription-based journal) are a critical factor. Authors should be aware of unscrupulous publishers that use author-pay models and take undue advantage by charging publication fees in exchange for few or no author services such as peer review, editorial review or editing. Such journals have been termed 'predatory' journals. Resources are available to help identify such journals [1] and to define best practices [2].

20.1.1 Access Control via Subscription or Membership

Journals that rely on subscription or member-based revenue generally permit article access only by those individuals and institutions who have paid for access (journal-wide, collection-wide or pay-per-view of an individual article), with a few exceptions as noted below. Access control requires maintenance of subscriber accounts and databases in concert with membership databases where necessary, subscriber access via user names and passwords or Internet protocol (IP) addresses, secure servers for financial transactions and responsive user support. Libraries and institutions that purchase subscriptions require COUNTER reports (Counting Online Usage of Networked Electronic Resources. http://www.projectcounter.org/) to measure the number of full-text (HTML or PDF) downloads per journal, to determine their cost per article download, for purposes of making purchasing decisions. Subscription-based journals require sales staff to maintain and grow relationships with libraries and institutions.

Websites of scholarly journals generally offer at least the following information free of charge: the tables of contents and collection lists, abstracts, search functionality, facility to register one's email ID to receive alerts that list contents of new issues published and information pages including instructions for authors. Some journals offer content free of charge as well. A fundamental shift in the publishing model occurred when the US National Institutes of Health (NIH) required that researchers funded by NIH submit their accepted papers to PubMed Central and make them freely available no more than 12 months after publication [3]. The UK Medical Research Council [4] and the Wellcome Trust [5] have similar policies that apply 6 months after publication; other funding organizations too have adopted similar policies. As a result, many journals with traditional subscription or membership models now provide free access to research content at varying times, such as 6 or 12 months after publication. In addition, some subscription-based journals make content that is published online ahead of print freely available, and some make content considered to be critical to public health freely available. Many publishers with access control provide free journal access to registered institutions within the poorest developing countries via the WHO programme HINARI [6].

Finally, because most readers and researchers use the Google search engine at some point in their online research, Google's requirement that at least some information be freely available in order for page content to be indexed has meant that journals wishing their content to be readily discoverable must provide either a free author summary (such as an abstract) or a free first page of the article PDF. This requirement provides a strong incentive for publishers to make such content freely available.

20.1.2 Advertising

Just as some journals generate revenue by publishing advertisements in their print journals, some journals accept paid advertisements on their websites. However, online advertising revenues are typically based on page views and/or click-throughs, and revenues are less than those obtained from print advertising.

As online advertising has become ubiquitous throughout the Web, some scholarly journals have permitted advertisements not only on home pages and information pages but also on abstract and full-text article pages. Some websites display advertisements only for readers that have not authenticated via user name, password or IP address, in an effort to recoup lost revenue because of free access. Journals may display advertisements to readers before the reader lands on the article (interstitial advertisements). However, the popular press practice of targeting advertisements to content is generally discouraged in scholarly publishing. Some basic science journals hyperlink product mentions (such as equipment, test kits and reagents) in text to the product site, ostensibly as a service to readers, but this practice has not become established in medical journals.

Many journals sell advertisements on table of content alerts, RSS feeds and the like. Authors may want to learn a journal's advertising policy before submitting, if the journal makes the advertising policy publicly available.

20.1.3 Reprints

Journals with controlled access to articles often sell reprints of articles, individually via pay-per-view and/or in bundles, e.g. to pharmaceutical companies. For some journals, these sales provide a substantial amount of revenue [7]. Though some authors have proposed that journals should provide authors' royalties for such sales, in parallel with book royalties, this practice has not become established in medical publishing.

Many publishers with access-controlled websites provide authors with a specific number of free e-prints (i.e. a printable file which can be downloaded on a specific number of occasions) to authors for accessing and sharing their article.

20.1.4 Copyright and Creative Commons

Many journals have a copyright policy similar to those used by book publishers, in which authors transfer copyright for their published works to the publisher at the time of publication. This means that authors who wish to reuse any portion of their publications (text, tables or figures or reprint the work) must request permission from the publisher to do so and, in some cases, pay usage fees if permission is granted. Authors should be aware of journals' copyright policies and also their fair use policies or the extent to which readers can share or copy published works (*see* Box 20.1 for an example). The work of authors who are US federal employees is not covered by the Copyright Act, and therefore they do not transfer copyright [8]. Similar laws may exist in other countries.

Box 20.1 An Example of Copyright Language Required of Authors
Copyright transfer/publishing agreement. In consideration of the action of the American Medical Association (AMA) in reviewing and editing this submission (manuscript, tables, figures, video, audio, and other supplemental files for publication), I hereby transfer, assign, or otherwise convey all copyright ownership, including any and all rights incidental there to, exclusively to the AMA, in the event that such work is published by the AMA.

An alternative to this policy is a Creative Commons licence used by some publishers such as PLoS (Public Library of Science) [9]. This licence allows authors (creators) to '... retain copyright while allowing others to copy, distribute, and make some uses of their work—at least non-commercially. Such license also ensures that licensors get the credit for their work they deserve. Every Creative Commons license works around the world and lasts as long as applicable copyright lasts (because they are built on copyright)' [10].

Publishers with copyright transfer policies take the perspective that they protect authors' content by controlling reuse, whereas publishers that use the Creative Commons licence allow authors to retain rights to use their content and encourage dissemination of scholarly content. Authors should be aware of any transfer of copyright and any restrictions placed on their published content particularly if they intend to reuse it in any way. (*See also* Chap. 10.)

20.2 Drafting the Electronic Manuscript

Electronic publishing has many benefits when drafting manuscripts but also some pitfalls of which one should be aware. A brief overview of the pros and cons of electronic drafting is provided below.

20.2.1 Authoring Tools

While Word and similar word processing software perhaps remain the most common manuscript drafting tools, wikis such as Google Docs and similar tools enable simultaneous drafting in multiple locations with version control and identification of who is responsible for which revisions. When authors create a new document in Word, they should be aware that the properties' feature remains a part of the document throughout its life and can provide information about the provenance of the manuscript.

20.2.2 Drafting and Note Taking

In the age of online research and reading, taking notes on relevant work is generally done electronically and may involve copy and paste of specific information. However, this practice can make it all too easy for authors to inadvertently reuse others' text. Authors must ensure that text and other content are not reused without specific attribution such as quotation marks. Similarly, when writing a new manuscript, authors may be tempted to start with their previous manuscript draft or add portions of an existing manuscript related to the new topic. Such a practice makes duplicate publication a serious possibility, and authors should be careful to ensure that no overlap exists, e.g. using the merge function on Word to identify areas of overlap.

The reuse, inadvertent or otherwise, of text of one's own work or that of others without attribution is not acceptable and is considered duplicate publication or plagiarism, respectively. (*See also* Chaps. 23 and 24.) Journal editors increasingly use software such as CrossCheck or iThenticate to screen submitted or accepted manuscripts for plagiarism and duplicate publication. A journal's detection of an overlapping sentence or two in a manuscript may suggest authors' lack of attention to the issues listed above and result in a request for revision that should be heeded. However, detection of large blocks of text lifted from other sources will likely result in a request for explanation and possibly considerably more, depending on the egregiousness of the problem and the point at which the overlap is detected. Some academic institutions purchase use of tools such as CrossCheck for authors to identify any problems with overlapping text in their manuscripts before journal submission or publication. The free tool http://etblast.org can also be used to search for overlapping work, but the text that can be searched is limited to free online databases such as Medline.

20.2.3 References and Citation Management Tools

Citation management tools enable easy tracking of relevant research and save time when numbering references and generating reference lists (*see* Chap. 9). A comparison of options is available at http://en.wikipedia.org/wiki/Comparison_of_reference_management_software. Tool capabilities range from tracking references only to organizing journal articles. Journals vary in their required reference style, and many citation management tools enable an author to easily change from one style to another. Many journals offer citation download options formatted for a variety of citation management systems for their articles.

Some journals require that the citation manager tracking system that enables easy renumbering of references be turned off and changed to standard numbering at the time of submission or revision, to avoid inadvertent renumbering. Before submission, authors should verify that their citations are correct, ideally verify any corrections to the cited articles to ensure that the points made in the manuscript are still accurate and verify that the cited articles have not been retracted (unless the manuscript refers to the retracted article per se).

Journals vary in their reference requirements; some require inclusion of the PubMed ID (PMID) as part of the citation, and some use software to check citations against PubMed to ensure the citations are correct and to facilitate linking of the published references. Others require inclusion of digital object identifiers (DOIs; *see* http://en.wikipedia.org/wiki/Digital_object_identifier or section on *Unique article identifiers* below) as part of the references. Citation of websites requires ensuring the website URLs accessible; the date on which they were accessed should be provided (*see* Chap. 9).

20.2.4 Tables and Figures

Journals increasingly expect authors to submit tables and figures in publication-ready formats, by following specifications and providing high-resolution images that will display well on the Web. Some journals provide specific instructions regarding figure creation that may be helpful [11, 12]. Of greatest importance is being aware of the journal's standards for figures and figure manipulation. (*See* Detection of figure manipulation, below, and Chap. 4 on 'The Results Section' including tables, figures, numbers and statistics.)

20.2.5 Supplemental Content and Data Deposition

Supplemental figures and tables can be provided as part of research submissions, and some journals permit submission of audio files. Related documents, including related manuscripts, protocols and guideline checklists such as STROBE or CONSORT (*see also* Chap. 18), can also be provided at the time of submission and can help speed the review process. Biomedical journals often post online-only supplemental content without additional copyediting, and authors should be aware that they are responsible for the copyediting and appearance as well as the accuracy of supplemental content. Some journals include a disclaimer to this effect. Supplemental content intended for publication should undergo peer review along with the rest of the manuscript. While the trend has been for journals to include more supplemental information online over time, the *Journal of Neuroscience* found the exponential growth in supplemental material too large to justify the investment of additional time by its reviewers and hence no longer publishes it [13]. (*See also* Chap. 21.)

Many journals recommend that data be deposited in a suitable online repository, but few medical journals currently mandate data deposition [14]. (*See also* Chap. 19.)

The National Information Standards Organization (NISO) and National Federation of Advanced Information Services (NFAIS) are developing standards for supplemental material in collaboration with stakeholders [15]. Authors, along with editors and reviewers, should determine which data are central to the study and which are truly supplemental. Additional considerations are whether data should be displayed in a format accessible to all (e.g. as PDF file) or in a format more useful for future analyses (e.g. as a spreadsheet) and how data will be preserved over time (how the data will be accessed if and when the interface necessary to use the file format is no longer available).

20.3 Submitting the Manuscript

20.3.1 Submission Components

Most peer-reviewed journals have some form of electronic submission and tracking system. These systems enable tracking of manuscripts and correspondence with authors and reviewers and provide efficiencies that benefit authors. However, submission systems differ in their organization and requirements and can often be time-consuming for authors to complete. Authors should check the journal's online system requirements before beginning the submission process to ensure that they have all the necessary information at hand.

Authors should provide a cover letter in addition to the manuscript itself. Journals often have requirements as to the information that should be included in the cover letter, such as an attestation that the manuscript has not previously been published and is not under consideration at another journal. Authors may wish to succinctly explain why their manuscript is suitable for that particular journal. Regardless, the author should ensure that the cover letter is appropriate for the journal to which they are submitting. Naming the wrong journal or editor in the cover letter does not give the manuscript the best first impression!

Many systems require basic information about co-authors and attempt to unify records that belong to the same author/reviewer. E-mail addresses are often used to identify unique individuals, and authors should be sure to enter co-author data accurately. Efforts are under way to develop an author identification number; such an identifier could be of great benefit for authors with common names but also require substantial investment in and maintenance of a massive database. Researcher ID (http://www.researcherid.com) and ORCID (Open Researcher and Contributor ID, http://about.orcid.org/) are two such efforts currently under way.

Some journals may require authorship forms, conflict of interest declarations and other related information at the time of submission. Some journals enable authors to indicate possible reviewers and indicate what reviewers the authors prefer not to review. Journal editors are not obligated to follow these recommendations.

Finally, journals may request that authors provide keywords for their manuscript. If the journal does not provide a closed taxonomy from which the author may select relevant terms, authors should use standard medical taxonomies (e.g. Medical Subject Headings [MeSH] from US National Library of Medicine or SNOMED) as much as possible to enhance indexing and retrievability of their manuscript (*see* Chap. 21).

20.3.2 Unique Article Identifiers

Authors need to be familiar with a variety of unique article identifiers. Traditional print articles are identified via citation using year, volume, issue and page, but these parameters are less relevant in the age of preprints, online ahead-of-print publication and online-only publications.

The DOI is one commonly used unique article identifier, created by the publisher and deposited for a fee with CrossRef. DOIs can also be used to designate chapters, figures, videos, audio or any other discrete types of content. The DOI resolver (http://doi.org) can identify multiple instances of an article with a particular DOI. The PubMed ID (PMID) is a free unique article identifier generated when an article is indexed in PubMed but requires that a journal be listed in PubMed.

20.3.3 Deposition of Manuscripts in Publicly Available Repositories

Some funding agencies (the NIH, Wellcome Trust and others) require that the final accepted version of the manuscript be deposited in a publicly available database. The PubMed Central identification number (PMCID) is generated when an article is deposited in PubMed Central (and is a different number from the PMID). Authors of publicly funded research often need to provide the PMCID to funders and/or institutions as proof that they have deposited their work in PubMed Central. Some journals deposit the accepted manuscript or published article in PubMed Central on the author's behalf and provide the author with the PMCID.

20.4 Journal Policies and Services

20.4.1 Detection of Duplicate Publication and Plagiarism

Journals may use software such as CrossCheck, interfacing with their manuscript submission systems, to detect duplicate publication or plagiarism. CrossCheck includes a database of articles provided by several participating publishers against which the manuscript is checked. Publishers pay a fee to CrossRef, the parent company, to participate. CrossCheck identifies matching text, and editors determine the threshold of matching text that they believe indicates that further investigation is necessary. However, simply identifying a match does not determine that duplicate publication or plagiarism exists; it simply flags the manuscript as requiring additional investigation, which is then up to the editor to investigate and pursue with the author. A free online tool, http://eTBlast.org, enables one to enter text to compare against the PubMed database and search results obtained using Google, but more extensive matching is not possible (*see* Chaps. 23 and 24).

20.4.2 Detection of Figure Manipulation

To try to prevent publication of manipulated figures, some journals provide specific guidelines for authors. While guidelines vary by journal, many of the basic elements are the same, requiring that any changes to figures be superficial and not alter the fundamental data or presentation [16].

The standards for *JAMA Network* journals, for example, are as follows:

> 'Digital adjustments of brightness, contrast, or colour applied uniformly to an entire image are permissible as long as these adjustments do not selectively highlight, misrepresent, obscure, or eliminate specific elements in the original figure, including the background. Selective adjustments applied to individual elements in an image are not permissible. Individual elements may not be moved within an image field, deleted or inserted from another image. Cropping may be used for efficient image display but must not misrepresent or alter interpretation of the image by selectively eliminating relevant visual information. Juxtaposition of elements from different parts of a single image or from different images, as in a composite, must be clearly indicated by the addition of dividing lines, borders, and/ or panel labels' [17].

Some journals have implemented checks for figure manipulation [18]. Authors are advised to check journal policy when submitting images.

20.4.3 Prior Publication and Prior Release of Data

One special instance related to duplicate publication is prior release of data. Whereas medical journals do not disapprove of the presentation of study results as abstracts at official scientific meetings, other forms of prepublication release may prevent the content from being considered by a scholarly journal. This policy is intended to discourage authors from releasing their study results before the content has undergone peer review because the data and implications might change in the course of review and revision, and there is little point in republishing content that is already available. Journals have also acknowledged that this policy helps preserve the newsworthiness of their content [19]. This policy is popularly referred to as the Ingelfinger rule, after the editor at the *New England Journal of Medicine* who first established the policy [20].

20.4.4 Embargo Policy

Many journals publish online content at a specific date and time and use an embargo, i.e. require that authors delay releasing information about the work until that date and time [21]. Journals also may release pre-published content and news releases to journalists in advance of the embargo, so that journalists need not write and publish quickly to avoid being 'scooped'. This arrangement is made with the understanding that journalists also must adhere to the embargo.

20.4.5 Article Dissemination and Promotion

Journals have several ways of highlighting or enhancing the online presence of an article, and authors may consider this potential benefit when submitting a manuscript (*see* Chap. 16) and certainly after the article has been accepted for publication. Besides traditional methods such as related editorials or commentaries placing the article in perspective, many journals offer email alerts and RSS feeds to alert readers to new content. Authors may be able to receive alerts whenever publication events regarding their article take place, including corrections, letters to the editor, comments and citing articles. Some journals use podcasts, video, blogs, Twitter, Facebook and other ways to further promote article content. Authors may want to use social media outlets themselves to help disseminate their content, but they should adhere to the journal's embargo policy. It is also important for information about the study to be consistent irrespective of the online channels used.

20.4.6 Measures of Journal and Article Impact

A full discussion of measuring journal and article impact is beyond the scope of this chapter. However, authors should be familiar with the most common measures being used and debated.

Impact factor. The impact factor, developed by Eugene Garfield at the Institute of Scientific Information, is the number of citations a journal receives during a year to articles published in the two previous years, divided by the number of 'citable' articles published in those same years (e.g. impact factor of a journal for the year 2014 is the average number of citations received by papers published in 2012 and 2013 divided by the number of 'citable' papers published in the journal in the years 2012 and 2013). The numerator includes all citations to any articles published in the 2-year period, whereas the denominator includes only the articles published in the 2-year period that are considered 'citable' as defined by ISI. Citable articles include research articles, reviews and other longer articles, whereas editorials, commentaries and letters to the editor are generally excluded. Other types of articles may be less easily categorized.

Another nuance of impact factor citations is that articles published online ahead of print are considered 'published' for purposes of the ISI denominator only when they appear in print, so articles published online ahead of print begin to accrue citations before they actually become citable.

The impact factor has proven to be susceptible to manipulation and has several limitations [22]. The impact factor has taken on meaning far beyond its intended use and value, with institutions and even some governments relying on it to judge the importance of an author's published work and reward accordingly; such use may not be appropriate.

Other measures have been developed to try to create more transparent measures that are less susceptible to manipulation and for other purposes, such as measuring the impact of an author or an article. These include the H index, developed to enable scientists to calculate a single number based on their most cited papers and the number of citations they have received in other publications [23], the Eigenfactor score and the Article Influence score [24]. A new metric being developed and standardized by COUNTER is the usage factor, which is intended to incorporate article accesses as another measure of journal impact [25].

Another transparent approach to article impact is altmetrics, which includes a range of ways in which individuals refer to articles [26]. Some journals make article-specific metrics freely available to readers [27] or to authors only. Article-level metrics generally include online article accesses and citations but may also include links from Twitter, Facebook and other social media, blogs and online commenting.

20.4.7 Publication Versioning

Publishing electronically creates many versioning options, including preprints such as the physics preprint server arXiv (http://arxiv.org/), posting of author manuscripts immediately after acceptance but before copyediting, posting unformatted but copyedited versions, publishing the fully redacted edited final proof and publishing subsequent corrected versions of the article. As another permutation, some print journals publish articles online ahead of print, either because of print lags in publishing or to coordinate publication of an article with presentation of the study at a scientific meeting, but in that case, the online and print versions of the article are usually identical. The different versions are united using one DOI, the common identifier. The benefit of prepublication posting is more rapid time to publication and faster dissemination of research, but the critical quality step of copyediting is particularly important in medical publishing where publishing inaccuracies could lead to substantial harm.

Journals have begun experimenting with other publishing models. In 2006, *Nature* tried open peer review, but nearly half of the articles received no comments at all. The editors concluded that 'feedback suggests that there is a marked reluctance among researchers to offer open comments' [28]. A number of more recent examples illustrate the importance of post-publication peer review [29]. In an entirely new model, *PLoS Computational Biology* selected articles in 2012 for an experiment in which they published the standard peer-reviewed archival version on their website as well as a version on Wikipedia that could be edited and updated over time [30]. *PLOS Computational Biology* has continued publishing these dual articles, referred to as Topic Pages in the journal [31–33].

20.4.8 Archival Repositories

Two basic types of repositories exist for scholarly articles. First, user-created repositories such as Mendeley, Zotero and many others enable researchers to organize and access key articles important to their work. Such repositories permit reprint storage, although publishers' policies as to sharing content vary based on their copyright and fair use policies.

The second type is journal-created repositories. Over time, some journals cease to publish, and their content is no longer hosted by their publisher. To ensure that content continues to be available, archival repositories host the content for a fee. Organizations such as CLOCKSS (http://www.clockss.org/clockss/Home) and Portico (http://www.portico.org/digital-preservation/) provide such a resource.

20.4.9 Corrections

The various forms of online publishing and versioning make transparent communication and documentation of corrections essential. Official published corrections are associated with the published article in PubMed and often linked online to the original article on journal websites. These formal corrections are essential for correcting major errors including author names and other article metadata, data errors and interpretation. Correcting the full-text and PDF versions of the article and/or appending the correction to the PDF help to ensure that the reader has access to the latest version of the article. Smaller errors such as typos can be fixed in the online version of the article only. Some journals note the date of the update to the article at the bottom of the files (HTML as well as PDF).

20.4.10   Retractions

Articles may need to be retracted for several reasons. According to a study analysing retractions from 1998 to 2008 [34], 40% of retractions were for honest errors or non-replicable findings, 28% were for research misconduct (plagiarism or data fabrication or falsification), 17% were for redundant publication and 5% were for unstated or unclear reasons. The retractions were most likely to be issued by the authors (63%), followed by editors (21%) and journals (6%); by contrast, publishers (2%) and institutions (1%) issued few retractions. In 7% of retractions, it was unclear who retracted the paper.

When an article is retracted, the journal should publish a notice of retraction online, submit the retraction notice to electronic databases such as PubMed and provide a link from the retraction to the article and vice versa. The article PDF and HTML files should both be modified to indicate clearly that the article was retracted.

20.4.11   Letters to the Editor and Online Comments

Most scholarly journals publish letters to the editor in response to articles. Many journals batch readers' letters for a particular period of time after publication, select those they believe are most appropriate for publication and response and send them to the author to reply. Authors are then given an opportunity to reply, and the letters and reply are then published simultaneously. For journals indexed in PubMed, letters to the editor are also indexed in PubMed and linked to the article to which they reply.

Some journals permit online comments in response to an article. Online comments may be moderated or not, and conflict of interest disclosure may be required. Authors publishing in journals that permit commenting will likely want to be alerted whenever new comments in response to their articles are posted, if possible, and may respond to the comments online. Online comments are not indexed in PubMed. However, PubMed Commons is an initiative to foster comments on articles within PubMed. PubMed Commons intends to offer an interface for journals to upload PubMed Commons comments on their articles to their journal sites.

20.5   Summary

The electronic world of journal publishing is evolving so rapidly that any static information is sure to soon become out-of-date. However, authors should be aware of the latest developments in electronic publishing and informed about journal business models, reader access, copyright options, various ways to measure article and journal impact and the way in which journals display reader feedback. Authors should be aware of their responsibilities in manuscript and supplemental file submission and data deposition. Finally, the publication process does not end on the publication date; an author engaged via social media and commenting venues can help ensure that the work gains maximal exposure, and the author is able to clarify any questions that emerge.

References

1. Clark J. How to avoid predatory journals—a five-point plan. BMJ Blogs. http://blogs.bmj.com/bmj/2015/01/19/jocalyn-clark-how-to-avoid-predatory-journals-a-five-point-plan/. Accessed 9 Sept 2015.
2. World Association of Medical Editors, Committee on Publication Ethics, Directory of Open Access Journals, Open Access Scholarly Publishers Association. Principles of transparency and best practice in scholarly publishing. http://www.wame.org/about/principles-of-transparency-and-best-practice. Accessed 9 Sept 2015.

3. National Institutes of Health. Public access policy. http://publicaccess.nih.gov/. Accessed 25 Apr 2015.
4. Open access policy. Medical Research Council. www.mrc.ac.uk/research/research-policy-ethics/open-access-policy/. Accessed 25 Apr 2015.
5. Open access policy: position statement in support of open and unrestricted access to published research. www.wellcome.ac.uk/About-us/Policy/Spotlight-issues/Open-access/Policy/index.htm. Accessed 25 Apr 2015.
6. HINARI. http://www.who.int/hinari/en/. Accessed 25 Apr 2015.
7. Lundh A, Barbateskovic M, Hróbjartsson A, Gøtzsche PC. Conflicts of interest at medical journals: the influence of industry-supported randomised trials on journal impact factors and revenue—cohort study. PLoS Med. 2010;7:e1000354. https://doi.org/10.1371/journal.pmed.1000354.
8. JAMA. Authorship responsibility, financial disclosure, acknowledgment, and copyright transfer/publishing agreement. http://jama.jamanetwork.com/data/ifora-forms/jama/auinst_crit.pdf. Accessed 25 Apr 2015.
9. Open-access license: no permission required. PLOS. http://www.plosone.org/static/license.action. Accessed 25 Apr 2015.
10. About the licenses: what our licenses do. Creative Commons. http://creativecommons.org/licenses/. Accessed 25 Apr 2015.
11. Figures. PLOS Medicine. http://journals.plos.org/plosmedicine/s/figures. Accessed 2 Jun 2015.
12. Figures in accepted manuscript. JAMA. http://jama.jamanetwork.com/data/ifora-forms/jama/jamatechreqfigures.pdf. Accessed 2 Jun 2015.
13. Announcement regarding supplemental material. http://www.jneurosci.org/content/30/32/10599.full. Accessed 25 Apr 2015.
14. PLOS. Editorial and publishing policies: sharing of materials, methods, and data. www.plos.org/policies/#sharing. Accessed 2 Jun 2015.
15. NISO/NFAIS Supplemental Journal Article Materials Project. http://www.niso.org/workrooms/supplemental. Accessed 25 Apr 2015.
16. Rossner M, Yamada KM. What's in a picture? The temptation of image manipulation. J Cell Biol. 2004;166:11–5. https://doi.org/10.1083/jcb.200406019.
17. Image integrity. Archives of dermatology instructions for authors. http://archderm.jamanetwork.com/public/instructionsForAuthors.aspx#SecFigures. Accessed 2 Jun 2012.
18. Data Integrity. About JCB. http://jcb.rupress.org/site/misc/about.xhtml. Accessed 25 Apr 2015.
19. Relman AS. The Ingelfinger rule. N Engl J Med. 1981;305:824–6.
20. Anonymous. Definition of 'sole contribution'. N Engl J Med. 1969;281:676–7.
21. PLOS embargo policy. http://www.plos.org/about/media-inquiries/embargo-policy/. Accessed 25 Apr 2015.
22. Amin M, Mabe M. Impact factors: use and abuse. Elsevier Perspectives in Publishing October 2000; revised 2007. http://www.elsevier.com/framework_editors/pdfs/Perspectives1.pdf. Accessed 25 Apr 2015.
23. Hirsch JE. An index to quantify an individual's scientific research output. arXiv:physics/0508025v5. 29 Sept 2005. http://www.cs.ucla.edu/~palsberg/hirsch05.pdf. Accessed 25 Apr 2015.
24. About Eigenfactor.org. http://www.eigenfactor.org/about.php. Accessed 25 Apr 2015.
25. Usage factor: introduction to release 1 of the COUNTER code of practice for usage factors. http://www.projectcounter.org/usage_factor.html. Accessed 2 Jun 2015.
26. Priem J, Taraboreilli D, Groth P, Neylon C. Altmetrics: a manifesto. 26 October 2010. http://altmetrics.org/manifesto/. Accessed 25 Apr 2015.
27. PLOS. Article level metrics. Overview. http://article-level-metrics.plos.org/alm-info/. Accessed 25 Apr 2015.
28. Nature's peer review trial. Nature 2006. https://doi.org/10.1038/nature05535.

29. Winker M. The promise of post-publication peer review: how do we get there from here? Learn Publish. 2015;28(2):143–5.
30. Wodak SJ, Mietchen D, Collings AM, Russell RB, Bourne PE. Topic pages: PLoS computational biology meets Wikipedia. PLoS Comput Biol. 2012;8:e1002446. https://doi.org/10.1371/journal.pcbi.1002446.
31. Topic Pages. PLoS Comput Biol. http://topicpages.ploscompbiol.org/wiki/Topic_Pages#cite_note-TopiPageCollection-4. Accessed 26 Aug 2015.
32. Ravenhall M, Skunca M, Lassalle F, Dessimoz C. Inferring horizontal gene transfer. PLoS Comput Biol. 2015;11:e1004095. https://doi.org/10.1371/journal.pcbi.1004095.
33. Inferring horizontal gene transfer. Wikipedia. https://en.wikipedia.org/wiki/Inferring_horizontal_gene_transfer. Accessed 26 Aug 2015.
34. Wager E, Williams P. Why and how do journals retract articles? An analysis of Medline retractions 1988–2008. J Med Ethics. 2011;37:567–70.

Editorial Process and Peer Review

Farrokh Habibzadeh

21.1 Manuscript Flow in Editorial Office

Nowadays, most journals use an online submission system. When you submit a manuscript to a journal, you will receive an acknowledgement. If you have not received an acknowledgement, the submission process is most likely incomplete, and you should try to ascertain the problem. One possibility is that the acknowledgement e-mail has gone to the spam folder of your e-mail. If not, contact the journal's editorial office, and make sure your complete submission has been received.

The manuscript handling system will also inform one of the journal editors or another member of the editorial staff of the arrival of a new submission. Then, the manuscript is assigned to a handling editor who assesses it for various points.

Submission to open-access journals that receive a publication fee has an extra step. During submission, you need to provide information on whether you or your institution can pay for the publication fee (for some journals, it is as much as US$4500). If you or your institution cannot pay the publication fee, you may explain the reasons and ask for a waiver. In some journals, say *PLOS One*, the waiver request is evaluated independent of the scientific review process, i.e. the scientific editor is not aware of the waiver decision, which is usually made within just a few days. However, in some journals, the submission process is pending upon the decision for waiver—you cannot complete the submission, unless you receive a positive response for the waiver request or accept to pay the publication fee (or a discounted value).

F. Habibzadeh
The International Journal of Occupational and Environmental Medicine
Research and Development Headquarters, Petroleum Industry Health
Organization, Tehran, Iran
e-mail: Farrokh.Habibzadeh@theijoem.com

© The National Medical Journal of India 2018
P. Sahni, R. Aggarwal (eds.), *Reporting and Publishing Research in the Biomedical Sciences*, https://doi.org/10.1007/978-981-10-7062-4_21

21.1.1 In-Office Evaluation of the Manuscript

In the journal office, the manuscript is first evaluated for its completeness, relevance and appropriateness—whether all pages exist; whether it contains all the cited tables, figures and graphs; whether it fits the scope of the journal; and whether all the requirements mentioned in the journal's information for authors are met (e.g. length of the manuscript, number of references, tables and graphs, format of references, etc.). Therefore, you need to read the information for authors of the journal before you submit your manuscript. Lack of adherence to the instructions would be construed in various ways. As an example, if the format of the references in your manuscript is according to another journal's instructions, it may be assumed that you had previously submitted your manuscript to that journal and that it was rejected. This opinion, though it might be wrong, would have a negative impact on the handling editor—after all, editors are also human! If no obvious problems are found in the primary assessment of the manuscript, then it is screened in the editorial office.

Although we should generally follow the guidelines mentioned in journals' instructions for authors, since a couple of years ago, some journals have used a more author-friendly scheme—'your paper, your way'—where the authors can submit their manuscripts primarily without strict formatting or referencing requirements. Authors may submit their manuscript as a single file in MS Word or PDF format. Figures and tables can be placed within the text. References can be presented in any format (e.g. Vancouver, Harvard, etc.), as long as the style is consistent. When a manuscript reaches the revision stage, the authors will be asked to provide the necessary items such as editable source files. Currently, all journals published by Elsevier provide this option.

Editors are busy people looking for a short, clear, precise title; a good abstract; good design and methods; clear conclusions; brevity; and your adherence to the instructions. The title of a manuscript is the first level of contact of the editor with the manuscript; a good title is therefore of paramount importance. After that, a good abstract is the most important part, as it can serve to attract the editor's attention (and later on the reviewer's). In some journals where submission rates are high, a manuscript may be rejected solely based on its abstract, no matter how good the rest of the manuscript is. If the message to be conveyed is clear and concise, then the handling editor can easily evaluate the manuscript and, if reasonably acceptable, will send it for peer review. On the other hand, if the editor is unable to find a clear message, it is even harder to find appropriate reviewers for the manuscript. In this way, the manuscript would get delayed in going out for a review, resulting in further delay in making a decision on its publication in the journal.

Brevity is also important. Manuscripts that are unnecessarily long are difficult to understand, particularly if they are not well structured. Given the competition for limited journal space, well-written and concise manuscripts have the best chance of being accepted. Therefore, it is important to stick with Billings' rule: 'Have something to say; say it; and stop as soon as you have said it' [1].

21.1.2 Major Reasons for In-Office Rejection of a Manuscript

The main cause for in-office rejection of submitted manuscripts is the lack of relevance of their topics to the journal and its readership. For example, if you submit a manuscript reporting a novel chemotherapy for breast cancer to a journal on occupational medicine, the manuscript would most likely be rejected, whereas it would most likely be accepted and published in a prestigious journal on clinical oncology or even in high-impact general journals such as *New England Journal of Medicine*, *The Lancet* or *JAMA*. Another important cause for in-office rejection is the lack of a clear statement on the research question or hypothesis. An inappropriate format of the manuscript (e.g. submitting a 'case report' in the format of an 'original article') is another reason for in-office rejection. Some journals do not publish some types of manuscripts at all (e.g. case reports); therefore, these submissions will be rejected on the fly.

Some journals may accept only solicited articles for a particular section of the journal, say review articles. If you submit uninvited manuscripts for such sections, it is very likely that your submission will be rejected without any further processing. Methodological flaws (e.g. use of inappropriate methods to answer the research question or test the hypothesis, obvious problems with sampling, data analyses and inappropriate measurements) are among the other reasons for in-office rejection. Failure to obtain ethical clearance from an institutional review board or non-registration of submitted clinical trials in accepted trial registries could also result in outright rejection of a manuscript.

Poor reporting of research findings is another ground for rejection. It is difficult for a journal to manage a manuscript with 12 figures and 17 tables! Therefore, it would be wise to take a look at the target journal to see how many figures, tables, references, etc. they usually publish in each article. Manuscripts that contain already reported material (redundant publication) or plagiarized ones are also usually rejected in-office.

21.1.3 Pre-Peer-Review Editing of Manuscript

In some journals, where the submission rate is low and there is enough staff, manuscripts detected during office screening to have repairable problems are sent back to authors with comments (prior to peer review). The authors are asked to revise their manuscripts and resubmit for further processing. In some journals, the manuscript is also edited for clarity and readability before it is sent for peer review. This pre-peer-review process would increase the chance of acceptance as the manuscript becomes more understandable by reviewers. However, journals with a high submission rate rarely follow such a process.

If the manuscript survives the in-office evaluation process, it is sent for external review. Almost 25–50% of submitted manuscripts may be rejected in the office. This process would take around 10 days, and thus, if you do not receive a rejection letter within 2 weeks of submission, you may consider it as a good sign—your manuscript has possibly survived the in-office evaluation process.

21.2   Peer Review

What does peer review mean? According to the *American Heritage* Dictionary, 'peer' means 'a person who belongs to the same age group or social group as someone else' [2], and 'peer review' means assessment of a manuscript (or another product) by a person or persons of similar expertise (peers) as the author(s). In journalology, this term refers to evaluation of a manuscript by external reviewers. By 'external' we mean those outside the editorial office and editorial board, presumably increasing the chance of independent evaluation of the manuscript [3].

21.2.1 Goals

The process has three major goals: (1) to help the author(s) improve their manuscript, (2) to help the editor make an appropriate decision to publish or reject the manuscript and (3) to help the editor improve the quality of what will be published. However, peer review is inefficient, as Fiona Godlee, the editor of *BMJ*, once said, the process is 'expensive, slow, subjective and biased, open to abuse, patchy at detecting important methodological defects, and almost useless at detecting fraud or misconduct' [3]. Nevertheless, in the absence of a better process, editors of scientific journals use it extensively.

21.2.2 Types

Generally, there are three types of peer review—double-blind, single-blind and open-review systems. In double-blind review, neither the authors nor the reviewers are informed of each other's identities. Some journals use double-blind peer review since many people believe that it would decrease bias and give a fair chance of review. However, for several reasons and in light of the results of some studies that show that blinding reviewers is difficult [4, 5], the single-blind review system— where reviewers know the authors' identity, but the authors are not aware of the reviewers' identities—is currently more extensively used. This system is used successfully by many good journals such as *The Lancet*. The open-review system is used by fewer journals, *BMJ* being one of them. In this system both reviewers and authors are aware of each other's identity. The system is completely transparent. However, it is very important that no matter what review system is used, authors and reviewers should not contact each other directly—all communications should be done through the editorial office.

21.2.3 The Process

The manuscript is generally sent to two reviewers (and sometimes to a statistical reviewer too, depending on the complexity of statistical treatment of the data). They are usually given around 3 weeks to complete the review and send their comments to the editorial office. Reviewers are generally asked to comment on the following: the originality of the manuscript, its relevance to the scope of the journal and its importance to the journal's readership, whether the methodology used is appropriate to answer the research question or test the research hypothesis, whether the presentation of results is appropriate, what sections of the manuscript are better published only on the web (questionnaires, movies of the technique used, raw data, etc.), appropriate use of statistics and so on.

The reviewers of a manuscript expect good research design and methods, simple tables and figures, logical organization, brevity, appropriate use of statistics and balance in the introduction and discussion.

When reviewers' comments arrive, they are summarized and compiled by the handling editor, who with the help of other editors (or editorial board members) makes a decision about the manuscript. The editor-in-chief is then informed of the decision and, after examining all the evidence, decides what to do with the manuscript. The decision ranges from 'accept as is' (which is rare) to 'revision' or 'rejection'.

21.3   If Your Manuscript Is Accepted …

This is good news and a time to celebrate (and continue working on your other manuscripts!). You need to wait till the proofs of your article are sent to you. The proof is usually a PDF file looking almost identical to the final version of the article to be published in the journal. Do not pay attention to the page numbers as they will be changed in the final layout. Sometimes, the quality of figures in the proof is inferior to those that will be published in the print version. Do not forget that this is your final chance to pick up any errors that may have crept into your article. Therefore, read the proof carefully; pay attention to spellings, words, numbers, tables, references and whatever you think is important. At this stage, you cannot do any substantial editing. The only acceptable corrections are pointing out a misspelt word, incorrect number, an omitted verb, etc. However, if you find a major problem, say omission of a figure or table, you can mention it, as probably this error occurred in the production section and the journal would thus feel obliged to correct it. Asking for major edits at this stage may delay publication of your article, as the manuscript would then have to be returned to the editorial office to be re-examined by an editor; some journals may in fact charge you for this extra work.

If you find any problems in the proof, point these out clearly; you may use the annotations tool in the PDF reader software to insert comments or edit the text. Alternatively, you may list the exact points where attention is needed; specify the exact place (page, column, paragraph and line) where the changes should be made; also indicate the change. The article lines in some proofs are numbered; this makes it much easier to indicate the place where changes should be made. There is usually a deadline for sending the proof back to the production department or journal office (around 48 h). If you do not return the proof or your comments within the timeframe, it is assumed that you agree with the publication of the article as is (silence is a sign of acceptance!).

After your article is published, some journals will send you one or a few copies of the journal or reprints of your article. Journals also send you a form for reprint request. If you need more reprints, you can buy as many copies as you like. Currently, most journals provide a PDF reprint free of charge to the corresponding author to be used for non-commercial use.

21.4   If the Journal Asks for Revision

If the journal asks you to revise your manuscript, then do whatever the reviewers ask for, as long as it does not jeopardize the scientific argument and quality of your article. In fact, it is not necessary to comply with all the comments of reviewers; you can provide reasonable answers why you do not agree to all or some of the comments—you may provide some scientific reasons, a reference, and show the editorial office that you are right in the calculation of the sample size, dosage of drugs, etc. As mentioned earlier, those who reviewed your manuscript are presumably your peers and have (at least) the same scientific background as you. However, in the real world, that may not always be the case. Sometimes, reviewers may misinterpret parts of your manuscript. Often, this is because the manuscript lacks clarity. In such instances, the reviewers' comments may not be correct. You should attempt to further clarify to the editor what you wish to say.

Occasionally, the suggestions of the two reviewers may be contradictory (e.g. one reviewer suggests omission of subgroup analysis, while the other suggests a more detailed subgroup analysis). This does not happen often, because the editors take care to remove such suggestions from the reviewers' comments, before these are conveyed to the authors. Nevertheless, in the event, you may choose to follow one of these and explain the situation to the editor in the cover letter, or better still within the responses to reviewers' comments; it may help to indicate why you chose a particular option.

You should answer all the reviewers' comments point by point and clearly. Indicate if you have complied with the suggestion, or provide appropriate reasons if you have not. In the revised version of the manuscript, indicate the changes you have made; you may highlight the revised text, write the changes in another colour, underline the changes or turn on the 'track changes' option of your word processor. No matter what you do, the revised parts should be clearly recognizable. One of the important points is to remember to make changes throughout the manuscript—text, tables, legends to figures, abstract, etc. Many authors just change the text and forget to correct other parts of the manuscript (e.g. abstract), leading to discordance between the content of various sections.

In addition to the comments of the reviewers, you may have to deal with some editorial queries too. Those usually include a request for further clarification of the text, raw data for redrawing the graphs or reconfirming the statistical analyses, figures with higher resolution, more details about references which may happen to be incomplete, any funding sources, conflicts of interests, etc. The editorial office may occasionally ask you to provide copies of some of the references you cited in your manuscript or copies of the consent forms signed by the participants. The journal office usually asks you to make the necessary revisions within a certain period. It is, therefore, necessary to stick to this schedule; if this is not possible, explain why you cannot do so, and ask for more time—this should be done before the deadline.

After the revised version of the manuscript and the necessary explanations arrive at the editorial office, these receive the attention of the handling editor. The revised version of the manuscript along with your answers is usually re-evaluated in the editorial office itself. However, sometimes, the journal may consider it necessary to send the manuscript back to reviewers again.

If the revisions and clarifications are acceptable, you will receive an acceptance letter—you already know what will happen next. The editorial office may accept publishing the revised version in another format; for example, the journal may indicate that your manuscript that has been submitted as an 'original article' is acceptable for publication as a 'brief report' or 'correspondence'. It is of course your right to accept the proposal or not.

Sometimes, the revisions and answers are not acceptable. Here, the editorial office may ask you to revise the manuscript more carefully, and you need to redo the work with greater diligence. Finally, despite all your efforts, the manuscript may sometimes be rejected.

21.5   If Your Manuscript Gets Rejected

This is an unpleasant situation but inevitable in the course of your career. If it is of any comfort to you, let me confess that after I have rejected some of the manuscripts, I have occasionally felt that I may have taken an incorrect decision.

There are many reasons why your manuscript may get rejected; however, you have two options: to file a plea and ask the editor to re-evaluate your manuscript—where in most instances, the original verdict will stay—or to submit your manuscript to another journal. Here, you should look at the glass as half full—now, you can revise your manuscript according to the comments of reviewers and submit it to a more appropriate journal (do not forget to change the style, references, etc. of your manuscript, if necessary, to match the requirements of the second journal).

Some journals such as *BMJ* and *The Lancet* have several affiliated journals. During your primary submission, to such journals, you are given an option to indicate whether, if the manuscript is rejected, the system may pass your manuscript (and the reviewers' comments) automatically to another affiliated journal (of lesser repute). The new journal can then process your submission more easily and in a shorter time. Some other journals may ask you to also submit the comments of reviewers (if any) with your new submission. Although that is optional and you are not obliged to do so, such submissions may help in faster evaluation of your manuscript.

The time from submission to first verdict varies from journal to journal, but it is usually 6–12 weeks. However, the time from acceptance to publication varies widely for different journals and, at times, even between various sections in a journal. For some sections in certain journals, it could be as long as 18 months. For original articles, it usually takes 2–6 months. Therefore, it is important to select the target journal appropriately.

Some journals provide another route for publication—fast-track publication where the authors ask for a rapid processing of their manuscript; sometimes, the editor may decide that a submitted manuscript is suitable for fast-track publication (when the manuscript discusses a topical and controversial topic or something that has public health implications). In such cases, the journal endeavours to complete all the above-mentioned processes in a shorter period. This process is usually expensive, and the authors may be asked to pay for it. The accepted articles will usually be published first online and then in print.

With more experience (and receiving more rejection letters!), you will progressively master the process and learn to survive peer review. But, do not forget that neither revisions nor rejections are personal and all that is done is aimed at improving the quality of your published work.

References

1. Billings JS. An address on our medical literature. BMJ. 1881;2:262–8.
2. Peer. Merriam-Webster online Dictionary. http://www.merriam-webster.com/dictionary/peer. Accessed 7 April 2014.
3. Godlee F, Jefferson T, editors. Peer review in health sciences. 2nd ed. London: BMJ Books; 2003.
4. Godlee F, Gale CR, Martyn CN. Effect on the quality of peer review of blinding reviewers and asking them to sign their reports: a randomized controlled trial. JAMA. 1998;280:237–40.
5. Justice AC, Cho MK, Winker MA, Berlin JA, Rennie D. Does masking author identity improve peer review quality? A randomized controlled trial. PEER Investigators. JAMA. 1998;280:240–2.

Conflicts of Interest

Christine Laine

Conflicts of interest in biomedicine have perhaps existed in some form since the dawn of medicine with healers more apt to recommend therapies whose use would lead to some benefit for the healer, whether directly through financial gain or indirectly through gains in reputation and prestige. However, over recent decades, conflicts of interest have grown in frequency, degree and their potential to bias the medical literature, and, consequently, medical practice [1]. For this reason, the management of potential conflicts of interest has become a critical component in the communication and publication of biomedical science. Editors, publishers, researchers, peer reviewers and funders are among the involved stakeholders who must be aware of conflicts of interest and cooperate in managing conflicts in an ethical and transparent manner.

22.1 What Is Conflict of Interest?

The potential for conflict of interest arises when an individual has a relationship with an entity that has a stake in the results of research or other scholarly work that could inappropriately influence the design, conduct, reporting or interpretation of that work [2]. For example, consider a researcher who is conducting a clinical trial of a new drug and also owns shares in the company that produces that drug. The researcher stands to gain financially if the drug fares favourably in the trial and becomes a popular treatment option for the condition under study. This relationship has the potential to subtly (or not so subtly) influence the decisions that researcher must make in conducting the trial and interpreting the results [3]. For example, the

C. Laine
Annals of Internal Medicine and American College of Physicians,
Philadelphia, PA, USA
e-mail: claine@mail.acponline.org

© The National Medical Journal of India 2018
P. Sahni, R. Aggarwal (eds.), *Reporting and Publishing Research in the Biomedical Sciences*, https://doi.org/10.1007/978-981-10-7062-4_22

researcher might be less motivated to uncover potential adverse events than a researcher who did not have financial ties to the drug manufacturer or be inclined to use as a comparator a placebo instead of a drug already known to be effective in the particular condition. It is the presence of conflicts that matters, and not the individual's opinion about whether or not his or her behaviour is influenced by those relationships.

While financial conflicts of interest tend to receive the most attention, financial relationships are not the only factors that have the potential to introduce bias and hence are included under conflicts of interest. Intellectual passion, personal relationships, political views, religious beliefs and academic competition all have the potential to colour how someone conducts or interprets scholarly work. Yet, it is much more difficult to objectively define and identify these nonfinancial conflicts than it is to identify whether someone owns equity in or receives funding from a certain company or has some other relationship that involves the transfer of funds. For that reason, discussions and policies around conflict of interest tend to call for detailed financial disclosure with less focus, if any, on nonfinancial relationships. However, many policies for disclosure of conflicts of interest recognize that there may be nonfinancial relationships that reasonable readers would want to know about. An example of such a policy is that of the *BMJ* [4]. Of note, a uniform disclosure form developed by the International Committee of Medical Journal Editors (ICMJE) includes several specific questions about a variety of financial relationships and a single question about nonfinancial relationships that states, 'Are there other relationships or activities that readers could perceive to have influenced, or that give the appearance of potentially influencing, what you wrote in the submitted work?' [5]. It is in an individual's best interest to err on the side of full disclosure when reporting nonfinancial sources of potential conflict of interest. When this is not done and such factors become known after the fact, it can create the perception of deliberate deception, a situation that is best avoided.

Another type of conflict of interest that can be financial or nonfinancial relates not to the individual investigators or authors, but rather to the institutions they work for. A 2009 report of the Institute of Medicine includes examples of how these relationships, which often generate substantial benefit to an institution even if no direct benefit accrues to a specific faculty member, can lead to problems and bias in research [6]. For this reason, it is important that individual investigators make themselves aware of institution–industry relationships and disclose them when submitting work for publication.

22.2   Do Conflicts of Interest Really Matter?

While some investigators argue vehemently that financial relationships do not influence their research, ample evidence suggests otherwise. A 2003 systematic review identified 37 articles published during 1980–2002 that contained original data on financial relationships [7]. The review found that one-quarter of investigators had industry affiliations and two-thirds of institutions had a financial stake in an entity that sponsored research at that institution. Eight of the included articles explored the relationship between industry funding and study outcome in a total of 1140 studies and showed a positive association between industry funding and results that were favourable to the funder. Additional studies have observed similar relationships between conflicts of interest and results of published research [8–11]. Further, poor handling of potential conflicts of interest is among the reasons for a lack of public trust in the biomedical research enterprise.

22.3   Strategies to Address Conflicts of Interest

Since real-life situations clearly document that conflicts of interest can bias medical research, what is the solution? Some advocate avoidance of potential conflicts by creating a firewall to separate academia and industry. However, such a separation would not only be difficult to implement in current times but could also hinder scientific process as industry–academia collaborations have become an increasingly important source of discovery of new healthcare interventions [12, 13]. In addition, there is evidence that researchers who collaborate with industry are more productive than those who do not [14]. Thus, while individual researchers may choose to eschew any relationship with industry, many will find that such relationships are necessary and beneficial. Thus, the biomedical research enterprise must develop methods to manage conflicts of interest responsibly. The strategies that medical journals and other stakeholders use to manage conflicts of interest include disclosure, exclusion and methodological transparency.

22.3.1 Disclosure

Within the sphere of biomedical publication, disclosure is the most common strategy for managing conflicts of interest. The rationale is that conflicts of interest represent a potential source of bias and, if consumers of the medical literature know that conflicts exist, they can consider these when deciding whether and how to apply research findings to their practice [3]. A decade ago, there was substantial variability in the way that the academic community approached potential conflicts of interest. Many journals either did not ask about conflicts or did so without specifying the sorts of relationships the editors were interested in knowing about. Some journals provided these disclosures to readers by including them with the published article, whereas others simply filed them for record.

In 2001, the ICMJE strengthened its policy on conflicts of interest by requiring authors to disclose specifically whether or not they had financial or personal relationships with entities that might bias the work, to specify these relationships when these existed, and to disclose these relationships to study participants [15]. This statement also recommended that editors err on the side of full disclosure to readers of authors' declared potential conflicts of interest.

In 2009, motivated by great variation from journal to journal and confusion among stakeholders regarding the relationships that warranted disclosure, the ICMJE developed a uniform disclosure form [16]. The Committee members agreed to use the form and invited non-member journals to also adopt it. The form has been updated based on feedback from users [17], and currently, hundreds of journals use it. The form is available at www.icmje.org [5]. Authors submitting to journals that ask for disclosure without providing further guidance might find it useful to refer to the ICMJE form when assembling their disclosure statements.

22.3.2 Exclusion

As noted previously, the complete exclusion of industry–academia relationships is not feasible in current times. Some journals do have policies that prohibit publication of certain types of articles by authors who have certain types of conflicts of interest. For example, the *BMJ* and BMJ Group will not consider some non-research content if authors have competing interests [4]. Other journals, such as *Annals of Internal Medicine*, on the other hand, do not summarily exclude consideration of articles based on the presence of potential conflicts of interest but admit that the presence of conflicts does weigh heavily in decisions about the publication of non-research articles [18].

In 1990, the *New England Journal of Medicine* implemented a policy that excluded review articles and editorials authored by individuals with a financial relationship with an entity that could benefit from an intervention discussed in the article [19] but amended this policy in 2002 to permit exceptions [20]. This journal-to-journal variation in policies that use exclusion to manage conflicts of interest makes it imperative that authors consult information for authors or contact editorial offices when considering submission of a non-research article that includes authors with potential competing interests.

22.3.3 Methodological Standards and Transparency

A third strategy for limiting bias related to conflicts of interest is strict adherence to methodological standards and transparency. Such standards exist for articles such as those reporting original research articles and systematic reviews but not for articles such as those reporting narrative reviews and commentaries. This is the rationale that underlies why the exclusion policies described above generally apply to these latter article types but not to the former. When authors with potential conflicts of interest prepare work for submission to peer-review journals, they should adhere carefully to reporting standards for the type of work they are reporting (www.equator-network.org). Such rigor and transparency of reporting will enable editors and reviewers to detect whether the conflicts disclosed are likely to have biased the work. When methods are not carefully reported, reviewers and editors will be likely to worry whether a bias actually exists.

22.4   Resources from Professional Organizations

Several organizations concerned with the integrity of scientific publication provide guidance about the proper handling of conflicts of interest by authors, editors and peer reviewers. Authors who have relationships that present the potential for conflict of interest should become familiar with such guidance. These sources include the ICMJE's 'Recommendations for the Conduct, Reporting, Editing, and Publication of Scholarly Work in Medical Journals' (www.icmje.org), the Council of Science Editors' 'White Paper on Promoting Integrity in Scientific Journal Publications, 2012 Update' (www.councilofscienceeditors.org), the World Association of Medical Journal Editors' policy statement on conflict of interest (www.wame.org/conflict-of-interest-in-peer-reviewed-medical-journals), the Federation of American Societies for Experimental Biology guidelines [21] and the Committee on Publication Ethics recommendations (www.publicationethics.org).

A position statement on responsible research publication developed at the 2nd World Congress on Research Integrity in July 2010 includes declaration of conflicts of interest to be among the international standards expected of authors [22]. This policy statement emphasizes that, in addition to disclosing personal relationships with entities that represent potential conflicts of interest, authors should declare the role of the funding source in the design, conduct, analysis, interpretation and reporting of the work. In addition, this statement notes that sources of potential conflict of interest include the relationship of author(s) to the journal, such as if someone submits work to a journal for which he or she serves in an editorial role.

The International Society for Medical Publication Professionals, an organization whose membership consists largely of professionals working for the pharmaceutical industry, developed guidelines for good publication practice for communicating industry-sponsored medical research [23]. These 2009 guidelines emphasize the importance of full disclosure of potential conflicts of interest and suggest that authors favour more rather than less disclosure when they are uncertain about what they need to disclose.

22.5   Other Considerations

While authors are typically the focus of discussions about potential conflicts of interest, it is important that the biomedical research community keep in mind that conflicts may apply to others involved in publishing, including peer reviewers, editors and publishers. Journals should have processes in place for the disclosure and management of potential conflicts of interest among these stakeholders too. The ICMJE, the World Association of Medical Editors, the Council of Science Editors and the Committee on Publication Ethics all offer guidance on this issue. If authors believe that a conflict of interest on the part of a peer reviewer, editor or publisher influenced the decision on their work, they should raise the issue accordingly with the editor, publisher or journal owner.

The Internet makes it possible to quickly and easily gain access to information on activities and relationships of researchers and other stakeholders in biomedical research. It is increasingly common for information on the Internet not to correspond exactly with information that an individual author discloses related to a specific article. Often the discrepancy is easily explainable. For example, an author may report no relevant conflicts on a journal disclosure form, but a prior publication available on the Internet lists relevant relationships with industry because the journal publishing the current paper asked about conflicts only during the past 3 years and the prior publication was from the previous decade when the authors did have active relationships with industry that have since ceased. It is prudent for biomedical researchers to be familiar with information relevant to their potential conflicts of interest that is accessible on the web and be prepared to explain any apparent discrepancies.

22.6   What to Do When Policies Are Not Followed?

Despite the best intentions of those involved in scholarly scientific publication, there will be occasions where potential conflicts of interest are managed inadequately and a piece of work is published without appropriate attention to relevant conflicts of interest. In such cases, it is the responsibility of the journal to correct the literature and to inform the universities and other institutions employing individuals who misreported conflicts of interest. The Committee on Publication Ethics provides flow charts and case examples that are useful guidance when such circumstances develop (www.publicationethics.org).

22.7   Summary

Conflicts of interest can and have adversely influenced the quality of research. Bias associated with poorly managed conflicts of interest can harm study participants and subsequent patients through its effect on biased interpretation of published research. Poor management of conflicts of interest also damages public trust in biomedical research. Thus, it is essential that all involved in the conduct and reporting of biomedical research adhere to practices that aim to minimize the adverse effects of potential conflicts of interest within the research enterprise. Conflicts of interest are ubiquitous in today's world in which academia–industry collaboration is responsible for many advances in the care of disease and maintenance of health. The presence of potential conflicts of interest does not indicate scientific misconduct, but the inappropriate disclosure or management of these conflicts does.

References

1. Campbell EG, Gruen RL, Mountford J, Miller LG, Cleary PD, Blumenthal D. A national survey of physician–industry relationships. N Engl J Med. 2007;356:1742–50.
2. Author Responsibilities—Conflicts of Interest. http://www.icmje.org/recommendations/browse/roles-and-responsibilities/author-responsibilities--conflicts-of-interest.html. Accessed 28 Aug 2015.
3. Davidoff F. Where's the bias? Ann Intern Med. 1997;126:986–8.
4. Declaration of competing interests. http://www.bmj.com/about-bmj/resources-authors/forms-policies-and-checklists/declaration-competing-interests. Accessed 28 Aug 2015.
5. ICMJE Conflict of disclosure form. http://www.icmje.org/conflicts-of-interest/. Accessed 1 May 2015.
6. Lo B, Field MJ, editors. Institute of Medicine (US) Committee on Conflict of Interest in Medical Research, Education, and Practice. Washington, DC: National Academies Press (US); 2009.
7. Bekelman JE, Li Y, Gross CP. Scope and impact of financial conflicts of interest in biomedical research: a systematic review. JAMA. 2003;289:454–65.
8. Friedman LS, Richter ED. Relationship between conflicts of interest and research results. J Gen Intern Med. 2004;19:51–6.
9. Tereskerz PM, Hamric AB, Guterbock TM, Moreno JD. Prevalence of industry support and its relationship to research integrity. Account Res. 2009;16:78–105.
10. Kjaergard LL, Als-Nielsen B. Association between competing interests and authors' conclusions: epidemiological study of randomized clinical trials published in BMJ. BMJ. 2002;325:249.
11. Djulbegovic B, Lacevic M, Cantor A, Fields KK, Bennet CL, Adams JR, et al. The uncertainty principle and industry sponsored research. Lancet. 2000;356:635–8.
12. Drazen JM. Revisiting the commercial–academic interface. N Engl J Med. 2015;372:1853–4.
13. Zerhouni EA. Translational and clinical science—time for a new vision. N Engl J Med. 2005;353:1621–3.
14. Gulbrandsen M, Smeby JC. Industry funding and university professors' research performance. Res Policy. 2005;34:932–50.
15. Davidoff F, DeAngelis CD, Drazen JM, Hoey J, Højgaard L, Horton R, et al. Sponsorship, authorship, and accountability. Ann Intern Med. 2001;135:463–6.
16. Drazen JM, Van der Weyden MB, Sahni P, Rosenberg J, Marusic A, Laine C, et al. Uniform format for disclosure of competing interests in ICMJE journals. Ann Intern Med. 2010;152:125–6.
17. Drazen JM, de Leeuw PW, Laine C, Mulrow CD, DeAngelis CD, Frizelle FA, et al. Toward more uniform conflict disclosures: the updated ICMJE conflict of interest reporting form. Ann Intern Med. 2010;153:268–9.
18. The Editors. Publishing commentary by authors with potential conflicts of interest: when, why, and how. Ann Intern Med. 2004;141:73–4.
19. Angell M, Kassirer JP. Editorials and conflicts of interest. N Engl J Med. 1996;335:1055–6.
20. Drazen JM, Curfman GD. Financial associations of authors. N Engl J Med. 2002;346:1901–2.
21. Brockway LM, Furcht LT. Conflicts of interest in biomedical research—the FASEB guidelines. FASEB J. 2006;20:2435–8.
22. Wager E, Kleinert S. Chapter 50: Responsible research publication: International standards for authors. A position statement developed at the 2nd World Conference on Research Integrity, Singapore, 22–24 July 2010. In: Mayer T, Steneck N, editors. Promoting research integrity in a global environment. Singapore: Imperial College Press/World Scientific Publishing; 2011. p. 309–16. ISBN: 978-981-4340-97-7.
23. Battisti WP, Wager E, Baltzer L, Bridges D, Cairns A, Carswell CI, et al. Good publication practice for communicating company-sponsored medical research: GPP3. Ann Intern Med. 2015;163:461–4. https://doi.org/10.7326/M15-0288.

Redundant Publications

23

Nithya Gogtay

23.1 Introduction

Studies on healthcare issues often consume a large amount of time, effort, money and resources to complete. The success of such a study is measured by its end product, namely, a published paper, and its eventual impact on human health. Biomedical scientists are under intense pressure to publish for several reasons as follows: to sustain research funding; to secure a promotion; to continue to be recognized and acknowledged as an expert within a peer group; to get invited to workshops, conferences or meetings; to serve on academic bodies or other decision-making committees; and to secure patents. This intense pressure can sometimes push scientists to publish the same piece of work more than once or, worse still, publish another person's work as their own.

A redundant publication, also referred to as a duplicate, repetitive or multiple publication, has been defined by the International Committee of Medical Journal Editors (ICMJE) as 'the publication of a paper that overlaps substantially with one already published in print or electronic media' [1]. Redundant publications have a spectrum that ranges from publishing an identical copy of a previously published paper right through to publishing sliced copies. These redundant papers add little or no new information to the existing literature. They represent poor scientific and publication ethics, poor academic conduct and often border on scientific fraud.

The scientific and editorial communities have taken several steps to deal with this issue.

N. Gogtay
Department of Clinical Pharmacology, Seth GS Medical College and KEM Hospital, Mumbai, India
e-mail: nithyagogtay@kem.edu

© The National Medical Journal of India 2018
P. Sahni, R. Aggarwal (eds.), *Reporting and Publishing Research in the Biomedical Sciences*, https://doi.org/10.1007/978-981-10-7062-4_23

23.2   Historical Perspective: The Ingelfinger Rule

The first steps to prevent duplicate publications were perhaps taken at the *New England Journal of Medicine* (*NEJM*) by Franz Joseph Ingelfinger in the late 1960s. A gastroenterologist by training, Ingelfinger served as the editor of *NEJM* during 1967–1977. He noted with concern that the post-World War II era was marked by an increase in the number of scientific journals, the frequency of scientific matter appearing in trade publications before publication in academic journals and increased scientific coverage in the lay press. He perceived this to be a serious threat to his journal's capacity to publish original research and ability to educate its readers. In 1969, he formulated and implemented at the *NEJM* what would later come to be known as the Ingelfinger rule. It prohibited authors submitting papers to the *NEJM* from speaking to the media until after publication of the paper; for those who violated this rule, their papers stood rejected and were not published [2]. Today, most journal editors have adopted this rule and insist on a declaration by authors that the work has not been sent or submitted elsewhere for publication.

23.3   Definitions

The ICMJE's comprehensive definition of a redundant publication is not the only one. They have also been defined as publications that share the same, similar or overlapping data, hypotheses, methods, results, discussion or conclusions [3]. They are often characterized by failure to include cross-references to the main article, and may or may not have the same authors. At times, the order of authorship of the original publication differs from that of its clone [4, 5].

Another type of redundant publication is one where the data are sliced into subsets and published as separate papers rather than the entire study being published as a single article [6]. Each article resulting from the salami slice, referred to as the 'least publishable unit' or 'minimum publishable unit', then provides only minor incremental understanding that could have easily been part of the main or index article.

The addition of a small amount of new data to previously published data is yet another type of redundancy which may make the study look new [4, 7]. Table 23.1 gives a list of criteria for redundant publications used by the editors of a group of cardiothoracic journals [8].

Table 23.1 Criteria for redundant publication

• Similar hypothesis
• Similar sample size
• Identical or almost identical methodology
• Similar results
• At least one author in common in both manuscripts
• No new information or new information of little relevance

Adapted from reference [8]

23.4   Problems with Redundant Publications

Redundant publications, besides constituting unethical research conduct, are also inappropriate for a variety of other reasons. From a journal's perspective, such papers overburden and waste the time of already beleaguered peer reviewers, use journal pages that could have been devoted to truly original publications and result in the editors spending time, energy and effort on punitive action and reprimand. From readers' perspective, they overload medical literature and waste their time. It is also unfair to those researchers who do not resort to this deception as academic position and merit continue to be judged by the number of published papers, thereby favouring those with a larger number of publications [9–12]. This phenomenon also inflates the importance of some research findings and can distort the results of meta-analysis and thus impact adversely on the practice of evidence-based medicine. Tramer et al. [13] specifically analysed the implications of covert redundant publications on the assessment of therapeutic efficacy of anti-emetics by analysing data from randomized controlled trials. They found that 17% of published studies represented duplicate publications, and this led to the duplicate inclusion of results for 28% of patients. Even more disconcerting was that those studies with the most positive findings were the ones more likely to be duplicated. They further showed that an analysis that included the redundant publication led to a 28% overestimation of the therapeutic effect of these drugs when compared with an analysis that included only the original work [13]. This also led to a lower estimate of the number of patients that would need to be treated for one patient to benefit; this has a direct effect on patient care!

23.5   Extent of Redundant Publications

Fang et al. analysed 2047 biomedical and life science research articles indexed by PubMed that had been retracted as of 3 May 2012 and found that only 21.3% of retractions were attributed to error. In contrast, 67.4% of retractions were attributable to misconduct—fraud or suspected fraud (43.4%), duplicate publications (14.2%) and plagiarism (9.8%) [14]. In another study, retractions accounted for 0.02% of articles included in the database of biomedical literature, and redundant publications accounted for 17% of these retractions [15].

Some studies have looked at the prevalence of redundant publications in different medical specialties. In a study of papers published in the *Journal of Urology* during 2006, the problem was found to affect 3.8% of papers [16]. In another analysis, studies in radiology had a very low rate of redundant publications (0.02%), whereas the rate for papers in surgery was 11% [4]. The true extent of the problem in biomedical literature probably lies between these two extremes.

23.6   Patterns of Redundant Publications

At least two papers have attempted to classify the patterns of duplicate publications. In a study of systematic reviews in *Anesthesia and Analgesia* from 1989 to 2002, von Elm et al. analysed 103 duplicate papers and their main articles ($n = 78$) and identified six distinct patterns [17]. Pattern 1A had an identical sample and outcome(s) to the main article and mostly did not carry a cross-reference to the main paper. Pattern 1B was similar to 1A, the only difference being that rather than one article, two or more articles were put together to create the duplicate; duplicates with this pattern were more likely to have been sponsored by the pharmaceutical industry. In pattern 2, the main paper and the duplicate had the same study sample but reported different outcomes. Patterns 3A and 3B primarily pertained to duplicates having different sample sizes (larger and smaller, respectively) relative to the main paper but with a similar outcome, while pattern 4 had both sample size and outcome different from the main article [17]. Pattern 1A constituted a *copy*, pattern 2 *the least publishable unit*, pattern 3A a *meat extender* and 3B *disaggregation*. The study also showed that duplicate articles were published soon after the original article (median 1 year) and in journals with a similar impact factor; furthermore, the number of citations received by the original article and the duplicate article was similar.

Bailey used a classification based on similarity: Level 1 where 10% or more of the contents were identical, Level II where the contents were very similar but not exact duplication, Level III where the data were salami sliced, Level IV where the sample size was increased without a change in the conclusion or intervention and Level V where the same message was published for a different readership [18].

23.7   Why Do Redundant Publications Occur?

There are several disparate (overt or covert) reasons for duplicate publications. These range from inexperience to deliberate acts. Authors may try to reach a wider audience through publishing in two journals with widely different readerships. Alternatively, they may want to increase the number of their published papers in an attempt to secure research grants or promotions. In the early stages of a researcher's career, inexperience or ignorance (including lack of guidance or supervision by senior co-authors) may also play a role.

Occasionally, authors may have nothing to do with an apparent redundant publication; a journal editor may think it more appropriate to publish the data in two papers rather than one long one and may have suggested this to the authors.

Decreasing research budgets coupled with pressure to publish also does not help [3, 19]. In today's research environment, there is little likelihood of an immediate scientific discovery, and it may take several years of hard labour to reach a major breakthrough or have publishable findings. This leads to 'undue' pressure on scientists to show results in the form of publications.

23.8 When Are Redundant Publications Acceptable?

There are occasions when it is acceptable to publish the same paper in two (or more) journals simultaneously or closely following each other. But this must always be done with full agreement of all the journals concerned and the authors.

Journal editors will consider publishing abstracts that have been presented at conferences, meetings or workshops in either oral or poster format or are being considered for printing in conference proceedings. The International Committee of Medical Journal Editors (ICMJE) permits the posting of results in clinical trial registries prior to full publication as a paper, as long as the results are in the form of a table or a structured abstract. The registry should always carry a statement indicating the current publishing status of the full paper, and if published, the complete citation should be provided in the registry [1].

Guidelines formulated by international agencies, government organizations or professional bodies need to reach the widest possible audience and are intentionally published in more than one journal. Authors/editors of such guidelines usually decide which journal would be considered primary (or 'index') and those that would be considered secondary. Complete transparency among all the parties is paramount, and readers are informed of the multiple publications through a note in each journal.

Another acceptable 'repetitive' publication of a paper applies to republication in another language. This may serve to increase the readership and reach of the information. Again, complete transparency among all parties must be ensured.

It is generally agreed that certain norms, as listed below (adapted from the ICMJE), should be met for acceptable 'repetitive' or 'multiple' publication:

1. The authors should have received approval from editors of both the journals (the one with index publication and the other with the secondary publication); the editor of the secondary publication must have seen an exact copy of the primary or index publication.
2. The index publication should precede the secondary publication by at least a week unless specifically worked out between the editors; this preserves the respect for the former version.
3. The secondary publication should be true in all respects to the index publication.
4. The secondary publication should be targeted for a different group of readers; it is important to consider whether an abbreviated version may be sufficient for this readership.
5. The title page should clearly indicate that it is a secondary publication and it should carry a footnote providing a full reference of the primary publication. Further, the title should indicate whether the secondary publication is a complete or abridged republication or a complete or abridged translation. The ICMJE recommends that the permission for the secondary publication be free of charge. The National Library of Medicine (NLM) indexes only the primary language version and does not cite or index translations.

23.9   Searching for Redundant Publications

23.9.1 The Use of Electronic Search Engines and Databases

From discovery through serendipity, the detection of redundant publications today has moved to electronic resources that specifically address this problem. *eTBLAST* is a text similarity-based information retrieval and search engine that has been developed by the Innovation Laboratory at the Virginia Bioinformatics Institute and is available free at http://invention.swmed.edu/etblast/index.shtml [20]. It searches citation databases and databases that contain full text such as PubMed. A hybrid algorithm is used to conduct a search at two levels; the first is based on keywords and the second on sentence alignment. *eTBLAST* then returns a quantitative similarity score with a higher score indicating greater similarity.

Another useful resource is *Déjà vu*, a database funded by the Hudson Foundation and the Human Services Office of Research Integrity through a grant from the National Institutes of Health. It contains citations that are very similar to those in Medline—many of which could represent duplicate publications and possible plagiarism. The citations are computationally identified but manually curated (titles and abstracts). The final arbiter is the user [21]. Although this database might deter some authors, it also contains false positives. The latter can jeopardize and harm the careers of honest scientists [22].

23.10   Dealing with Redundant Publications

23.10.1   The Committee on Publication Ethics (COPE) Guidelines

The COPE has flowcharts on its website to help editors deal with suspected misconduct; this includes redundant publications that may be detected while a manuscript is under review or after it has been published.

In brief, redundancy detected before publication is classified as no significant overlap, minor overlap and major overlap. If there is no significant overlap, the editor can discuss the issue with the reviewer and then proceed with the review process. If there is minor overlap, the author is contacted in neutral terms, the journal's position explained and disappointment expressed where appropriate. The author is asked to look again at the article and either cross-reference or delete the overlapping parts; the journal editor can then decide whether or not to proceed with the review and inform the reviewer appropriately. If there is major overlap, the corresponding author is contacted in writing, ideally with a copy of the signed author declaration/statement and evidence of redundancy. Further action depends upon the nature of the author's response. If the journal considers it unsatisfactory, all other authors are written to, the journal's stand explained and the article rejected. The author's superiors may be notified and the author apprised of this. The final action taken is then communicated to the reviewer. Should the author fail to respond after repeated attempts, the journal writes to the head of the author's institution and requests contact with the author.

When duplication or redundancy is detected after publication, the principles of dealing with it are broadly similar. If the degree of overlap is determined to be major, the published paper might be retracted and the authors' superiors advised. The journal's readers also need to be informed of the action taken [23].

23.11 Minimizing Redundant Publications

Detection of redundant publications is a laborious process for both reviewers and editors. Clear communication between the author and the editor (particularly for inexperienced authors) can help minimize the problem.

Authors should inform the journal, before submitting a manuscript or in the accompanying letter, of any potential areas of overlap and redundancy with papers they have previously published or intend to publish in the future.

Authors should ask themselves: Are we really reporting new knowledge? Is our information enhanced by reporting in two or more smaller papers? Would the overall impact be strengthened by combining the papers, rather than publishing in slices? [24]. Have we identified cases or subjects included in our group's other published studies and made sure that they are appropriately referenced? [24].

In addition, we need to modify the academic system that leads authors to indulge in this practice. Promotions can be based more on the quality of published papers, rather than the number of publications. The relative contribution an author has made to a publication should also be taken into account. The evaluation of teaching work (and skills) could be another criterion for promotion. These measures may help address the all-pervasive 'publish or perish' syndrome that currently exists in our institutions [10, 25, 26].

23.12 Summary

Publication misconduct in the form of redundant publications is a common problem and a widely debated issue. The goal of medical journals is to educate, provide high-quality scientific content and thereby serve the best interests of patients. Redundant publications strike at the root of the scientific publication structure, which is based on credibility, trust and presumed scientific honesty and integrity. While elimination of the problem seems unlikely, prevention is possible and a far better option than policing and reprimand [26]. This requires promotion of awareness on the issue and cooperation and communication among authors, reviewers and editors.

References

1. International Committee of Medical Journal Editors. Recommendations for the conduct, reporting, editing, and publication of scholarly work in medical journals. http://www.icmje.org/recommendations/. Accessed 30 April 2015.
2. Toy J. The Ingelfinger rule: Franz Ingelfinger at the *New England Journal of Medicine* 1967–77. Sci Editor. 2002;25:195–8.
3. Benos DJ, Fabres J, Farmer J, Gutierrez JP, Hennessy K, Kosek D, et al. Ethics and scientific publication. Adv Physiol Educ. 2005;29:59–74.
4. Schein M, Paladugu R. Redundant surgical publications: tip of the iceberg? Surgery. 2001;129:655–61.
5. Rivara FP, Christakis DA, Cummings P. Duplicate publication. Arch Pediatr Adolesc Med. 2004;158:926.
6. Elstein AS, Cadmus C, Pitkin R, Mundy D, McDowell C. Salami science: are we still allowing it? Sci Editor. 1998;21:200.
7. Tobin MJ. AJRCCM's policy on duplicate publication: infrequently asked questions. Am J Respir Crit Care Med. 2002;166:433–4.
8. Angell M, Relman AS. Redundant publication. N Engl J Med. 1989;320:1212–4.
9. Cho BK, Rosenfeldt F, Turina MI, Karp RB, Ferguson TB, Bodnar E, et al. Joint statement on redundant (duplicate) publication by the editors of the undersigned cardiothoracic journals. Ann Thorac Surg. 2000;69:663.
10. Angell M. Publish or perish: a proposal. Ann Intern Med. 1986;104:261–2.
11. Relman AS. Publish or perish—or both. N Engl J Med. 1977;297:724–5.
12. Alfonso F, Bermejo J, Segovia J. Duplicate or redundant publication: can we afford it? Rev Esp Cardiol. 2005;58:601–4.
13. Tramer MR, Reynolds DJM, Moore RA, McQuay HJ. Impact of covert duplicate publication on meta-analysis: a case study. BMJ. 1997;315:635–40.
14. Fang FC, Steen RG, Casadevall A. Misconduct accounts for the majority of retracted scientific publications. Proc Natl Acad Sci U S A. 2012;109:17028–33. https://doi.org/10.1073/pnas.1212247109. Erratum in: Proc Natl Acad Sci U S A. 2013;110:1137.
15. Wager E, Williams P. Why and how to journals retract articles? An analysis of Medline retractions from 1988–2008. J Med Ethics. 2011;37:567–70.
16. Hennessey KK, Williams AR, Afshar K, MacNeily AE. Duplicate publications: a sample of redundancy in the Journal of Urology. Can Urol Assoc J. 2012;6:177–80.
17. von Elm E, Poglia G, Walder B, Tramer M. Different patterns of duplicate publication: an analysis of articles used in systematic reviews. JAMA. 2004;291:974–80.
18. Bailey BJ. Duplicate publication in the field of otolaryngology–head and neck surgery. Otolaryngol Head Neck Surg. 2002;126:211–6.
19. Johnson C. Repetitive, duplicate and redundant publications: a review for authors and readers. J Manipulative Physiol Ther. 2006;29:505–9.
20. Lewis J, Ossowski S, Hicks J, Errami M, Garner HR. Text similarity: an alternative way to search MEDLINE. Bioinformatics. 2006;22:2298–304. https://doi.org/10.1093/bioinformatics/btl388.
21. Errami M, Sun Z, Long TC, George AC, Garner HR. Déjà vu: a database of highly similar citations in the scientific literature. Nucleic Acids Res. 2009;37(Database issue):D921–4.
22. Rifai N, Bossuyt PM, Bruns DE. Identifying duplicate publications: primum non nocere. Clin Chem. 2008;54:777–8.
23. Committee on Publication Ethics Guidelines on Good Publication and Code of Conduct. http://www.publicationethics.org/resources/guidelines. Accessed 30 April 2015.
24. Bankier AA, Levine D, Sheiman RG, Lev MH, Kressel HY. Redundant publications in radiology: shades of gray in a seemingly black-and-white issue. Radiology. 2008;247:605–7.
25. Kassirer JP, Angell M. Redundant publication: a reminder. N Engl J Med. 1995;333:449–50.
26. Doherty M. The misconduct of redundant publication. Ann Rheum Dis. 1996;55:783–5.

Scientific Fraud and Other Types of Scientific Misconduct

Lorraine Ferris

24.1 Introduction

A study of 395 retracted papers by journals published in English and indexed in MEDLINE between 1982 and 2002 shows that 107 (27.1%) of these were retracted for scientific misconduct [1]. Similarly, Wager and Williams [2] report that 28% of the 312 MEDLINE English journal retractions (during 2005–2008 and a 1:3 random sampling of those during 1988–2004) were labelled as resulting from scientific misconduct. Many believe that more scientific misconduct in published articles goes undetected.

When discovered, findings of scientific misconduct damage the reputations of authors, tarnish entire fields of study and contribute to negative public opinion about science in general (and support for it). Moreover, undetected misconduct in published articles can divert the course of science and discovery and lead to waste of time, money and intellectual talent. Even more importantly, fraudulent conclusions in the field of medicine can expose the public and patients to increased risk.

Steen [3] studied retracted papers indexed in PubMed (during 2000–2010) involving human participants (or fresh human biomaterials) and highlighted how fraudulent published research (particularly clinical trials) poses potential risks to patients. These risks can be due to commission (e.g. exposing patients to risks of ineffective or dangerous treatment) or omission (e.g. withholding effective and safe treatment). Fraudulent research in the area of public health could prompt inappropriate changes to public health practices that put an entire population at risk.

Often in cases of scientific misconduct, an attempt is made to determine which author or authors of the implicated publication are to blame and which are not.

L. Ferris
World Association of Medical Editors (WAME), Toronto, ON, Canada

Research Oversight and Compliance, University of Toronto, Toronto, ON, Canada
e-mail: lef@ices.on.ca

© The National Medical Journal of India 2018
P. Sahni, R. Aggarwal (eds.), *Reporting and Publishing Research in the Biomedical Sciences*, https://doi.org/10.1007/978-981-10-7062-4_24

However, it is not always possible to establish who is responsible. Also, when a paper is retracted, the formal notice refers to the publication itself and, at times, reasons for the retraction; it may stop short of naming the authors responsible.

Huth summed up authorship responsibility clearly: 'The lesson is that if you are a co-author, you take responsibility for the paper on which your name appears, but this responsibility includes what your co-authors have done and written as well' [4]. While many find this definition of universal responsibility to be impractical, especially for large research endeavours such as large multi-country and multisite studies, Kennedy asks a difficult question: 'If the benefits of authorship are enjoyed jointly and severally by all the authors, shouldn't the liability be shared in the same way?' [5].

24.2   The Purpose of This Chapter

This chapter offers some steps authors can take to help prevent and identify scientific misconduct before a paper is submitted for publication. Some of these steps are already required by a few journals; where they are not, authors are advised to adopt these precautions in their research practice. Fortunately, many of these steps also contribute to a paper's scientific soundness and integrity, and following them should improve the quality of the work. While it is not possible to address all aspects of scientific misconduct here, those most relevant to this chapter will be discussed.

Unfortunately, it is not possible to offer an exhaustive list of steps for preventing scientific misconduct. Some journals may have additional steps or stipulations, and some subspecialties or fields of study may have specific requirements. However, this chapter offers important information that should be of help to most authors.

Authors will have different expertise and different responsibilities with respect to the paper (and the research process). It is not realistic to assume, for example, that an author with expertise in designing randomized controlled trials should be able to identify data suppression when reviewing complex and technical data analysis plans and outputs. Moreover, a corresponding author has responsibilities additional to those of other authors (and these could vary from journal to journal). In this chapter, these differences are recognized where appropriate; however, where no particular author is associated with a step, the research team should appoint one of its members to be responsible for that step.

This chapter is intended to be relevant for all types of peer-reviewed publications (e.g. empirical, review, opinion papers), and therefore some of the information will not apply to every paper submitted for publication.

24.3   Definitions

Scientific misconduct (sometimes called research misconduct) is either intentional or due to recklessness [6]. Most definitions emphasize that it involves serious departure from the relevant scientific community's commonly accepted practices when proposing, reviewing, conducting or reporting research findings. The definition of scientific misconduct is not all embracing [7], and in the United States, the Code of Federal Regulations limits the definition to fabrication, falsification and plagiarism [6]. Despite there being no universal definition, 'there are some flagrant acts that everybody would agree are misconduct, and we need broad definitions to begin the process of deepening understanding of what constitutes misconduct' [7]. Honest errors or honest differences about conducting research or reporting/disseminating research findings do not constitute scientific misconduct [6, 8].

Table 24.1 provides definitions used in this chapter for various categories of scientific misconduct relating to submitted or published papers. On p. 244 are some additional comments about Table 24.1:

Table 24.1 Definitions of various categories of research misconduct concerning the publication of papers

Category of research misconduct	Definition
Fabrication	Making up data or results and recording or reporting them [6]
Falsification	Manipulating research materials, equipment or processes or changing or omitting data or results such that the research is not accurately represented in the research record [6]
Plagiarism	Appropriation of another person's ideas, processes, results or words without giving appropriate credit [6]
Using intellectual property or research data that does not belong to the authors	Using 'intellectual property' without permission from the owner who has the legal right to exclude others from using it or transferring it without the owner's permission. In biomedical sciences, 'intellectual property' often concerns property such as inventions, methods, techniques, patents, composition of materials, computer programmes or copyright, but it can also be something less tangible related to human creativity. There are different types of legal protections given to various kinds of intellectual property. Using 'research data' without permission from those who own or co-own it. 'Research data' is information that is collected, observed or created for research purposes and includes, for example, questionnaires, transcripts, audiotapes/videotapes, slides, samples/specimens, laboratory/field notebooks and data files
Failing to disclose relevant conflicts of interest	Failure to disclose material conflicts of interest or failure to follow journal rules about disclosing conflicts of interest
Inappropriate assignment/ non-assignment of authorship	Inappropriate assignment of authorship credit: including as authors those who do not meet authorship criteria, failing to include as authors those who meet the authorship criteria, naming an individual who did not consent to be an author and submitting a paper without all the authors agreeing on it

Note: A finding of scientific misconduct may depend on the seriousness of the act and whether it falls within the definition of scientific misconduct used

- Fabrication, falsification (including altering and/or suppressing data) and plagiarism are uniformly seen as serious scientific misconduct.
- Other definitions in Table 24.1—such as failing to disclose relevant conflicts of interests, using inappropriate rules of authorship, failing to obtain appropriate research ethics approvals—are also serious acts that are seen by some as scientific misconduct or as academic misconduct/violations, depending on their severity. In the biomedical sciences, these acts are widely and increasingly being considered scientific misconduct (again, depending on their egregiousness).
- Duplicate publication, another form of misconduct, is discussed in detail in Chap. 23 on 'Redundant publications'.

24.4   Steps for Preventing and Identifying Scientific Misconduct

Good communication among authors is essential in a well-functioning team and helps avoid misunderstandings about the responsibilities of each author. It can also foster a collegial environment that allows authors to raise questions or concerns about the scientific soundness and scientific integrity of the work. Special care is needed in situations with power imbalances, such as when there is a mix of new and experienced researchers or authors or research trainees and their supervisors. The US National Academy of Sciences issued an excellent report on being a responsible scientist that provides examples of the type of challenges that face trainees and junior faculty on research teams [9]. Concerns about the integrity of the work from any author should be addressed before submission of a paper. Obviously, no author should ever commit—or be pressured to commit or not report—scientific misconduct.

24.4.1 General Steps

The following are some general guidelines to avoid and prevent scientific misconduct:

- All authors and those contributing to the research process (e.g. technicians, research assistants, trainees) should be educated about research integrity and research misconduct. At a minimum, this education ought to include the following: the principles of research integrity; professional and scientific standards with respect to the ethical conduct of research and the research process, including collecting, treating and reporting data; writing to avoid plagiarism; conflicts of interest; authorship and giving credit to others; what is scientific misconduct and examples; and what to do if scientific misconduct is suspected. Everyone in the research process should understand the concept of equipoise [10].

- Authors should prepare a description of their contribution to the paper and clearly articulate their direct responsibilities to the research work and the paper. These statements should be shared with the other authors and agreement on their accuracy reached. Some journals require author contribution statements as a mechanism to show who takes public responsibility for the work. Even if a journal does not require it, contribution statements should be included in the paper. It is also advisable for the team to have an internal and more detailed contribution statement before the research is undertaken and during paper preparation; this document should be updated as and when appropriate (and this may be several times during the life of a research project).
- Authors must declare any conflicts of interest they may have (or which a reasonable person believes should be declared) before the research is undertaken (*see also* Chap. 22 on 'Conflicts of Interest'). Steps can then be taken to reduce the impact (or perceived impact) on the integrity of the study (e.g. a conflicted researcher/author ought not be responsible for data management, data analysis or data interpretation). There are different ways to capture conflict of interest information; these include adopting a checklist approach for the life cycle of research ending with publication [11]. See below the section on 'Failing to Disclose Relevant Conflicts of Interest' for information regarding such declarations before submission of a paper.
- Identify early on an author (or authors) who will take responsibility for data integrity and accuracy of data analysis. This may be the senior most responsible author or someone else with the appropriate expertise. It is strongly advised that those in this role do not have (or be perceived to have) a conflict of interest in the study findings or with the research sponsor/funder. The individual(s) with this role should be clearly identified in the contribution statements included in the paper. Note that some journals may have specific requirements about who takes on this role and/or the need for an independent statistician.
- Authors supervising researchers must understand their responsibilities and identify who they supervised and for which part of the research process (this includes employees and trainees).
- Before starting research, the team should agree that they will conduct regular audits or get them done on their behalf. These audits would be carried out for accuracy (e.g. of the research record) and to ensure that the research protocol is being followed. Audits may deter wrongdoing, identify scientific misconduct and, more generally, improve the scientific soundness and integrity of the work.
- No one should agree to be an author if she or he has concerns about the integrity of the research or the paper. Researchers or authors should report misconduct to the relevant institution or institutional authority and, if warranted, to those that funded the research.

24.4.2 Fabrication and Falsification

Simply put, the main goal of research is to advance our knowledge or understanding through honest endeavours that provide answers and explanations. It is not surprising that fabrication and falsification are universally viewed as very serious acts of research misconduct.

Fabrication refers to making up data or results in the research record, whereas falsification is interference with the research record so that it is inaccurate (*see* Table 24.1). Intentionally suppressing data is a serious departure from commonly accepted practice and a form of falsification. Examples include reporting only data that shows a positive effect of an intervention and suppressing data that shows no effect or a negative effect or manipulating primary or secondary outcomes so that the findings show positive effects. Intentionally falsifying or fabricating image data is also research misconduct [12].

In smaller research teams, it may sometimes be possible for an author to know if someone has made up the data or the results or interfered with the research record. By contrast, large studies with large teams, especially if multiple sites in several countries are contributing to the research, pose a particular challenge. Regardless of the size or complexity of the research team, authors rely on the scientific honesty of everyone involved, as it is impossible for each and every author to be present when data are being collected, generated or analysed. However, authors can take the following precautions to detect fabrication or falsification prior to submission of the paper:

- Authors should agree that the original scientific protocol,[1] original data and the 'metadata' [13] (technical information about the data, such as when the data were collected, analytical methods/changes and software codes), statistical output and full research records will be retained, lock-boxed and stored together in a secured place. Approved protocol modifications or updates (never to be made during or after data clean-up or data analysis) should be stored with the original scientific protocol. Ideally more than one person (or more than one research site) should have a copy. This will make verification possible and may deter fabrication or falsification.
- Any changes to the planned analysis or any decisions made at the time of data analysis or interpretation should be carefully noted in the research record and become part of the metadata. Not only is this information needed for verification purposes, but it also allows for further scrutiny of the research process.
- Always review the original protocol (or, if relevant, the approved or modified protocol) before submitting the paper and ensure there have been no deviations from it. This includes a review of the inclusion/exclusion criteria and prespecified statistical analysis plan (including primary/secondary outcomes) to warrant that it is consistent with the paper being submitted. Any deviations should be examined carefully. Of course, deviations for scientific reasons are allowed (but must be documented as part of the research record).

---

[1]A scientific protocol should include at minimum the research question/hypothesis (or if appropriate, research aims), study design (including treatment/intervention(s), sample size and inclusion/exclusion criteria), methodology (with detail so that it can be replicated) and data analysis plan (including primary/secondary outcomes and clear definitions of each).

- Ensure that all those involved in data analysis, data presentation or image construction are fully aware of the relevant scientific and ethical standards. This includes the seriousness of data suppression, selective reporting, falsifying or fabricating image data as well as examples of them.
- Ensure that computers used for creating the research record are password-protected and password-locked after a time period of non-activity (and that the research record is automatically backed up).
- If possible, rigorously assess all images using forensic software as visual examination often fails to detect inappropriate data manipulation. There are some relatively accessible tools [14]. (Honest mistakes are often made when digital images are created, so careful review might prevent inadvertent errors.) Journals are often a source of important instructions about creating acceptable images (see, e.g. the *Journal of Cell Biology* that provides excellent instructions to authors and has strong editorial standards about detecting and dealing with image manipulation). (*See also* Chap. 20 'Electronic publishing').
- If the research is a clinical trial and registered in a publicly accessible database, review the public information to ensure there have been no deviations from that public record, either in the conduct or the reporting of the trial.

Authors who take responsibility for data integrity and accuracy of the data analysis have additional responsibilities. Those who lack all the required expertise to fulfil these responsibilities may receive assistance from other authors or a person who is not an author on the study. Any authors providing this kind of assistance should be identified in the contribution statements (or, if not authors, in the acknowledgement section). It is strongly advised that all who render assistance should have no conflicts of interest with the research question or findings (and be independent of the sponsor/funder). Therefore, the following steps should be taken:

- Authors with responsibility for data integrity and accuracy of the data analysis must be provided with access to the original protocol, original data, analysed data and metadata (including computer codes and other information needed to verify the results).
- Verify the results by reconstructing the study findings from the raw data. This approach ensures data integrity and the accuracy of the data analysis and assures that the paper honestly reports the study findings and clearly explains any deviations from the original protocol.

24.4.3 Plagiarism

Plagiarism is taking 'another person's ideas, processes, results or words without giving appropriate credit' [6]. The term 'plagiarism' includes a wide spectrum of issues with varying degrees of wrongfulness. The most serious type is blatant copying of an entire paper or of large portions of other people's written work. The Committee on Publication Ethics (COPE) has released an important discussion paper on what constitutes major and minor plagiarism [15] noting that it can range from copying entire papers or large sections of text to copying or close copying of less than 100 words (with or without citation). There is universal agreement about the most serious forms of plagiarism being unacceptable, but less unanimity regarding its minor forms. However, less serious instances of plagiarism are also important. If serious plagiarism is detected in a published paper, the journal editors will most likely take public action such as retracting the paper. For less egregious plagiarism, the editors may issue a correction or publish a letter of apology from the authors.

One of the challenges in dealing with plagiarism is that while the theft of another author's words is sometimes intentional, it can also be sloppiness or a lack of understanding about what is and is not allowed. However, journal editors may treat intentional and unintentional plagiarism in the same way depending on the definition they follow [16]. This is one reason why it is important for authors to take responsible steps to detect any plagiarism before a paper is submitted.

Steven Shafer has categorized plagiarism into 'intellectual theft, intellectual sloth, plagiarism for scientific English, technical plagiarism and self-plagiarism' and offers helpful definitions of each [17]. Someone committing 'intellectual theft' steals the ideas or words of an author without giving the latter due credit. An 'intellectual sloth' is someone who copies the words of an author that are in the public domain and are generic text, because they are 'simply too lazy' to provide the source and rewrite it in their own words. The example given by Shafer is of someone who copies generic text from Wikipedia without citing the source and who has just 'cut and pasted' text. 'Plagiarism for scientific English' occurs when someone tries to use grammatically proper English by copying text from a variety of published authors and ends up with a paper that includes sentences taken verbatim from many sources but contains no large blocks of text taken from a single source. Such copying may also occur by those who have full command of English. 'Technical plagiarism' refers to using word-for-word text and referencing the source but failing to use quotation marks. 'Self-plagiarism' is a term used to describe the reuse of an author's own words without citing where he/she first used those words (text recycling). Some text recycling may be acceptable, particularly if it relates to the methods section. However, many journals are becoming more concerned about it, especially if the amount of recycled text is more than 15–20% and is not in part due to text recycling of the methods sections. Currently, there are no agreed rules that specify the amount of recycled text allowed [17, 18]. Self-plagiarism is not the same as duplicate publishing. 'Duplicate publishing' is typically where the same or a very similar paper is submitted or published twice (a paper that substantially duplicates text in another paper, without citing the other paper, and where the two papers have one or more authors in common) [19]. (*See also* Chap. 23 on 'Redundant publications.)

Plagiarism can involve using someone else's ideas as one's own without giving credit to its creator or originator. Shafer's 'intellectual theft' definition includes the appropriation of ideas or words. Some people find it difficult to think of ideas as being something that can be plagiarized, especially given how science evolves by the free sharing of ideas and people building on the ideas of others. It is not always easy to identify who first expressed an idea or whether an idea is really so novel that others could not have arrived at it independently. Findings of idea plagiarism are quite uncommon, but when they do occur, the facts often reveal clearly wrongful acts. Miguel Roig provides a helpful definition of what is meant by an 'idea' with his examples of 'an explanation, a theory, a conclusion, a hypothesis, a metaphor in whole or in part, or with superficial modifications without giving credit to its originator' [20]. An example may be of a researcher who reviews a grant application and steals from it a novel theory to explain an aspect of his own study without getting permission from, or giving credit to, the grant applicant for the theory. Roig offers some excellent examples, including a reviewer who reads a paper or grant proposal describing a new methodology, then writes a negative evaluation of the paper or protocol and subsequently prepares a grant proposal using that same methodology without crediting its originator.

Authors can take the following precautions to increase the chances of detecting plagiarism before submitting a paper:

- Make use of free online tutorials that provide clear examples of how to avoid plagiarizing and that provide examples of plagiarism. There are several options, including one hosted by the [US] Office of Research Integrity written by Dr. Miguel Roig [20], which is an excellent resource. In addition, some universities have very helpful tutorials on the web. www.Plagiarism.org provides excellent educative material as well.
- When submitting an article, tell the journal if any co-authors have published a paper with possible overlap of text with the work currently being submitted. Provide copies of these other publications. Ensure the submitted paper references the first publication where the author's words are written (and if appropriate, use quotation marks so that the reader knows that the text has been copied word for word).
- Submit the draft paper to anti-plagiarism software. There are some excellent options, including some free plagiarism software [21] that is designed to detect the use of another author's text (*see also* Chap. 20 on 'Electronic publishing').
- Identify novel ideas and ask the author(s) that contributed them if anyone needs to be referenced or credited. This may not identify authors who intentionally take other's ideas without credit but remind ethical authors that original ideas need to be credited.

24.4.4 Using Intellectual Property or Research Data That Is Owned by Others

A research project is often conducted by many people and will likely include some who are involved in other research studies. Authors need to be sure that any intellectual property (such as novel methodologies) or data they receive is theirs to use. It is useful to verify this with the original owners of the data or intellectual property, and the written consent of the owner must be stated in their paper. It is a serious offence for authors to use intellectual property or research data that is not theirs to use. Any intellectual property or research data owned by others must be identified at the beginning of the research process so that permissions can be secured; however, authors should always review the matter before final submission of a paper and be confident that they have the right to use the data.

Conflicts in research teams can generate problems that go far beyond creating unpleasant and unproductive work environments. The breakdown in team functioning can lead to disputes about who actually owns the products of research. Taking intellectual property or research data that is not the authors' to use most often occurs in situations where people know one another. In fact, they often are, or were, on the same research team or worked in the same facility. For example, in a research team that is not functioning well, some team members may try to use the intellectual property or data before their colleagues do. Similarly, when there is a dispute over who owns intellectual property or data, someone who believes they have the right may use it before ownership has been fully determined. Another example can be of a researcher who brings data or intellectual property into a new research team whose members are unaware that the data/property is not owned by the researcher. It can also be the case that the individuals had never worked together but worked alongside each other in the same facility (e.g. laboratory) (*see also* Chap. 10 on 'Copyright issues').

Before submitting a paper, there are some precautions authors can take that will improve the chances that they have the right to use the intellectual property or research data in their study:

- Do not use intellectual property or data when there is a current dispute as to who owns it or when its owner has not given written permission for its use.
- If there is any doubt about whether the intellectual property or the research data can be used, seek guidance from those who can help (e.g. relevant research institute or university). For example, differences between commercial use and general research use might require clarification.
- Authors who bring intellectual property or data with them to a research project and/or research paper must confirm to the team that they either own it or are authorized to use it; if the latter, they must supply written permission from the owners.

24.4.5 Failing to Disclose Relevant Conflicts of Interest

Authors may have competing interests in the work or be reasonably seen by others as having such interests (*see also* Chap. 22 on 'Conflicts of interest'). Conflict of interest is an important issue, as having financial interests in the findings may impact on the integrity of the work and influence what research outcomes are reported [22]. A conflict of interest is defined as 'a set of conditions in which professional judgment concerning a primary interest (such as a patient's welfare or the validity of research) tends to be unduly influenced by a secondary interest (such as financial gain)' [23]. While financial conflict of interest is most often considered and reported, there could be other types of conflicts, such as personal relationships or institutional affiliations [24]. It is important for research teams to manage any conflicts of interest and to disclose them as required—especially at the time of submission of the paper. There are several instances where journals have taken action for undeclared and material conflicts of interest [25, 26], especially when these are paired with flaws that call into question the scientific merit of the work [27]. The following steps should help avoid conflicts of interest:

- Always review a journal's instructions for authors about declaring conflicts of interests and follow the rules. If in doubt, report the conflict of interest. If the journal does not request such declarations, do it anyway for reasons of transparency and honesty. (Conflicts of interest revealed after submission of the manuscript may call into question the integrity of the work.)
- Declare who funded the research and any role they might have had in the research process (particularly data collection, analysis and interpretation) and the publication. The ICMJE says that 'authors should describe the role of the study sponsor, if any, in the study design; collection, analysis and interpretation of data; writing the report; and the decision to submit the report for publication. If the supporting source had no such involvement, the authors should so state' [28].
- One author (usually the corresponding author) must ensure that all conflicts of interest are declared to the journal and included in the text of the manuscript.

24.4.6 Inappropriate Assignment/Non-assignment of Authorship

Authorship is for individuals who have contributed to the work. There are different conventions about who is an author, and most journals will include a statement on their policy (*see also* Chap. 15 on 'Authorship and acknowledgements'). The concept of authorship has evolved over time. For example, it is no longer acceptable that the academic or clinical head should be listed as a co-author when he/she has not contributed directly to a work or to be conferred authorship status for having obtained funding for a project. Over time, some practices have come to light that are unacceptable. Recently, there has been attention on 'ghost writers'—people who contributed substantially to a paper (including but not limited to writing the first draft) but who are not named as authors themselves [29]. Drug companies have been known to write (or hire a medical writer to write) a paper favourable to their interests but not list either the company or the hired writer as authors. Instead, the company would have found researchers with the credentials to be listed as authors, but contributions insufficient to truly confer them with authorship status [29, 30].

To conclude, take the following steps:

- Ensure that all individuals listed as authors—and only those individuals—meet the criteria for authorship and agree that the paper is ready for submission.

Journals may vary in the criteria they use, but a commonly used and cited source is the International Committee on Medical Journal Editors (ICMJE) Statement of Authorship [28].

- Include in the acknowledgement section of the paper anyone who provided important assistance with the paper but does not qualify as an author. If relevant, provide the source of funding for that assistance. (*See also* Chap. 15 on 'Authorship and Acknowledgements'.)

24.4.7 Failing to Have Appropriate Research Ethics Approvals

Studies involving people or animals require ethics approval. Authors need to ensure that they have the appropriate research ethics approval and that the research is conducted and reported as described in the protocol and other materials that led to that approval. Research ethics approval is a formal mechanism used to protect human or animal research participants. It involves a review of the protocol (including information and consent forms for potential participants, laboratory animal care, etc.) by people other than the researchers who are responsible for deciding if it is ethically acceptable. Ensure the following steps:

- Review the protocol (including what participants, or their agents, consent to) during the research process and again before manuscript submission. Ensure that the research ethics approval is appropriate and that the research is conducted as described in the documentation that led to the ethics approval.
- Review the documentation that led to the ethics approval to be sure the authors have a right to publish the research in the way it has been done. For example, if the protocol said that no hospitals will be identified, the authors must ensure that the readers of their paper cannot work out the identity of any hospitals.

24.5 Summary

It is a sad truth that the steps described in this chapter may not prevent all scientific misconduct or detect it before publication. Misconduct may occur simply because it goes undetected. It may also be that those in a position to detect misconduct condone the practice rather than condemn it.

Authors have a responsibility to themselves, to their field of study and to the public at large to understand what exactly constitutes scientific misconduct. They need to know what is unacceptable in our scientific communities so that they themselves do not commit scientific misconduct and so that they can prevent or identify it in the research of others.

Institutions for their part must support authors in putting the steps into practice. They need to create an environment that places scientific integrity above scientific productivity. Institutions need clear statements and actions that show they take research misconduct seriously, and they need to have an appropriate whistle-blower policy.

References

1. Nath SB, Marcus SC, Druss BG. Retractions in the research literature: misconduct or mistakes. Med J Aust. 2006;185:152–4.
2. Wager E, Williams P. Why and how do journals retract articles? An analysis of Medline retractions 1988–2008. J Med Ethics. 2011;37:567–70.
3. Steen RG. Retractions in the medical literature: how can patients be protected from risk? J Med Ethics. 2012;38:228–32.
4. Huth EJ. Responsibilities of coauthorship. Ann Intern Med. 1983;99:256–7.
5. Kennedy D. Next steps in the Schön affair. Science. 2002;298:495.
6. United States CFR Title 45: Public Welfare, Part 689 Research Misconduct.
7. Smith R. What is research misconduct. In: White C, editor. The COPE Report 2000: Annual Report of the Committee on Publication Ethics. London: BMJ Books; 2000. p. 7. http://publicationethics.org/files/u7141/COPE2000pdfcomplete.pdf. Accessed 25 May 2015.
8. Resnik DB, Stewart CN Jr. Misconduct versus honest error and scientific disagreement. Account Res. 2012;19:56–63.
9. Committee on Science, Engineering, and Public Policy; Institute of Medicine; Policy and Global Affairs; National Academy of Sciences; National Academy of Engineering. On being a scientist: a guide to responsible conduct in research. 3ed ed. Washington, DC: National Academies Press; 2009. http://www.nap.edu/catalog/12192/on-being-a-scientist-a-guide-to-responsible-conduct-in. Accessed 25 May 2015.
10. Chopra V, Davis M. In search of equipoise. JAMA. 2011;305:1234–5.
11. Rochon PA, Hoey J, Chan AW, Ferris LE, Lexchin J, Kalkar SR, et al. Financial conflicts of interest checklist 2010 for clinical research studies. Open Med. 2010;4:e69–91.
12. Parrish D, Noonan B. Image manipulation as research misconduct. Sci Eng Ethics. 2009;15:161–7.
13. TechTerms.com. Metadata. http://www.techterms.com/definition/metadata. Accessed 25 May 2015.
14. Institute for Basic Biomedical Sciences, Johns Hopkins Medical School. Scientific integrity in the age of photoshop: photoshop and the internet have become invaluable tools for preparing research publications—as well as potential instruments of research misconduct. http://www.hopkinsmedicine.org/institute_basic_biomedical_sciences/news_events/articles_and_stories/employment/2011_01_scientific_integrity.html. Accessed 25 May 2015.
15. Wager E. How should editors respond to plagiarism? COPE discussion paper. 2011. http://publicationethics.org/files/COPE_plagiarism_discussion_%20doc_26%20Apr%2011.pdf. Accessed 25 May 2015.
16. Shashok K. Authors, editors, and the signs, symptoms and causes of plagiarism. Saudi J Anaesth. 2011;5:303–7.
17. Shafer SL. You will be caught. Anesth Analg. 2011;112:491–3.
18. Akst Jef. When is self-plagiarism ok? The scientist [entry posted 9 Sept 2010]. http://www.the-scientist.com/blog/displya/57676. Accessed 25 May 2015.
19. Fact Sheet. Errata, retractions, partial retractions, corrected and republished articles, duplicate publications, comments (including author replies), updates, patient summaries, and republished (reprinted) articles policy for MEDLINE. http://www.nlm.nih.gov/pubs/factsheets/errata.html. Accessed 25 May 2015.
20. Miguel R. Avoiding plagiarism, self-plagiarism, and other questionable writing practices: a guide to ethical writing. http://ori.hhs.gov/avoiding-plagiarism-self-plagiarism-and-other-questionable-writing-practices-guide-ethical-writing. Accessed 25 May 2015.
21. Ochroch EA. Review of plagiarism detection freeware. Anesth Analg. 2011;112:742–3.
22. Bekelman JE, Li Y, Gross CP. Scope and impact of financial conflicts of interest in biomedical research: a systematic review. JAMA. 2003;289:454–65.
23. Thompson DF. Understanding financial conflicts of interest. N Engl J Med. 1993;329:573–6.

24. Ferris LE, Fletcher RH. Conflict of interest in peer-reviewed medical journals: the World Association of Medical Editors (WAME) position on a challenging problem. Neurosurgery. 2010;66(4):629–30. http://www.wame.org/about/wame-editorial-on-coi. Accessed 25 May 2015.
25. DeAngelis CD, Fontanarosa PB. Resolving unreported conflicts of interest. JAMA. 2009; 302:198–9.
26. Barberger-Gateau P. Failure to report financial disclosure information. JAMA. 2009; 302:2433–4.
27. Garite TJ, Kim MH. Editors' note on notice of retraction. Am J Obstet Gynecol. 2011;205:396–7.
28. ICMJE. Defining the role of authors and contributors. http://www.icmje.org/recommendations/browse/roles-and-responsibilities/defining-the-role-of-authors-and-contributors.html. Accessed 25 May 2015.
29. McHenry L. Of sophists and spin-doctors: industry-sponsored ghostwriting and the crisis of academic medicine. Mens Sana Monogr. 2010;8:129–45.
30. Ross JS, Hill KP, Egilman DS, Krumholz HM. Guest authorship and ghostwriting in publications related to rofecoxib: a case study of industry documents from rofecoxib litigation. JAMA. 2008;299:1800–12.

Podium Presentation: Planning, Preparation, and Delivery

25

Rakesh Aggarwal and Gourdas Choudhuri

There are several forms of podium presentations, the most common being the oral delivery of a research paper at a scientific meeting. Other types include invited lectures, orations, and nonscientific talks. This chapter focuses on the oral paper presentation and touches briefly on the other forms.

25.1 Planning a 10-min Oral Paper Presentation

25.1.1 Abstract Preparation

A podium presentation of a scientific paper starts with preparing and submitting the abstract (*see also* Chap. 7). Professional societies or conference organizers often allow authors to indicate at the time of abstract submission whether they would prefer their paper to be considered for a podium or poster presentation. Some scientific papers are particularly suited for a poster presentation, especially if they contain a lot of pictorial data. Though the final decision usually rests with the organizers, you must indicate your choice if you believe that your data are more suited to a particular form of presentation.

The abstract must be clear and concise. The upper word limit, decided in advance by the conference organizers, must be adhered to along with any other

R. Aggarwal (✉)
Journal of Gastroenterology and Hepatology and Department of Gastroenterology,
Sanjay Gandhi Postgraduate Institute of Medical Sciences, Lucknow, India

G. Choudhuri
Department of Gastroenterology and Hepatobiliary Sciences,
Fortis Memorial Research Institute, Gurgaon, India

© The National Medical Journal of India 2018
P. Sahni, R. Aggarwal (eds.), *Reporting and Publishing Research in the Biomedical Sciences*, https://doi.org/10.1007/978-981-10-7062-4_25

instructions. Brevity dictates that an abstract contain only essential information. It should be grammatically correct, and make sparing use of abbreviations and acronyms. It must stand on its own and follow the IMRAD (Introduction, Methods, Results, and Discussion) structure of the scientific research paper. An abstract must emphasize what was done, how it was done, what was found, and how the authors interpret it. In view of the word limit, the introduction must not exceed a couple of sentences and should indicate the rationale for the study. Methods should be provided only in generic terms, and specific details should be kept for the final presentation. However, to enable the reviewers and readers to assess the appropriateness and the validity of the conclusions drawn, you should give sufficient details about the study design and composition of control and study groups. Take special care with the results; they are the most important section of the abstract and should take the most space. Always provide the actual number of observations (and not just percentage values). In addition to measures of central tendency (mean or median), also give the measures of dispersion (standard deviation or range). Confidence intervals should be expressed when appropriate and always include the main statistical results (e.g., p values, correlation coefficients). The discussion section is limited to a couple of sentences at most, so there is only room for stating your study's conclusions and none for discussing the work of others.

The draft abstract must undergo several rounds of editing, not only by all the co-authors but also by one or two peers who were not involved in the work. The latter provides useful criticisms and suggestions, which frequently add to the quality of the abstract. Don't be alarmed if your first draft bears little resemblance to the final abstract!

While preparing the abstract, always keep in mind that the work you cover will have to be presented in 10 min. Authors are often tempted to compress several years of work into one abstract, and this is impossible to present in a single podium presentation. Look closely at your draft to see whether (1) it is addressing several questions; (2) it is addressing a very complex question; or (3) it is based on non-standard methods, which require a detailed description. If the answer is "Yes," select just one aspect to focus on, i.e., one of several questions addressed, one aspect of a complex question, or the standardization of a new technique. The presentation will then be able to cover this aspect completely, rather than briefly touching on several issues.

Before submission, stop and consider whether the abstract is appropriate for the forum to which you are submitting it. It may not be a good idea to submit an abstract based on clinical work to a society whose members are primarily basic scientists, or vice versa. It is difficult to make the concepts in a paper understood to an unfamiliar audience in the limited time available for presentation.

A good abstract reports on a study that has already been completed and not on work in progress, so avoid using phrases such as "the results will be presented" or "the results will be discussed." Ensure that the abstract length does not exceed the specified word limit by using the word/character count feature on your word processing program.

25.1.2 Printing and Mailing the Abstract

Nowadays, most abstracts are submitted online. Use a simple font such as Times Roman, although the conference organizers might change it for their abstract publication. If a printed abstract is requested, use a laser printer or a good quality inkjet printer—with no erasures or smudges. Again select a simple font, such as Times Roman or Helvetica, as more ornate fonts are difficult to read. The conference organizers often photograph or scan the submitted abstract, so make sure the paper is unfolded, wrapped in polythene, and mailed in a rigid envelope.

25.1.3 Designing the Talk: When and Where to Begin

It is common for the preparation of a podium presentation to be left to the week immediately preceding the actual event. Once the acceptance letter arrives, waste no time and start right away, particularly if you are not a seasoned presenter.

The first step is to review your abstract and make sure that the data and conclusions are still valid. Abstracts are usually based on data that have only recently become available; occasionally, data that have subsequently become available may prove the original conclusion to be incorrect. If this is the case, consider withdrawing your abstract, or request the organizers to accept a modified version.

The presentation format allows only 10 min (sometimes just 6–8 min) to describe your objectives, methods, results, and conclusions. It is an imperative that you present only the bare essentials, while not compromising on scientific reliability and validity. Thus, you will need to condense your data substantially. Go through your abstract as well as data, and try to summarize your main results into a few tables. As described above, focus on one or two aspects and a few key messages. Also, in a podium presentation, it is far better to present the data as charts and graphs, rather than tables.

Podium papers are conventionally presented with supporting projection slides, so the next step is to decide on the number of slides and what needs to be included in the spoken text, since the time available is limited and punctuality is of utmost importance. You will create a bad impression if you fail to finish your talk in the stipulated time.

25.1.4 Optimum Length of Text

One can speak no more than 100 words per minute without affecting comprehensibility. So you should be able to speak roughly 1000 words in 10 min; this length is no more than three to four pages of A4-size sheets, typed double space using a 12-point font. The length of the text will be proportionately shorter if the time allotted is less than 10 min.

This is a daunting task. In the short span of 10 min armed only with a short text and a set of slides, you have to gain the interest of the audience and inform them about a study that is far more familiar to you than it is to them.

25.1.5 Preparing the Text

It helps to begin with a draft of the full typescript of your paper, complete with tables and figures. The usual length of a scientific paper is 2000–3500 words with four to five tables and/or figures. The first draft of your talk should be 40–50% longer and edited back to the final length of 1000 words. You may allocate words to different sections of the IMRAD format as follows: 150 for introduction, 350 for methods, 350 for results, and 150 for stating the conclusions. Of course, there may be minor variations in this distribution depending on the nature of the work.

The next step is to prune and polish the draft of your speech. Imagine that you are telling a friend, who does not know your work closely, what you set out to study and why. Use spoken language with short sentences and simple words, as we do in our daily lives. Take particular care to orient those who may not be familiar with your subject. The task of shortening the length of your text involves two processes— removal of some sections of the text entirely and modification of language to reduce verbosity and complexity.

Removing parts of the text is difficult for beginners. Each section, when looked at individually, appears important. Try to see the bigger picture, keeping your audience in mind. The methods is usually the section where one can most easily remove details. For instance, if your audience consists of endocrinologists, there is little need to define the diagnostic criteria for diabetes beyond indicating which set of guidelines or criteria you used. Consider the need to describe the steps involved in a polymerase chain reaction or enzyme immunoassay; you could just say how you modified a standard procedure, rather than describe the whole procedure. Is it important to describe the demographic profile of patients in detail? Is it important to describe the results of simple tests, such as haemoglobin and blood counts, if these have no relation to the primary question being addressed? The answer to many of these questions will be "No." Using simpler words would take less time to deliver the text. Cut long sentences to shorter ones. For long phrases that are used repeatedly, an acronym can be used. (See Chap. 14 for more guidance on brevity and precision.)

Placing the results of two related experiments together may allow you to describe their results in one sentence, rather than in two. You do not have to read out everything that appears on your slide. For instance, if you are presenting the results of a drug trial, and your slide has a table showing the demographic details of patients and controls (e.g., age, gender distribution, duration of disease, disease severity, etc.), you need not read out all the values. Suffice it to say: "The two groups were similar." Sentences in the active voice are always shorter than those in the passive voice.

Lastly, a colleague who does not know your work closely may be able to look at the whole presentation far more dispassionately than you can.

25.1.6 Number of Slides

A good rule of thumb is one slide per minute of time allotted. Thus, 10–12 slides are the optimum number for a 10-min presentation. Of course, this number may need revision based on the nature of data in the slides and the time needed to describe them. Slides that are simple pictures may need little description, but those with a complex flow diagram could take longer than a minute. The total number of slides has to be divided among various sections, with a larger share reserved for the methods and results sections and only one to two slides for the introduction and conclusions.

Planning and preparation of the slides and text should go hand in hand. The introduction should end with a hypothesis or aims. The methods, in particular the study design and treatment protocols, are shown much better as flow diagrams than as text; this format needs fewer slides and is largely self-explanatory. Results should more often be displayed as graphs and figures, rather than tables. These should be followed by conclusions. A detailed discussion, an integral part of a written paper, is rarely included in a podium presentation.

A useful tip is to make the slides yourself instead of asking someone else to do it; this will familiarize you with everything that is in them. If someone else must make them on your behalf, do try and give the finishing touches. Time spent with the slides is time well spent!

25.1.7 The Final Speech

After preparing the draft speech, planning the audiovisual aids, and pruning and polishing the text down to 1000 words, align the visuals with the text. Many presenters mark in the margins of their text the exact places where the slides should change. Alternatively, one could type the text corresponding to each slide in a separate paragraph. Rehearse your talk, preferably with drafts of your slide material, to get a feel of how it sounds, how long it takes to complete, and where you need to pause. The aim should be to narrate a story to the audience, not to read out a document to them. Rehearsals are the most important aspect of preparing for an oral presentation—and that is something even the most seasoned presenters do not ignore.

The initial rehearsals should be self-rehearsal. In their simplest form, they involve sitting alone and reading out your text with the drafts of your slides in front of you and noting how much time it takes. Then ask yourself the following questions: Does the text read smoothly? Are there any points where the text lacks coherence? Are there any complex sentences? Am I stuttering or stalling at a complex word or stumbling over a succession of consonants? Am I finishing in time—and if not, by how much time is my talk overshooting?

Computer programs have made rehearsal easier. Many presentation programs for making slides (e.g., Microsoft PowerPoint) allow you to type your text as notes for each slide. As you expose each slide, the corresponding text appears in a corner of the screen; you can then rehearse by reading the text aloud. A better way to detect flaws is to record the speech within the PowerPoint program (or on an audio tape recorder) and to listen carefully to the replay.

After the self-rehearsals, your next step is to rehearse in front of a colleague who is frank and critical. Request your colleague to point out shortcomings in your presentation and identify the points that you are failing to convey.

The opening and closing sentences are the most important and need to be memorized. However, avoid the temptation to memorize the entire text verbatim; this may sound easy but carries the risk of you being rendered speechless by an unexpected distraction (such as failure of the slide projector).

This is also the time to think of the possible questions that may be asked after your presentation and to arm yourself with possible replies.

25.1.8 A Few Final Tips

Once your slides and text are done, you are ready for your podium presentation. However, there are still a few things to do. Verify that there is no typing error. If you propose to use the same slide twice, make sure you have two copies of it in your presentation, rather than going back and forth through the slides. Guard against a sudden technical snag by copying the presentation to multiple devices. Also e-mail the computer file to an address from which you can retrieve it remotely. And finally, if you travel to the conference venue by air—make sure your pen drive (or disk) stays with you and doesn't go into the baggage hold.

25.2 Planning Invited Talks and Lectures

The other common forms of podium presentation differ in several ways from that of giving a scientific paper:

- The speakers are usually more senior and more adept at presentations
- The invitation is based not on submission of an abstract but on several years of consistent work in a particular area
- The audience is more aware of the topic to be covered and likely to be more receptive
- The time allotted for the speaker is usually longer than that for an oral scientific paper
- The sequence of material to be presented can be more flexible

Several principles that apply to a 10-min paper also apply to these talks. Punctuality and clarity are virtues that need to be emphasized. It is important to know your audience well in advance—Are they experts in the field who are looking for the latest information, or are they novices? Remember that slides and text prepared for a talk for one kind of audience may not be appropriate for another.

A talk should be divided into three parts: the introduction, the main body, and the conclusion. These three sections are best summarized in the maxim: "Tell them what you are going to tell them, tell them, then tell them what you told them." The introduction should introduce the subject to the audience, the main body should describe the topic in detail, and the conclusion should reemphasize the main points covered in the talk.

It is useful to break the main body of your talk into several sections, each dealing with one concept or idea, and then to deal with each of these sequentially. These sections should follow an order—at times, various ideas have a natural or intuitive order; if they don't, start with simpler concepts, and then go on to more complex ideas. It may help to end each important section with a summary slide. The concluding part of your talk should provide a few simple take-home messages; usually, this is all that will remain with your audience once they leave the hall.

25.3 Delivering the Talk

25.3.1 Animation

Body language or animation is what sets an oral presentation apart from a written paper and makes the former live, vibrant, and engaging to the audience. Animation encompasses the speaker's gait, posture, facial and body expressions, gesticulations, and the overall style of presentation.

Establishing a rapport with the audience begins as soon as the speaker rises from his or her seat in the hall and starts walking up to the podium. The audience closely notice a speaker's dress, gait, enthusiasm, mannerisms, and expressions. You should wear formal attire that is appropriate for the occasion. A T-shirt, tattered jeans, or slippers may compromise the audience's respect for you! Take a seat in the first row—it takes less time to walk to the podium.

As a speaker, remember that the audience is keen to know something about you, in addition to learning about your work. It is expected that, when called, you walk up to the podium confidently and spend a little time adjusting your microphone and checking that the pointer is working. It is essential that you look at and make eye contact with your audience. It is unfair on the gathering for a speaker to begin by saying: "May I have the lights off please?" A presenter who takes cover in a dark hall, and provides only a vocal backdrop to a sequential projection of slides, can hardly complain if the audience slip into a siesta.

Another oft-neglected aspect is the posture. It is embarrassing to see a speaker slouch over the podium, speak with hands in his pockets, fling his arms about, or brandish a pointer as if it were a saber. Make a mental note of "negative" postures, and consciously avoid them. A relaxed straight posture, with hands by your sides or resting on the podium, is the default position—and it makes a far better impression on the audience. Of course, a few gestures and some facial expressions are welcome, but the motto should be "underplay but never overdo."

Remember that slides or other audiovisual aids are, as the term implies, only aids and not a substitute for a good speech. These are assets, which, when used skillfully, can enhance your presentation; they are not props to clutch at or a replacement for inadequate preparation.

25.3.2 Speech Modulation

Modulation is the ability to vary or regulate one's speech. Imagine or recall a talk in which the speaker goes on and on in a flat and monotonous tone; a lack of modulation makes a speech boring. Various techniques are needed to hold the attention of the listener: speech must be punctuated, the amplitude and pitch of the voice must be varied, and the words or phrases that matter must be delivered with just that little extra thrust or emphasis. Some speakers let their voice drop or tail off at the end of each sentence—a habit that frustrates the audience as they strain to catch those last important words in every sentence. (This sometimes happens when speakers turn their heads away from the microphone towards the screen behind them.)

One needs to learn how to speak clearly and audibly, articulating each word well and delivering the speech at the right pace. A close friend or colleague can be a major asset in pointing out if the flow is smooth, the sentences punctuated, and the words clear and comprehensible. The next stage of rehearsal could focus on variations in loudness and pitch, adding punch to the keywords and terms, while going over the superfluous phrases quickly and in softer tones. All this needs to be done subtly, without sounding dramatic. Most people today prefer a simple conversational tone to old-fashioned theatrical oratory, especially in a scientific meeting. Solid data backed by simple logic delivered in a conversational tone can be far more convincing than a slipshod delivery of information accompanied by histrionics.

While some have an innate ability to speak better than others, anyone can become a good and effective speaker with practice and experience. There is no substitute for rehearsal; so do not hesitate to rehearse time and again, especially in the early phase of your career. Having a colleague criticize you and point out your deficiencies is an essential aid for acquiring this skill.

25.3.3 Time Management

Exceeding the allotted time is unpardonable. It speaks of a poor ability to discern what is important, a lack of proper preparation, and a failure to consider your audience. In an oral presentation, brevity and lucidity are far more important attributes than detail and completeness; the interested listener can often get all the information he or she desires from another source.

The attention span of the audience is limited, especially by the end of the day when there have been several speeches already. The audience are usually willing to give a new speaker no more than 3 min to decide whether his talk is worth listening to or descend into reverie. If you can hold their attention till then, you can have them for another 4–5 min—time enough to share your results and conclusions. If your speech stretches beyond this point, and the red light comes on or the chairperson starts reminding you to conclude, the audience has either deserted you or is about to do so. In your own interest, it is better to wind up gracefully while the audience is still on your side. To retrieve the situation and finish on time, cut the flab rather than rush through your slides!

25.4   Question and Answer (Q&A) Session

It is not uncommon to find a speaker who, having delivered a lucid and elegant talk, fumbles for words, gets angry and argumentative, or goes completely mute on being asked a few simple questions. If this happens, the positive impression generated during the talk disappears into thin air.

Make sure you prepare in advance for the Q&As. Encourage your colleagues to ask you questions that are likely to be asked at the final presentation; rehearse the answers to those questions. The answers should be brief and to the point. If the questioner asks you something that you have already stated in your talk, refrain from showing your irritation or impatience for two reasons: one, that your speech had failed to hold his or her attention, and, second, that more people are watching your response and conduct than that of the questioner. It is wise to retain your cool and rephrase the reply in brief; do not rub in the fact that you had already mentioned this.

Answer questions in a tone that is appreciative and friendly, rather than indignant, condescending, or dismissive. Show your gratitude to the audience for attending your talk, listening at least to most parts of it, and evincing interest in your work.

Some questions may be beyond the scope of your work or presentation. And you may not know the answers to some. At such times, it is better to admit that the answers are beyond or besides the objectives and results of your study; hazarding a wild guess can risk exposing your ignorance. Sometimes, a question by a senior person may be intended more to show his knowledge and make his presence felt, rather than eliciting an answer; thus, more may be gained by encouraging him to provide the answer himself. Keeping an open-minded attitude is desirable; the audience does not take kindly to overconfident (and arrogant) speakers who insist on having the last and final word.

25.5   Summary

Despite advances in the speed and ease of communication and an explosive increase in the number of medical journals, oral presentation of scientific papers at conferences retains its place as an important means of sharing knowledge. The presentation could alternatively be a long-awaited opportunity for a researcher to share with his peers the results of years of his hard work as a prestigious oration in a conference. In either case, the speaker is usually the most knowledgeable person on the subject of his or her talk. And, for their part, members of the audience have already shown a positive intent in the speaker and his work, having decided to attend the session. However, the outcome of a podium presentation can vary from the audience listening with rapt attention and leaving with a few clear take-home messages to regretting the time wasted in attending the session while erasing any memory of the talk. The difference between a successful presentation and a flop is the effort the speaker makes in planning the talk, articulating it well, and holding the attention of the audience during the presentation. Fortunately, these skills can be honed: it is never too early to begin, nor too late to learn, from this never-ending apprenticeship.

Suggested Reading[1]

https://www.ted.com/talks/abraham_verghese_a_doctor_s_touch
https://www.ted.com/talks
https://www.ted.com/talks?topics%5B%5D=medicine&topics%5B%5D=medical+research&sort
=newest

---

[1] Try listening to some talks (links below) on the Iinternet, and see how some speakers can be lucid and impressive.

The Poster

26

Sita Naik

Poster presentation of research data at scientific meetings developed at the end of the Second World War in 1945. It was a response to the burgeoning scientific output, particularly in North America. In India, posters were introduced to medical meetings and conferences during the late 1980s, but they are yet to find widespread popularity.

26.1 Origin of Posters

Traditionally, scientific breakthroughs were presented by reading out papers before a select peer group, such as the Royal Colleges in the UK and their equivalent organizations in other countries. Scientists who sought admittance to these select groups were voted in by its members—a practice that still exists for several 'clubs'. These groups did not allow their platform to be used by non-members, particularly the young, new entrants into science. As science grew and diversified, the scientists' need for regular interaction led to the inception of more specialized societies such as the American Medical Association and the American Physiological Society. These organizations held annual conventions where both members and non-members read out papers on new discoveries.

Over the years, the number of scientific papers submitted to a meeting increased, and it became difficult for all the papers to be delivered orally during the limited time of a conference. Eventually, simultaneous sessions, or parallel sessions, were introduced, usually by dividing papers into defined subspecialty areas. After the Second World War, North America witnessed a rapid growth in science, boosted in

S. Naik
Apollo Hospitals Educational Foundation, Hyderabad, India

© The National Medical Journal of India 2018
P. Sahni, R. Aggarwal (eds.), *Reporting and Publishing Research in the Biomedical Sciences*, https://doi.org/10.1007/978-981-10-7062-4_26

part by financial incentives given to young men who had missed out on their education because of the war. The increase in parallel sessions led to constraints on venue facilities, and delegates interested in subjects that were being presented in different halls had to choose which session to attend. The concept of presenting data as poster displays helped overcome this difficulty. Today, most original data presented at biomedical meetings around the world are poster presentations.

In most big meetings, posters are displayed in large halls, arranged in clusters according to topics. The meeting/conference programme allots 1.5–2 h everyday for poster viewing, at a time when there are no oral presentations. The presenting author is expected to be available by her display to answer any viewer queries.

26.2 Advantages and Disadvantages of Posters

The static poster format offers several advantages over the linear- and IMRAD-constrained 7–10-min oral presentation. The limitations of time are removed, and viewers can move back and forth between sections of the paper and spend more time looking at the parts that interest them. The format is ideal for studying illustrative matter when compared to the length of time a slide is flashed on screen. A poster exhibit is also of particular advantage to a nervous and apprehensive presenter, who may find a podium presentation quite daunting but feel more at ease in a less formal one-to-one situation. By contrast, podium presentation is suited to persons with an outgoing personality, with prior experience and good public-speaking skills—talents that require studious cultivation. For a person who lacks proficiency in English (a second or third language for many in India), a podium presentation is an added handicap. In such a situation, presenting a poster may be an attractive alternative. A poster can also be more informative than a talk especially for those seriously interested in that work, since it allows for easier interaction with the presenter.

Posters have some disadvantages as well, the biggest being that the audience is not captive, and conference delegates are attracted to the most eye-catching displays. Thus the appearance of a poster is as important as its content, and the aesthetic aspects of composition, layout, colour scheme, etc. need much attention. These requirements might well make the poster format more expensive than slides.

26.3 Objectives and Qualities of a Good Poster

The primary objective of a poster is to accurately and precisely inform the audience of the results of a piece of scientific research. Paper is the medium normally used, but some posters are on bromide, board or vinyl. A poster must generate interest among peers about its subject and achieve the end result—criticism and feedback from the author's peers, which may in turn provide ideas for further work. To achieve these ends, a poster should be as informative and attractive as the best that accompanies museum displays and as persuasive as those used in advertising campaigns!

26.4   Planning a Poster

Planning is the most crucial step in making a poster. First read the 'instructions to presenters' provided by the conference organizers, and become thoroughly acquainted with all the specifications—size of poster boards, location at the venue, the viewing time, suggestions for layout and any additional information that the organizers may want included in the poster.

Next, decide on the amount of information to be included. 'Information-packed' posters are not the most impressive as crowding of material may obscure the principal messages and turn away prospective viewers. Limit the poster to two or three key ideas, and convey these effectively. Although the presenter is on hand during the set-viewing times, the poster must be complete in itself so that visitors at other times can comprehend it independently. The skill in planning a good poster lies in conveying a clear message in a limited space. It is important to always keep your target audience in mind. For instance, a microbiologist presenting a new test for diagnosing tubercular meningitis would tailor his/her display according to whether the conference was for microbiologists or neurologists. Details of laboratory tests would be more appropriate for a gathering of microbiologists, whereas a group of neurologists would be more interested in case selection and clinical outcomes.

The first thing in making the poster is to select those tables and figures that support the results related to your key ideas. The poster is a visual and pictorial medium, so present as many results as possible with graphs, photographs and line drawings. A poster can include a wide variety of pictorial materials including samples of any devices that you may have used, computer printouts, outputs of machines that produce graphic data (such as electroencephalography, electrocardiography) and images (X-rays, ultrasonography, echocardiography, gamma camera, autoradiograph, histopathology, electron micrograph, etc.).

Wherever possible, graphs should be preferred over tables to represent the data. The graph type should be carefully selected so that the maximum possible information can be conveyed for quick comprehension. Long tables with many rows and columns are not appropriate in a poster; if a table must be included, use only the essential columns and exclude the less important data.

When you have selected the figures to support your results, finalize the 'Methods' section keeping your target audience in mind (*see above*). After allotting space for the results and methods sections, you will know how much space is available for the usually less detailed 'introduction' and 'discussion' sections.

26.4.1 Layout

At this stage, read the 'instructions to presenters' carefully to find out the size and aspect ratio of the poster. Sketch a scale plan of your poster on a piece of paper to get an idea of how to arrange the material.

A poster includes title, authors' names and affiliations and the main body with scientific contents. Sometimes, the organizers may want you to include the poster number or a copy of the abstract, a strategy that discourages authors from enlarging the scope of the poster beyond that of the submitted abstract. This can be placed in the left upper corner or as instructed by the conference organizers.

Leave space across the top of the total allotted space for displaying the title (and the abstract, if required by the organizers; Fig. 26.1). The instructions may specify a point size for the title. The space remaining will form the main body of the poster. The progression of information should be from top to bottom and from left to right. The space located immediately below the title and at eye level (measuring about 2 ft or 60 cm vertically) should contain the most important information with less important material placed at the bottom of the poster.

26.4.2 Title

The title should be brief, informative and attractive and convey the main points of interest in your study (Fig. 26.2). Since people will be walking through a hall full of posters, catchy titles are more likely to attract prospective viewers.

26.4.3 Abstract

If the instructions ask for the submitted abstract to be included in the poster, try and place the text in the left upper corner and to the left of the title. It need not be very prominent as a copy will be printed in the conference abstract book.

Fig. 26.1 Suggested layout for a poster 6 ft (1.8 m) in width and 3 ft (0.9 m) in height. A 6–8 inch band at the top can be used for the title and the remaining space for the main content

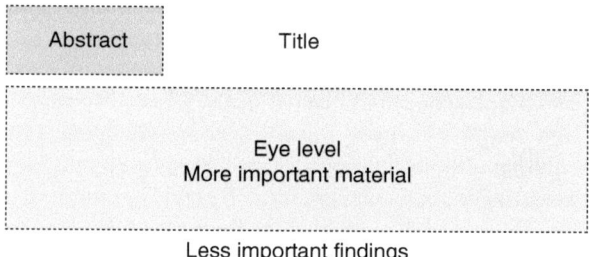

Fig. 26.2 Examples of poster titles of different lengths and their qualities

A lengthy but informative title:

Development, standardization and evaluation of a new polymerase chain reaction (PCR)-based test for the definitive diagnosis of tubercular meningitis

A shorter and yet more informative and attractive title:

A new, rapid and accurate test for diagnosis of tubercular meningitis

26.4.4 Text

Manuscripts are composed in full sentences arranged in paragraphs. This style of writing is unsuitable for a poster as the viewer will struggle to find the core message. Plan your text as short, clear, simple and separate statements, preferably in bullet points, rather than complete sentences. This format allows the viewer to quickly scan the text for the key messages.

The text of a poster should be arranged under distinct sections of introduction (or background), objectives, methods, results and conclusions. If required, a section could have subsections. This allows a viewer to select the sequence in which he/she would like to view the poster or to spend more time on some subsections.

The 'Methods' panels should inform the viewer exactly what you did. For clinical studies, posters should include details about the number of patients and controls, diagnostic criteria, exclusion and inclusion criteria and the plan of study. For experimental studies, include details of the procedures used; quote the method if it has been used before and highlight any modifications; and list standardization of methods, selection of controls and sources of all reagents (and acknowledge the source of any reagents that are not commercially available). Finally, include information on the statistical methods used for each part of the study, and, in the case of clinical studies, state the power of the study.

26.4.5 Lettering and Organization of Text

A good poster conforms to the 'law of tens', i.e. ten or fewer panels, with ten or fewer lines per panel, and visible from a distance of 10 ft. Since the poster is usually viewed from a distance of 3–5 ft (1–1.5 m), it is important to use a font size large enough for all text and figures to be clearly visible at this distance. Do not have so many figures that you need to reduce the font size or squeeze them together; doing so will clutter your poster and make it hard to read. It is better to edit out some information. Be focused and do not lose sight of the few key ideas that you wish to emphasize.

The title should be in a larger font than the rest of the text; a 48–96-point size is acceptable. The text matter should be at least 24 point or larger in size. Use a sans-serif font (a typeface without the fine horizontal extensions or tapered lines at the terminal strokes of letters, e.g. Arial, Helvetica, Tahoma, Verdana) as these are more legible and appear less cluttered; serif fonts (which have the terminal extensions, e.g. Times New Roman, Book Antiqua, Perpetua) are easier to read as running text matter but are not suitable for the text in a poster (Fig. 26.3). It is advisable to use the same font throughout the poster.

Make sparing use of 'bold', 'italics' and 'underlined' fonts. Large sections of text in 'bold' or capital letters are difficult to read (Fig. 26.4).

Fig. 26.3 Appearance of text in serif and san serif fonts, and their relative uses

Arial (San Serif)

Chest pain
Nerve
Heart
Lungs

Sans serif fonts lack the fine extensions at the extremes of letters. These are bolder, easier to read and appear less cluttered, particularly when used for short text strings.

Times New Roman (Serif)

Chest pain
Nerve
Heart
Lungs

Serif fonts have fine extensions at the extremes of letters. These extensions make long stretches of such text easier to read (as in printed matter). However, such fonts are not good for short text.

Fig. 26.4 Comparison of text written in capital letters with the same text written in lower case letters. The latter is easier to read and understand

Text in all capitals

A NEW, RAPID AND ACCURATE TEST FOR DIAGNOSIS OF TUBERCULAR MENINGITIS

Text in lower case letters

A new, rapid and accurate test for diagnosis of tubercular meningitis

26.4.6 Peer Input

It helps to prepare a rough output, and then request comments from your colleagues and friends. You may put up your draft poster on the wall of the seminar room or the coffee room of your department—wherever you feel a large number of people would see it. Encourage everyone to give you feedback. If you value the opinion of someone from outside the department, request that person to visit your draft poster. Even those not involved with the subject may give very useful inputs regarding aesthetics, layout etc.

26.5   Preparation and Transport

Conventionally, text matter was placed on a large chart paper using either a lettering stencil or paste-on letters. Today, most of the text and diagrams are generated using computer programmes and large-sized inkjet or laser printers. It is important to know the features and limitations of the hardware and software you have access to while preparing the material. If you need assistance using such equipment, take help from a colleague who is in the know or seek the help of a professional. Good-quality paper and a high-resolution inkjet or laser printer will give you a good-quality poster.

The final appearance can be enhanced by selecting pleasing colour combinations for the background and lettering or by adding borders and an institutional logo to the text panels. The colours used in diagrams should be consistent throughout. For example, diagrams of control and treated groups should use the same colour for each group throughout. The choice of colours is a matter of personal preference; however, lighter shades are generally preferred.

It is not unknown for preparation of a poster to be left until a few days before the presentation is due. Remember, it takes time to make a good poster. If you start at the last moment and find that your images are not of the best quality, there may not be time to obtain better ones. While making a poster, it helps to prepare a complete first draft, and then slowly make incremental improvements. If you start early, you will be able to prepare a draft in time and get feedback from your co-authors and peers.

Plan how you are going to carry your poster. It may need special packaging, such as a cylindrical tube of an appropriate size. Always carry the poster in your hand baggage—a poster lost or damaged in the baggage hold will surely induce a state of misery. And, finally, having taken it on board the aircraft, don't leave it in the over-head locker.

26.6   The Final Display and Presentation

It helps to visit the poster area a day before the scheduled display. Locate and have a look at the board that has been allotted to you. (Don't be overly surprised if the size of the board differs from that specified in the conference brochure.) Always carry your own backup supply of tape, Velcro, mounting pins, scissors etc. You might consider inviting experts and peers in your area of research to view your poster. Be sure to give them your poster number and the times it will be displayed.

Mount your poster well in time, and ensure that you are available during the time allotted for viewing. You will be expected to answer all queries. One of the visitors might be a judge, and your absence could rule you out of the running for the best poster award! Visitors may also provide valuable suggestions and ideas for future research work. Senior people in the field often go around the poster area seeking prospective candidates for jobs in their institution—your visitor might offer you a position in his group.

Appendix: Links to Some Useful Resources

1. International Committee of Medical Journal Editors (ICMJE). Recommendations for the Conduct, Reporting, Editing, and Publication of Scholarly work in Medical Journals
   www.icmje.org/icmje-recommendations.pdf
   These guidelines review best practices and ethical standards in the conduct and reporting of research and other material published in medical journals and help authors, editors and others involved in peer review and biomedical publishing create and distribute accurate, clear, reproducible and unbiased medical journal articles. Authors should use these recommendations along with individual journals' instructions to authors and guidelines for the reporting of specific study types (e.g. the CONSORT guidelines for reporting of randomized trials).

2. World Association of Medical Editors (WAME). Definition of a peer-reviewed journal/authorship
   www.wame.org/about/policy-statements#Definition%20PR
   This policy statement defines a peer-reviewed journal and enumerates the criteria for authorship of articles for publication.

3. World Association of Medical Editors (WAME). Conflict of interest in peer-reviewed medical journals
   www.wame.org/about/conflict-of-interest-in-peer-reviewed-medical
   This policy statement defines 'conflict of interest' and explains it in the context of reporting and publishing research. It also delineates the responsibilities of various stakeholders such as authors, editors and reviewers. WAME has also published an editorial on COI, which can be accessed at *www.wame.org/about/wame-editorial-on-coi*.

4. International Committee of Medical Journal Editors (ICMJE). Form for declaring conflicts of interest
   www.icmje.org/downloads/coi_disclosure.zip
   Credibility of published research depends largely on how transparently conflicts of interest are handled during the planning, implementation, writing,

© The National Medical Journal of India 2018
P. Sahni, R. Aggarwal (eds.), *Reporting and Publishing Research in the Biomedical Sciences*, https://doi.org/10.1007/978-981-10-7062-4

peer review, editing and publication of scientific work. To allow authors to report their conflicts of interest in a simple and effective manner, ICMJE has developed a form which can be completed, stored and transmitted electronically.

5. Committee on Publication Ethics (COPE). Flowcharts designed to help editors follow COPE's Code of Conduct and implement its advice when faced with cases of suspected misconduct

   http://publicationethics.org/files/u2/All_flowcharts.pdf

   COPE provides advice to editors and publishers on publication ethics and, in particular, on how to handle cases of misconduct in research and publication. It has developed a set of flowcharts that are designed to help editors follow COPE's Code of Conduct and implement its advice when faced with cases of suspected misconduct of different types. These flowcharts can be downloaded individually or as a complete set.

6. World Association of Medical Editors (WAME). The registration of clinical trials

   www.wame.org/about/policy-statements#Trial%20Reg

   This policy statement supports registration of all clinical trials at their inception. It also explains the advantages of registration in the wider context of research and patient safety.

7. Committee on Publication Ethics (COPE). International standard for editors and authors

   http://publicationethics.org/resources/international-standards-for-editors-and-authors

   During the 2nd World Conference on Research Integrity in Singapore in 2010, COPE helped develop two position statements setting out international standards for responsible research publication for editors and authors. These statements have been published as part of the proceedings of this conference under a Creative Commons licence and have also been published by several journals.

8. CONSORT (CONsolidated Standards of Reporting Trials) 2010 Statement

   www.consort-statement.org/downloads/consort-statement

   This statement is an evidence-based, minimum set of recommendations for reporting randomized trials. It provides a standard way for authors to prepare reports of trial findings, facilitating their complete and transparent reporting and aiding their critical appraisal and interpretation. The recommendations include (i) a 25-item checklist that focuses on reporting how the trial was designed, analysed and interpreted and (ii) a flow diagram that displays the progress of all participants through the trial.

   The CONSORT 2010 Explanation and Elaboration [E&E] document is also available on this website.

9. World Association of Medical Editors (WAME). Impact factor

   www.wame.org/about/policy-statements#Impact%20Factor

   This policy statement advises journal editors to educate their readers, authors, administrators and the scientific community in general about the impact factor and its relevance, as also about other measures of journal and article quality.

10. World Association of Medical Editors (WAME). Ghost writing initiated by commercial companies

    www.wame.org/about/policy-statements#Ghost%20Writing

    This policy statement addresses the issue of integrity of the published record of scientific research. This depends not only on the validity of the science but also on honesty in authorship. Editors and readers need to be confident that authors have undertaken the work described and have ensured that the manuscript accurately reflects their work, irrespective of whether they took the lead in writing or sought assistance from a medical writer. This document advocates for transparency about authorship and public accountability of scientific publications.

11. EQUATOR Network (Enhancing the QUAlity and Transparency Of health Research)

    www.equator-network.org/

    This online library contains a comprehensive searchable database of reporting guidelines for manuscripts with a variety of research designs. It also has links to other useful resources for writing and publishing health research.